# FORENSIC GENETICS RESEARCH PROGRESS

# FORENSIC GENETICS RESEARCH PROGRESS

**FABRICIO GONZALEZ-ANDRADE**
EDITOR

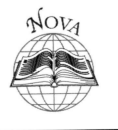

Nova Science Publishers, Inc.
*New York*

Copyright © 2010 by Nova Science Publishers, Inc.

**All rights reserved.** No part of this book may be reproduced, stored in a retrieval system or transmitted in any form or by any means: electronic, electrostatic, magnetic, tape, mechanical photocopying, recording or otherwise without the written permission of the Publisher.

For permission to use material from this book please contact us:
Telephone 631-231-7269; Fax 631-231-8175
Web Site: http://www.novapublishers.com

**NOTICE TO THE READER**

The Publisher has taken reasonable care in the preparation of this book, but makes no expressed or implied warranty of any kind and assumes no responsibility for any errors or omissions. No liability is assumed for incidental or consequential damages in connection with or arising out of information contained in this book. The Publisher shall not be liable for any special, consequential, or exemplary damages resulting, in whole or in part, from the readers' use of, or reliance upon, this material.

Independent verification should be sought for any data, advice or recommendations contained in this book. In addition, no responsibility is assumed by the publisher for any injury and/or damage to persons or property arising from any methods, products, instructions, ideas or otherwise contained in this publication.

This publication is designed to provide accurate and authoritative information with regard to the subject matter covered herein. It is sold with the clear understanding that the Publisher is not engaged in rendering legal or any other professional services. If legal or any other expert assistance is required, the services of a competent person should be sought. FROM A DECLARATION OF PARTICIPANTS JOINTLY ADOPTED BY A COMMITTEE OF THE AMERICAN BAR ASSOCIATION AND A COMMITTEE OF PUBLISHERS.

**LIBRARY OF CONGRESS CATALOGING-IN-PUBLICATION DATA**
Forensic genetics research progress / editor, Fabricio Gonzalez-Andrade.
 p. ; cm.
Includes bibliographical references and index.
ISBN 978-1-60876-198-2 (hardcover)
1. Forensic genetics. I. González Andrade, Fabricio.
[DNLM: 1. Forensic Genetics. W 750 F71249 2009]
RA1057.5F673 2009
614'.1--dc22
 2009033368

*Published by Nova Science Publishers, Inc.* ✢ *New York*

# CONTENTS

| | | |
|---|---|---|
| **Preface** | | vii |
| **Chapter 1** | Bringing Tissue Identification into the 21$^{st}$ Century: mRNA Analysis as the Next Molecular Biology Revolution in Forensic Science?<br>*Trisha L. Noreault-Conti and Eric Buel* | 1 |
| **Chapter 2** | Trace DNA Analysis<br>*Kaye N. Ballantyne* | 35 |
| **Chapter 3** | The Continuing Evolution of Forensic DNA Databases<br>*Simon J. Walsh, John S. Buckleton and Olivier Ribaux* | 51 |
| **Chapter 4** | Homicide Investigation: Anthropology and Genetic Analysis for the Crime Scene<br>*I. Roca, M. Beaufils, A. Esponda, G. Said and C. Doutremepuich* | 73 |
| **Chapter 5** | Influence of Humic Acid on DNA Analysis<br>*Davorka Sutlovic* | 91 |
| **Chapter 6** | Advances in DNA Typing in Sexual Assault Casework<br>*María de Fátima Terra Pinheiro* | 117 |
| **Chapter 7** | Analysis of Reduced Size STR Amplicons as Tools for the Study of Degraded DNA<br>*Miriam Baeta, Carolina Nuñez, Fabricio González-Andrade, Santiago Gascón and Begoña Martínez-Jarreta* | 133 |
| **Chapter 8** | The Study of Ancient DNA in Forensic Genetics<br>*Cecilia Sosa and Begoña Martínez-Jarreta* | 151 |
| **Chapter 9** | Forensic Mitochondrial DNA Analysis<br>*Luísa Pereira, Farida Alshamali and Fabricio González-Andrade* | 173 |
| **Chapter 10** | SNPs Technologies in Forensic Genetics: Approach and Applications<br>*Anna Barbaro* | 193 |

| | | |
|---|---|---|
| **Chapter 11** | Statistical Assessment of DNA Paternity Tests in Uncommon Cases: From the Routine to the Extreme<br>*Iosif S. Tsybovsky, Nikolay N. Kuzub*<br>*and Vera M. Veremeichyk* | 231 |
| **Chapter 12** | MtDNA Analysis for Genetic Identification of Forensically Important Insects<br>*Adriano Tagliabracci and Federica Alessandrini* | 245 |
| **Chapter 13** | Molecular Techniques for the Identification of Non-Human Species in Forensic Biology<br>*Antonio Alonso* | 265 |
| **Chapter 14** | Local DNA Databases in Forensic Casework<br>*José Luis Ramírez, Miguel Angel Chiurillo,*<br>*Noelia Lander, Maria Gabriela Rojas*<br>*and Marjorie Sayegh* | 277 |
| **Chapter 15** | In vitro Studies of DNA Recovered from Incinerated Teeth<br>*Paola León-Sanz, Carolina Bonett, Raúl Suárez,*<br>*Yolanda González, James Valencia, Ignacio Zarante* | 293 |
| **Chapter 16** | Promising Prospects of Chinese Medical Semiology on Forensic Genetics<br>*Ahmed Youssif El Tassa* | 307 |
| **Index** | | 317 |

# PREFACE

In addition to supplementing existing analysis techniques in serious crime cases, trace DNA can allow investigation of volume crime cases such as burglary or vehicle theft, where previously DNA evidence was not considered usable. However, despite the widespread use of trace DNA, at present there are very few specific validated methods. This has lead to controversy in the use of trace DNA, and particularly the low copy number amplification technique. It has been established that the use of existing methodology (developed for high-copy number samples) leads to significant levels of artefacts with trace DNA, including allele drop-out and drop-in, stutter, and allelic/locus imbalance. To minimize these, there are numerous modifications that can be made to existed methods to increase the success of trace DNA analysis. This book presents advances in the field of DNA research as an aid in Forensic studies and Genetics.

Chapter 1 - DNA analysis using advanced molecular biological tools is universally used to unlock identifying information contained in crime scene stains. These advances have allowed scientists to provide critical information to solve crimes and allow the criminal justice community to convict the guilty and exonerate the innocent. Scientific research continues to develop new automated technologies and methods to yield more information from limited samples allowing scientists to optimize time and effort. Although the changes realized over the last 20 years have been remarkable, only small changes have occurred in the identification of the tissue source of a biological stain. Considerable research has been conducted to offer an alternative to these classical identification methods through the use of mRNA analysis. The application of mRNA into the forensic laboratory has not yet taken hold, but offers a new approach that could unequivocally identify difficult to characterize stains and allow the use of molecular biological tools for the identification of stains found at a crime scene. The nature of the research in this chapter is to identify mRNA transcripts that will definitively identify the tissue of origin, determine if such transcripts survive the typical environmental insults that forensic samples may encounter, and develop rapid assays using small amounts of sample. The stability of RNA was evaluated over time using real-time TaqMan®-based PCR assays. Once RNA was shown to be stable in samples aged up to 4 years, 2-3 tissue-specific transcripts were identified for a variety of stains. In addition to specificity, the sensitivity of the assays was also determined using different sized stains. Once candidates were shown to be tissue-specific, the Plexor® One-Step qRT-PCR System was used to develop multiplex assays. This system allows the multiplexing of multiple RNAs in one assay, thus reducing the amount of sample needed and time of analysis. Through collaboration with Promega, a quick, one-tube seminal fluid-saliva screening assay was designed, since analysis of these fluids is a major task for all forensic laboratories. Additionally, a RNA/DNA co-isolation technique was developed which effectively extracts both nucleic acids, thus removing the requirement for separate extractions and allows DNA profiling from the exact stain in which RNA testing was performed. In conjunction with Promega, a likely outcome is a real-time PCR screening assay that determines with certainty whether a stain contains seminal fluid and/or saliva, an invaluable tool to the forensic community.

Chapter 2 - Trace DNA has become a large part of the average forensic laboratories' workload. Remarkably low DNA amounts (<100pg) have been successfully analysed to obtain profiles from a wide range of sample types. Touched objects constitute the most common source of trace DNA, but any type of biological material present in low amounts may be considered as trace, including minute blood deposits, saliva residue on partially consumed food, or even epithelial cells from the interior surface of condoms. In addition to supplementing existing analysis techniques in serious crime cases, trace DNA can allow investigation of volume crime cases such as burglary or vehicle theft, where DNA evidence had not previously been considered usable. However, despite the widespread use of trace DNA, at present there are very few specific validated methods. This has led to controversy in the use of trace DNA, and particularly the low copy number amplification technique. It has been established that the use of existing methodology (developed for high-copy number samples) leads to significant levels of artefacts with trace DNA, including allele drop-out and drop-in, stutter, and allelic/locus imbalance. To minimize these, there are numerous modifications that can be made to existing methods to increase the success of trace DNA analysis. These include reduced extraction volumes, increased cycle number, reduced PCR volume, and increased injection time for capillary electrophoresis. In addition, new research shows that the introduction of techniques such as whole genome amplification, molecular crowding, and post-PCR purification can significantly increase success rates with trace DNA. It is clear that each step of the analysis procedure (including collection, extraction, amplification and fragment detection) can, and should, be optimized with regards to trace DNA. However, the use of increasingly sensitive trace DNA analysis techniques must bring an increasing awareness of the potential for contamination, both within the laboratory and at crime scenes. In particular, this has implications for the analysis of trace DNA from cold cases, which were not collected or stored with highly sensitive DNA detection techniques in mind. Although it is certain that trace DNA will continue to be used within forensic biology, there may need to be modifications to a wide range of practices to ensure accuracy and reliability.

Chapter 3 - In terms of forensic-specific applications of DNA technology, few have had a more profound effect on the field than the launching of databases around the world. The expansion of this phenomenon has not only required an appropriate level of scientific sophistication, but also unprecedented legislative, political and financial backing. In practical terms DNA database implementation and operation has brought massive increases in case submissions and a demonstrable change in case and evidence profiles. Forensic DNA databases also remain high profile and retain some element of controversy, typically in relation to socio-legal issues. Despite this impressive impact, it is important to acknowledge that forensic DNA database applications are still young, still only partially developed and understood and still requiring of our attention, monitoring and effort to ensure an ongoing positive contribution.

Fresh complexities are emerging in the management and development of DNA databases. Some of these problems have been examined in detail in this chapter, and, new solutions that allow cross-comparison of database performance are discussed. These methods should assist, not only in identifying present strengths and weaknesses but also in enhancing future database performance and effectiveness. Effective and creative database management has to be seen as a key priority for the forensic community. Achieving it will require a concerted effort of oversight that scientists themselves must be prepared to participate in as it is crucial to maximising the benefits of their work.

Forensic science has traditionally focussed on the production of evidentiary outcomes – retrospectively, and with a view to confirming or refuting an already-held belief. DNA databases also offer, however, the potential for proactive forensic contributions to investigations. Delivering these requires functional and philosophical adjustments to the process by which forensic outcomes are produced. This chapter also outlines specific steps that need to be taken to progress beyond the traditional operational framework to one that is also conducive to effective policing and crime resolution.

Chapter 4 - Dr Watson has been replaced by Sir Jeffreys in 1985, day when a criminal case was elucidated thanks to genetic analysis; forensic laboratories have tried to decrease the DNA/cells quantity necessary to obtain a profile and to increase the analysis sensibility.

The DNA profile is put in evidence from each kind of tissue as epithelium, sperm, blood, bones and hairs. Two kinds of samples are realised: the samples of traces and those of comparison. The first step of the analysis is to investigate the stains or traces. Several techniques are used: chemical, cytological or visual. A specific organisation has been elaborated in the laboratory in order to eliminate the cross contamination and the contact between victim samples and suspect samples. This organization is present in the entire laboratory, for all the steps of the analysis. The second step is the extraction of the DNA from tissue. Since 2008, a new technique, the laser microdissection, is used in complement of classical method to analyse contact cells. This one is chosen as a function of the potential quantity of cells on the support. One to ten cells are sufficient to obtain a DNA profile. The laser microdissection permits to directly select and analyse the interest cells. The result is as efficient as it was with the classical one but on less than ten cells. With the reduction of the numbers of analysed cells, the number of DNA blend is reduced too. Since the use of the laser microdissection, the percentage of results has been significantly increased: results are obtained where no result was revealed with the classical technique of extraction.

The obtained profiles are compared either between them, or "trace" profiles with "comparison" profiles. A statistical analysis is realised for the "trace" profile corresponding to the "comparison" profile. Because of the importance of the results, quality assurance has to be present in the laboratory. One possibility is the accreditation ISO 17025 which permits to set the quality system and the methods after a checking and a control. All the used laboratory techniques are certified ISO 9001 and accredited ISO 17025 to assure the competency, the quality and the performance of the laboratory.

Nowadays, the analysis DNA becomes widespread and complementary to the other analysis for the investigators because of the numerous information it brings. To find one or several profiles thanks to a contact cells or sperm or blood permit to orient the investigation, to find a suspect and sometimes to understand the progress of the crime or the facts.

Chapter 5 - The identification process of dead bodies or human remains is now days conducted in numerous fields of forensic science, archeology and other judicial cases.

A particular problem is the isolation and DNA typing of human remains found in mass graves, due to the degradation process, as well as post mortal DNA contamination with bacteria, fungi, humic acids (HA), metals etc. In this study the authors investigated the influence of humic acid on the success of DNA extraction, quantification and typing by Real time - PCR and PCR methods.

It was reported that the humic acid if present in the amplification reaction mix inhibited the DNA amplification, but the addition of 50 mg PVPP to the reaction mixture before extraction, appeared to be optimum in overcoming that inhibition.

It was investigated the dose-response effect of humic acid on the Quantification Real Time PCR (QRT-PCR) inhibition and the efficiency of Taq polymerase increment in preventing inhibition by HA in DNA extracted from ancient bones. The addition 10 - 75 ng of synthetic HA (Fluka) can inhibit QRT- PCR while the addition of 100 ng of synthetic HA completely inhibits QRT- PCR. The addition of 1.25 Unit (U) of Taq polymerase per assay appeared to be the optimum amount in overcoming the HA inhibition. The best results were obtained when crude DNA extracts containing humic substances were quantified by QRT-PCR, with adding of 1.25 Unit (U) of extra Taq polymerase per assay.

It was investigated the possible mechanisms of HA interaction with human DNA, and kinetics of QRT-PCR inhibition were investigated. In QRT-PCR with pure human DNA and no HA added, $V_{MAX}$ was 40. With DNA sample containing 4 µg/ml of HA, $V_{MAX}$ was 30.30 while the addition of extra Taq polymerase to the same sample changed $V_{MAX}$ into 38.91, amplifying between 80 and 90% of input DNA. The $K_M/V_{MAX}$ ratio in all the samples remained constant, indicating that the mechanism of HA inhibition of QRT-PCR is uncompetitive by nature. Moreover HA shifts the human DNA melting temperature point ($T_m$) from 75°C to 87°C and inhibits DNase I mediated DNA cleavage, most probably affecting the enzyme's activity.

Chapter 6 - Sexual assault is usually a hidden crime where the only witnesses are the victim and the assailant. With this limited initial information, the physical and biological evidence collected from the victim, from the crime scene, and from the suspect will play a prior role in the objective and scientific reconstruction of the events. The obvious first step in finding semen evidence is interviewing the victim. During the investigation of sexual offences, intimate body swabs, clothing and bedding items are routinely submitted for examination. Biological material can accumulate under the fingernail hyponychium of both the victim and/or the suspect and has the potential to provide evidence and intelligence information. In addition to the hairs and debris that may be transferred in other types of violent crime, the rapist often leaves behind a personal biological signature that may include blood, saliva, and most importantly, semen. This semen evidence is frequently a cornerstone in the investigation and prosecution of the case. Bite marks perpetrated in the victim body is another type of sample that can be studied. The presence of a mixture (female/male) can be the unique probative evidence, being a very important statement in a court. The analysis of clothing damage can also be used to corroborate different versions of events. The two commonly used presumptive tests for semen are the Florence and the Brentamine tests. Moreover, prostate specific antigen can be used for forensic identification of semen stains. Confirmatory testing for semen involves the microscopy detection of spermatozoa and its DNA analysis. Identification of one or more intact spermatozoa is conclusive proof of the presence of semen and hence affirms sexual contact. However, the DNA profile identification of the perpetrator must be established. Traditionally, sperm cells are isolated from vaginal cell mixtures by preferential extraction methods. More recently the laser microdissection has proved to be a very powerful tool to isolate specific target cells from a more complex tissue. Autosomal STRs have been used for a long time for human identification and still are a valuable tool in forensic casework. Nevertheless, these markers have some limitations in the analysis of samples concerned to sexual assaults. Since a vast majority of crimes where DNA evidence is helpful, particularly sexual assault, involve males as the perpetrator, DNA tests designed to only examine the male portion can be valuable. A majority of the Y chromosome is transferred directly from father to son without recombination. Therefore, a match between a suspect and evidence only means that the individual in question could have contributed the evidence. A survey was done of alleged victims of sexual assault cases reported to the National Institute of Legal Medicine – North Delegation (Oporto-Portugal) in 2004-2008. Some parameters of interest were analysed, such as the cases that provided: a DNA profile different from the victim (autosomal STR, Y-STR or both); those with more than one perpetrator identified in a mixture; also those where a male profile was identified similar to the suspect one.

Chapter 7 - Polymorphic Short Tandem Repeats (STRs) markers have become a very useful tool in forensic analysis of human DNA. Multiplex PCR amplification of STR loci enables to obtain genetic information from almost any source of biological material. However, some forensic evidences, can be so extremely degraded (e.g. certain mass disasters, old and bad preserved remains, etc) that STR typing is unsuccessful. In these situations DNA typing can be challenging and it could be difficult to obtain quality profiles (ej: loss of signal of larger sized loci is frequently observed as a result of DNA fragmentation, etc.). Recent efforts have focused on the use of nuclear Single Nucleotide Polymorphism (SNP) markers as an alternative and more recently, on reducing the size of STR markers (miniSTRs). The development of miniSTRs is accomplished by simply moving the primer binding sites closer to the STR repeat region, and creating DNA fragments that are shorter than traditional STR markers. MiniSTRs markers have shown to be very successful at recovering DNA profiles from highly degraded samples The possibility of obtaining nuclear MiniSTRs profiles corresponding to conventional STR markers is also considered a great advantage as most of the National intelligence DNA banks are based on them. In this chapter the authors will review the development and use of miniSTRs loci in forensic genetics from its first application in the analysis of Branch Davidian fire in Waco to its incorporation in commercial kits. The authors will not only focus on autosomal miniSTRs but also on the recent development of miniY-STRs and miniX-STRs. Advantages and disadvantages of these markers in Forensics will be considered and compared to those of traditional STR markers. Finally, the authors will review potential applications and future perspectives of their use in Forensic Genetics.

Chapter 8 - The vertiginous progress in molecular biological techniques has enabled the retrieval and analysis of DNA from very diverse ancient specimens. This has broadened the spectrum of possibilities for Paleobiology and Genetic Anthropology and many exciting reports have come through. However, along with the technical progresses, the field has revealed certain peculiarities and drawbacks that on occasions could raise reasonable doubts on the authenticity of reported results. In this paper a review of the history of this challenging field is summarized. Since this is a vast and ever growing speciality, the authors will focus on the study of ancient DNA from human skeletal remains and on its Forensic applications. Particularities of bone diagenesis related to DNA preservation, features of ancient DNA molecules, unique characteristics, preservation conditions of skeletal remains, etc., are factors that make genetic typing of ancient bones and teeth a challenging task. The main technical issues on DNA analysis, such as molecular damage, exogenous contamination and presence of amplification inhibitors, are addressed in this chapter, emphasising in those practices that prevent from false-positive results and enable to demonstrate the authenticity of findings.

Chapter 9 - The introduction of mitochondrial DNA (mtDNA) investigation in forensic genetics allowed to obtaining results from ancient, residual and degraded samples, enlarging extensively the possibility of applying genetic analyses to difficult forensic cases. However, the particular characteristics of mtDNA brought some conceptual and statistical challenges to forensic genetics, namely: the uniparental (maternal) transmission implies lineage instead of individual characterization, so that mtDNA can be more informative in excluding rather than in including a suspect; the absence of recombination in mtDNA renders impossible to apply the product rule for estimation of match probabilities, so that evaluations are limited to the frequency of a certain haplotype in a database; most of mtDNA haplotypes are unique or very low frequent, implying that databases must have a considerable number of individuals in order to be informative; heterogeneity in mutation rates between mtDNA positions and heteroplasmy must be taken into account when evaluating if diverse haplotypes can come from the same individual. Typically, the mtDNA survey in forensic genetics is performed by sequencing two hypervariable regions in the control region or D-loop. Some databases, reporting haplotypes in diverse populations, are publically available for forensic purposes. Recently, information from other polymorphisms located in the coding region is being also added to forensic analyses, which allows to inferring more securely the haplogroup to which the haplotype belongs. This phylogenetic information can be very informative for quality purposes, helping in detecting possible mix-up of samples and in checking haplogroup defining polymorphisms. Lately, the mtDNA screening is being enlarged to the total control region (~1200bp), and in the near future to the complete molecule. Such amount of information, in such a short period of time, will challenge forensic genetics in maintaining its strict quality-control of sequences and in being efficient to updating online databases for match evaluation.

Chapter 10 - Single Nucleotide Polymorphisms (SNPs) represent the most common form of natural genetic variation in the human genome (approximately 90%) and are considered the major genetic source to phenotypic variability that differentiate individuals. Because SNPs occur frequently throughout the genome and tend to be relatively stable genetically, they serve as excellent biological markers for identification of genes in parts of the genome that may have some relation to a specific disease and even have influence on response to drug regimens.

In the last years the interest to SNPs is increased because they show a range of characteristics that make them well suited even to forensic analysis, including: abundance in the genome, Low mutation rates, reduced amplicon sizes (ability to analyze degraded DNA), relatively simple multiplex assays, potential for automation.

Single nucleotide polymorphisms may have in the near future a fundamental role in forensics, not only in specialized applications such as phylogeographical or ancestry studies (mtDNA, Y-SNPs) but also for the potential applications of autosomal SNPs either in the prediction of phenotypic traits than in real forensic caseworks applications.

Even if it is not likely that SNPs typing will totally replace STRs as the principal method for human identification, however new SNPs genotyping methods, chemistries and platforms are continuously being developed and considerable researches are still undergone to establish adequate scientific foundations for these applications.

Chapter 11 - Nowadays, more and more paternity investigations using microsatellite information are carried out in the laboratories all over the world. Tests were proceeded almost equally due to the basis of DNA-analysis – commercial multiplex kits PowerPlex16 System and AmpFlSTR Identifiler, distributed by American companies Promega and Applied Biosystems. Nevertheless, the practice of using these test-systems in parentage and forensic laboratories, complexity of some expert cases (deficient paternity, reverse paternity determination, occurrence of mutations, etc) have specific moments and need being studied and discussed in forensic community. Presented herein is comparative analysis of the paternity investigation results in 394 trio cases (mother, child, alleged father) and 77 duo cases (child, alleged father). Totally 1336 samples collected during paternity testing case work were analyzed using two nonaplex kits, developed in our laboratory. These kits form the universal panel of 17 STR loci (plus amelogenin), compatible to CODIS and test-systems by Promega and Applied Biosystems. The authors have demonstrated advantages of using this universal panel of 17 loci for resolving cases of disputable paternity. It is established that absence of the biological sample of mother in routine paternity testing reduces the level of random match probability at more than 800 folds. Values of paternity statistics were obtained for all 4 studied test-systems (CODIS – 13 loci, PowerPlex16 System and AmpFlSTR Identifiler – 15 loci and our kits – 17 loci) and compared. Our results underlined the necessity of inclusion of the mother in a paternity investigation, increase the number of analyzed STR loci and examination of more sets of genetic markers (Y- and X-chromosome, mtDNA) to match growing needs of routine expertise and clarify paternity in uncommon cases.

Chapter 12 - The determination of the time of death (post-mortem interval, PMI) has been the major topic of forensic entomologist. The method is based on the link of developmental stages of arthropods, particularly blowfly larvae, to their age. The major advantage against the standard forensic pathological methods for the determination of the early post-mortem interval is that arthropods can represent an accurate measure even in the later stages of the post-mortem interval when the classical methods fail.

Insect species have different developmental lifecycle timings and therefore, to utilise the correct developmental information, species need to be accurately identified. The misidentification of a specimen could produce a PMI estimate that, depending on the species and temperature, could be off by more than a week.

A technical difficulty faced by a forensic entomologist is that it is often difficult or impossible to identify the species of a maggot using classical methods. They require specialized taxonomic knowledge and although identification keys are available, only a few experts are able to identify the larvae of forensically important insects to species level. In addiction, differentiation at larval stages using morphological criteria is still not possible for some groups of insects. Definitive identification may be achieved by rearing larvae to adults but this can be time consuming and require larvae to be collected live and kept in conditions suitable for continued development.

Based on the above disadvantages of the morphological identification process, a forensic entomological investigation can benefit from molecular genotyping methods. There are several reports on the use of DNA techniques for identification of forensically important flies carried out on immatures insects stages and adult flies. As with so much of animal molecular systematics, mtDNA has played a leading role in insect genomic studies. High copy number, haploidy, and the availability of conserved mtDNA primers for more than a decade made it easy to obtain mtDNA sequence data from many previously unstudied insect species. The result was an explosive growth in mtDNA sequence data. Most forensic insect species-diagnostic papers focused on some portion of the genes for cytochrome *c* oxidase subunits one and two (COI+II). Coincidentally, the 5 end of COI is also the site of the proposed universal animal DNA barcode.

Suggested targets other than COI+II included randomly amplified polymorphic DNA (RAPDs), the gene for 28S ribosomal RNA, the ribosomal internal transcribed spacer regions, and NADH dehydrogenase subunit 5. Some authors have included more than one locus in a single analysis. However, there is no single agreed-upon locus for DNA-based identification of forensic insects, and it is not clear that there could be.

Chapter 13 - It seems clear that the biological remains from animals, plants, algae, fungi and microorganisms are becoming, increasingly relevant in the field of forensic biology and alternative disciplines such as other forensic sciences (forensic toxicology, forensic botany, forensic microbiology, ... ) and study at the molecular level could help with a broad variety of forensic studies of legal interest. There is currently a substantial number of technical protocols and genetic markers (nuclear DNA, mitochondrial DNA and chloroplast DNA) and various DNA databases that makes extremely reliable the genetic identification (at species, lineage, or individual levels) of non human species. This could overcome many of the limitation of classical non human species analysis based on morphological, biochemical or inmunological techniques. This issue outlines the different technologies and DNA markers currently used in the genetic identification of non-human species and its usefulness in a great variety of forensic cases.

Chapter 14 - Like many applications of molecular diagnostics, the field of forensic DNA typing is undergoing a period of growth and diversification. In contrast to strictly technological advances there have been a number of forensic-specific applications of existing techniques that have been raised in response to a particular research need, and that have had considerable impact on the field. The range of molecular markers and the analytical methods used in forensic genetics is continuously increasing. In Venezuela rising crime rates are outweighing state security systems, moreover, many mass disasters have recently occurred highlighting the necessity of implementing techniques for DNA analysis for the resolution of criminal cases, as well as the determination of genealogy and disaster victim identification. However, in this country despite having the human resources and training institutes and centers to conduct these tests, there has been a significant delay in the implementation of genetic technology in forensic science.

In response to these needs, in the last six years the authors have generated mitochondrial DNA (mtDNA) control regions, and autosomal and Y-chromosome Short Tandem Repeats (STR) databases from the admixed population of Caracas (capital city of Venezuela), and its use has allowed a better statistical analysis of forensic casework. Like many other countries, legislation is being adapted to technological innovations, and the creation of a Venezuelan forensic DNA national database is under discussion. In this work the authors highlight some of the most important cases analyzed, including disaster victim identification, criminal investigation, missing person cases and ancient DNA.

Firstly, the authors compare markers unbalance between mitochondrial DNA and chromosome Y in the Venezuelan population, confirming the colonization patterns reported for other Latin American countries; also the authors report in our population unique mtDNA haplotypes of phylogenetic significance. Second the authors describe the use of forensic genetic techniques and the databases in the identification of victims of an air disaster. Finally, the authors describe and discuss the experience of our attempts to recover the hypervariable sequences HVRI, HVRII, and HVRIII of the mtDNA control region from ancient hair samples of more than 140 years using technologies such as Phi29 DNA polymerase amplification protocols, and PCR analysis of reduced size fragments.

Although in our laboratory the number of forensic cases that has been processed has increased during the last five years, there is not yet a high output identification technology in place, and to this aim the authors are starting with the specific database for personal under high risk jobs, namely the Caracas Firefighters Squad. Finally, the authors are frequently testing standard methods used in forensic genetics, and each new case represents a new challenge for us and a contribution to the accumulated experience that is passed into other parts of the Venezuelan society. In this regard the authors acknowledge the outstanding contribution of the the Spanish and Portuguese Working Group of the International Society for Forensic Genetics (GEP-ISFG) without which these advances could not be possible.

Chapter 15 - Aim: To compare the quality of DNA extracted of molars and premolars teeth burned to temperatures between 300°C to 700°C, and provide the initial and detailed knowledge to handle the identification of incinerated bodies by dental DNA. This knowledge is advantageous to avoid delays in the scientific investigation of criminal caseworks.

Material and Methods: It included sixty-six teeth, upper and lower premolars and molars, of patients under extraction therapeutic, orthodontic treatment or periodontal disease. The samples were divided into six groups randomly, as follows: no burn teeth (control group); teeth incinerated at 300° C, at 400° C, at 500° C, at 600° C and at 700° C. The first group, control, was washed according the described protocol and using Alconox© at 1%. Samples were pulverized individually into a cryogenic impact grinder with self-contained liquid nitrogen. DNA was extracted by the organic of method phenol-chloroform-isoamilic alcohol. PCR was carried out using Amelogenin 10X first pair (2μM) fluorescein. Statistical analysis was tested three different models of logistic regression, which allow us predict about the appearance or absence of DNA on the variables sex, temperature, washing and tooth type.

Conclusion: It can isolate DNA of good quality in burned teeth, only when the heat reached 300° C or below, if the sample has not been handled or washed beforehand. The quality of the DNA will not vary with the gender, type of tooth or previous washes in the extraction process. It would recommend: do not wash to the teeth that have a high degree of destruction or where it suspects by their morphological features they have been exposed to heat above 300° C.

Chapter 16 - The present chapter starts by citing ancient semiologies, particularly by providing background knowledge on Chinese medical semiology. The intention is to stress their importance and value as assets to any Forensic Genetics researches performed today around the world. As an outcome, this chapter draws attention to the practical usefulness of Chinese Medical Semiology on Forensics and on Forensic Genetics.

It begins by presenting a discussion about the philosophical principles of typology in general and human typology in particular, and by portraying some analogies between nature and the human being. After a short introduction on the basic logics behind those universal principles, called *yin* and *yang*, literally *shadow* and *light*, which also could be resembled to *time* and *space*, each principle is compared to elements or phenomena from nature and human being, stressing the importance of this background towards Genetics and Forensic Genetics.

Inferred from the two fundamental principles (*yin/yang*) a categorization system is dialectically developed, transforming those two into five archetypes. Next, a peculiar typological system based on these five archetypes is then proposed to classify the five basic human races, classifying them according to the relative quantities of *yin* and *yang* they impart and to which they are connatural.

It is remembered that this approach of depicting nature is not exclusive to the East, given that in ancient Greece, a similar categorization method based in five elements was also traditionally used. The East called the five archetypes being: wood, fire, earth, metal and water, and the West labeled them as being: fire, air, earth, water and ether.

By contrasting an assertive, or direct approach on human typology performed throughout Western history to the moral, or indirect treatment of the same subject in ancient China, this article demonstrates the bio-ethical convenience of the later. When human types are primarily portrayed from a moral point of view, instead of an assertive, legal or a "normal" one, as the genome-wide association (GWA) studies tends to set down, *free will* embodied by each individual is appropriately emphasized as pre-requisite for a *free society*.

In: Forensic Genetics Research Progress
Editor: F. Gonzalez-Andrade

ISBN: 978-1-60876-198-2
© 2010 Nova Science Publishers, Inc.

*Chapter 1*

# BRINGING TISSUE IDENTIFICATION INTO THE 21$^{ST}$ CENTURY: mRNA ANALYSIS AS THE NEXT MOLECULAR BIOLOGY REVOLUTION IN FORENSIC SCIENCE?

*Trisha L. Noreault-Conti and Eric Buel*[*]
Vermont Forensic Laboratory, Department of Public Safety,
103 South Main Street, Waterbury, VT 05671, USA

## ABSTRACT

DNA analysis using advanced molecular biological tools is universally used to unlock identifying information contained in crime scene stains. These advances have allowed scientists to provide critical information to solve crimes and allow the criminal justice community to convict the guilty and exonerate the innocent. Scientific research continues to develop new automated technologies and methods to yield more information from limited samples allowing scientists to optimize time and effort. Although the changes realized over the last 20 years have been remarkable, only small changes have occurred in the identification of the tissue source of a biological stain. Considerable research has been conducted to offer an alternative to these classical identification methods through the use of mRNA analysis. The application of mRNA into the forensic laboratory has not yet taken hold, but offers a new approach that could unequivocally identify difficult to characterize stains and allow the use of molecular biological tools for the identification of stains found at a crime scene. The nature of the research in this chapter is to identify mRNA transcripts that will definitively identify the tissue of origin, determine if such transcripts survive the typical environmental insults that forensic samples may encounter, and develop rapid assays using small amounts of sample. The stability of RNA was evaluated over time using real-time TaqMan®-based PCR assays. Once RNA was shown to be stable in samples aged up to 4 years, 2-3 tissue-specific

---
[*] E-mail: ebuel@dps.state.vt.us

transcripts were identified for a variety of stains. In addition to specificity, the sensitivity of the assays was also determined using different sized stains. Once candidates were shown to be tissue-specific, the Plexor® One-Step qRT-PCR System was used to develop multiplex assays. This system allows the multiplexing of multiple RNAs in one assay, thus reducing the amount of sample needed and time of analysis. Through collaboration with Promega, a quick, one-tube seminal fluid-saliva screening assay was designed, since analysis of these fluids is a major task for all forensic laboratories. Additionally, a RNA/DNA co-isolation technique was developed which effectively extracts both nucleic acids, thus removing the requirement for separate extractions and allows DNA profiling from the exact stain in which RNA testing was performed. In conjunction with Promega, a likely outcome is a real-time PCR screening assay that determines with certainty whether a stain contains seminal fluid and/or saliva, an invaluable tool to the forensic community.

## INTRODUCTION

Twenty years ago forensic scientists offered a statistical interpretation of their biological stain analysis from a homicide or sexual assault case that could represent ten percent of the population. The prosecuting attorney was quite happy with this statistic as it ruled out ninety percent of the population as a possible donor. Alex Jeffreys changed all that in 1985 with his use of multi-locus probe restriction fragment length polymorphism (RFLP) analysis.

The application of DNA analysis to obtain the type of information that could link a particular individual to a crime scene stain has revolutionized the way forensic scientists analyze biological material. Since the early developments of DNA analysis, much effort has been made to improve the analytical capabilities of the forensic DNA typing laboratory. Methods have been developed to improve the extraction of DNA from a variety of sample types using robotics or other semi-automated procedures. Quantitation of total human DNA in extracts was once a labor intensive and semi-quantitative procedure using a slot-blot approach. This procedure was replaced by real-time polymerase chain reaction (PCR) assays which yield faster, more quantitative results with far less effort. Furthermore, improvements occurred within this technology to allow the simultaneous determination of the male component in addition to the total human DNA present in the sample.

The biggest change seen since the introduction of forensic DNA analysis is the rapid migration from RFLP analysis to PCR. PCR has revolutionized biotechnology and has allowed the forensic community to offer analyses that were beyond reach only a handful of years ago. The application of PCR has seen great changes throughout the years from a limited number of loci identified on hybridization strips to silver staining of short tandem repeats (STRs) on polyacrylamide gels to the use of multi-loci amplification analyzed semi-automatically on capillary electrophoresis instruments. These sweeping, fundamental changes have forever changed how forensic scientists approach biological stain analysis. Gone are the days where one speaks about absorption elution techniques to determine ABO blood type or where isoelectric focusing is used to sub-type an enzyme polymorphism. Today we have robots that can extract DNA from a stain for rapid instrumental analysis. Much has been accomplished to improve the "back-end" analysis of biological evidence.

The examination of biological evidence can be viewed as two separate steps. The "back-end" or the analysis of a particular stain as described above and the "front-end" of the analysis which involves the detection and identification of the tissue type of a potential body fluid stain. Evidence of a biological nature is routinely examined visually for stains which may then undergo presumptive and confirmatory testing. As described above, the analytical procedures to individualize a stain to a person have seen remarkable changes over the last 20 years. However, the front-end of the analysis, the presumptive and confirmatory testing of a biological stain, has not seen similar changes. A review of the progress made in the analysis of biological evidence was recently published by Fourney et al. (2007). This review details the advances seen in the two disciplines and points out the lack of significant progress in the screening of biological evidence. Traditional serological approaches for stain identification often involve a presumptive color test, followed by a confirmatory test that typically employs a specific antibody designed to complex with a known protein; such as hemoglobin for human blood and P30 or prostatic antigen for seminal fluid. Modest improvements have been made in the identification of some body fluids, but many of the tests still rely upon the fundamental antibody-antigen reactions used by the forensic community for years. These technical changes, dominated by the use of simple immunochromatographic tests, are less labor intensive than the classical Ouchterlony or crossover electrophoresis methods and have essentially replaced the older procedures.

Although these newly employed techniques offer a simplified and faster analysis, they still suffer from similar problems encountered with the classical tests. Major shortcomings of the broadly employed front-end methods include consuming portions of a perhaps limited sample, lack of acceptable confirmatory tests, limited capacity for automation and cross-reactivity with other fluids or species. For example, the traditional test for saliva involves detecting the presence of the enzyme amylase. While this enzyme is found in relatively high concentrations in saliva, it is also present at lower levels in other fluids which makes analysis of saliva via conventional methods problematic.

Over the past few years considerable work by many researchers has been conducted to change the very way forensic scientists identify the tissue source of a stain. With the advent of innovative molecular biological techniques, it is plausible to imagine the eventual replacement of the serological testing methods traditionally used to identify questioned stains with tests similar to those used for DNA analysis. As described above, the forensic community has embraced the use of PCR analysis for DNA profiling, making polymorphic enzyme assays used to differentiate individuals relics of the past. An analogous transition from the conventional biochemical approach to a molecular biological approach seems inevitable and could conceivably replace traditional tissue identification techniques. New tests that are tissue specific and designed to be multiplexed in a semi-automated approach would yield rapid results on a minimal amount of sample. Such testing could employ mRNA as the tissue-specific determinant to allow the identification of forensically important fluids/tissues by pinpointing the appropriate tissue-specific mRNAs. While the DNA of all tissues from an individual is essentially identical, the mRNA spectrum made by the different cells in each tissue is very different. Each tissue or cell type makes a unique constellation of mRNAs, some specific for only that tissue or cell type. Some body fluids, such as blood, contain cells as part of their function while other fluids, such as urine, contain cells that have been shed from their tissue of origin. Therefore, analysis of the "RNA profile" in a sample can uniquely identify the fluid or tissue of origin.

The purpose of this RNA-based stain identification research is to develop a simple mRNA extraction and analysis method to allow the quick, unequivocal identification of body fluid stains and tissues (for review, see Bauer, 2007). The proposed assays will be designed so that a single stain will amplify with only the corresponding mRNA(s) of its fluid/tissue type; a mixture, however, should amplify representing various fluids/tissues. The assays are designed to function more qualitatively than quantitatively, so although they may indicate which fluids/tissues are present, they may not give the exact ratio of each fluid contained in the stain. However, it is of greater concern to know what kind of mixture exists, than to know the exact amount of each fluid present. Furthermore, a major advantage to these assays is that a single test will be used to classify the sample as blood, semen, vaginal secretions, brain, heart, etc. which will drastically reduce the number of identification analyses performed prior to DNA profiling.

When molecular biologists began isolating mRNA for experiments, it was thought that mRNA was very ephemeral and that tissues needed to be processed rapidly in separate rooms with dedicated instruments and often with hazardous chemicals. However, due to the development of new techniques and the recent increase in knowledge concerning mRNA, it has been shown to be relatively stable. Groups have isolated mRNAs from blood, semen and saliva for research and diagnostic purposes. For blood, groups have isolated mRNA from dried blood spots for reverse transcription (RT) PCR and restriction or quantitation (Matsubara et al., 1992; Cao and Cousins, 2000; Zhang and McCabe, 1992; Watanapokasin et al., 2000). For semen, a number of groups have developed methods to detect hepatitis C viral mRNA or HIV mRNA in seminal fluid (Bourlet et al., 2002; Dulioust et al., 1998). Researchers have also isolated nuclear mRNAs such as calcium channel subunit mRNAs from the sperm in semen (Goodwin et al., 2000). In fact, mRNAs of a number of genes have been found in human spermatozoa (Miller, 2000; Richter et al., 1999). In addition, beta-hCG mRNA has been isolated from the prostate cells in human ejaculate (Daja et al., 2000). For saliva, mRNA of viruses such as measles has been detected (Jin et al., 2002). In terms of forensic analysis, Bauer et al. (1999) have detected mRNAs specific for epithelial (endometrial) cells in menstrual blood samples. They found that they could isolate mRNA after 6 months of room temperature storage and detect a number of mRNAs species. Bauer et al. (2003) have a subsequent paper where they studied 106 bloodstains stored up to 15 years. They found that mRNA levels as measured by laser-induced fluorescence capillary electrophoresis correlates with the age of the sample and that "mRNA suitable for RT-PCR can be isolated from samples stored up to 15 years". Various groups have demonstrated the stability of RNA in forensic stains by traditional RT-PCR and more recently, RT reactions coupled with real-time PCR (Juusola and Ballantyne, 2003; Alvarez et al., 2004; Bauer et al., 2003; Nussbaumer et al., 2006; Noreault-Conti and Buel, 2007). Furthermore, Setzer et al. (2008) addressed concerns on the stability, and hence recoverability, of RNA in forensic samples (blood, saliva, semen, and vaginal secretions) exposed to a range of environmental conditions from 1 to 547 days. The results demonstrate that RNA can be recovered from biological stains in sufficient quantity and quality for mRNA analysis.

In 2003, Juusola and Ballantyne, using RT-PCR to identify candidate tissue-specific genes for saliva, were able to demonstrate that RNA is stable in biological stains and can be recovered in sufficient quantity and quality for analysis. In that same year, Bauer and Patzelt (2003) showed that the detection of protamine gene expression in dried semen stains by RT-PCR provides evidence for the presence of sperm. More recent work from Juusola and

Ballantyne (2005) identified tissue-specific genes for the more common forensic casework samples: blood, saliva, semen and vaginal secretions. Furthermore, they developed a multiplex RT-PCR assay composed of eight genes which could be analyzed on a standard capillary electrophoresis platform; a more accurate and more sensitive detection method than agarose gel electrophoresis. Nussbaumer et al. (2006) reported the development of real-time PCR assays for body fluid identification using one gene each for blood, semen, vaginal secretions and saliva genes. The blood and semen gene transcripts were specific, but the vaginal secretion and saliva genes were variably expressed within and between different body fluids. In contrast, Juusola and Ballantyne (2007) chose to develop triplex real-time PCR assays that detect two body fluid-specific genes for blood, saliva, semen and menstrual blood in addition to a housekeeping gene; the idea being that the use of two markers in each assay would improve assay specificity and provide analytical redundancy by taking into account possible biological variation in gene expression levels between individuals. An approach to identify stable tissue-specific mRNA markers using real-time PCR verification of blood and saliva stains was reported by Zubakov et al. (2008); 5 mRNAs specific for saliva and 9 mRNAs specific for whole blood were identified. In a recent publication, Bauer and Patzelt (2008) expanded their work using real-time PCR and menstrual blood markers. In this report, samples were identified as non-menstrual by determining a cut-off value for the control marker GAPDH, below which negative results for the menstrual blood marker MMP-7 allow the conclusion that the sample was indeed not menstrual blood.

Technology in the field of multiplexing gene expression assays is rapidly improving. The Plexor® One-Step qRT-PCR System takes advantage of the specific interaction between two modified nucleotides to achieve quantitative PCR analysis. As part of the Plexor® One-Step qRT-PCR reaction, a reverse transcription step is performed in order to streamline the RNA analysis. It is possible to design assays to quantify multiple targets within the same reaction using primer pairs with a different fluorophore for each target sequence. The limiting factor in assay design is the dye capability of the real-time PCR instrument. However, since DNA quantitation is moving towards a molecular biological approach which utilizes three- or four-dye real-time PCR instruments, most labs could implement this technology without purchasing new equipment.

As the instrumentation necessary to perform mRNA analysis is in place in most labs, the next major obstacle to overcome prior to laboratories investing in RNA technology is the development of a straight-forward extraction procedure. A method that could co-purify RNA and DNA from a single sample with a minimal number of steps would be attractive to those seeking new technologies. A number of methods describing the simultaneous isolation of DNA and RNA have been reported (Alvarez et al., 2004; Bauer and Patzelt, 2003; Chomczynski, 1993). However, most of these have not been optimized to deal with the reduced quantity or quality of samples encountered in forensic casework. Alternatively, the co-isolation reports using forensically relevant samples (Alvarez et al., 2004; Bauer and Patzelt, 2003) require numerous time-consuming steps that would not benefit fast and simple stain identification assays. Making improvements to the extraction process to allow a streamlined approach is among the goals of our research and one which we envision developing with our commercial partner.

Change in a forensic laboratory can and does happen as witnessed by the revolution seen with DNA analysis. Changing any analytical approach requires documented external research detailing suitable methods and techniques and internal validation of published reports. The forensic laboratory must weigh the advantages and potential pitfalls of any new method and efforts required to bring such technology on-line in the face of pressures to maintain heavy caseloads and meet the demands of the criminal justice community. The research community has published considerable work on mRNA and has amassed a substantial body of information for the forensic community. Presently we understand that mRNA is stable in forensic stains and can be extracted in a sufficient quantity to be detected. Many markers have been identified as potential tissue determinants and a number of detection schemes have been described. This research has been published for many years but the general forensic community has not embraced mRNA for routine tissue identification. The analysis of mRNA is a radical change from the present approach, but the predominant reason for laboratory inactivity in this area is the lack of commercial support. The forensic community has become dependent upon commercialized products for forensic applications. This is not due to a lack of interest on the part of the forensic laboratory scientists to bring newly researched technologies on-line, but rather a realization that in the face of mounting casework, the efforts to bring published methods on-line in a laboratory is a very difficult task. A commercially available assay for particular mRNA transcripts could allow this technology to become a standard tool for forensic analysis.

Our laboratory is but one of many active in mRNA research and we have been fortunate to forge a relationship with a commercial organization to study the possibility of developing a product that could be useful for the forensic community. We intend to develop methods that broaden real-time PCR applications and to investigate a new technology that could radically change the analysis of biological stains and tissues. The biochemical approaches currently used in tissue identification are limited in scope and often imply, but not truly identify, the source fluid/tissue. We believe that the positive identification of fluids and tissues can be performed quickly and efficiently, and that tissues not routinely evaluated could be easily assessed by all laboratories so that an equality of testing could be realized across the country. The evaluation of mRNA through real-time PCR will be a technique that can offer a level of confidence and expand our knowledge of the materials we routinely examine. The nature of our research is to identify mRNA transcripts that will definitively identify the tissue of origin, determine if such transcripts survive the typical environmental insults that forensic samples may potentially encounter, and develop rapid assays to assess these molecules using small amounts of sample. The research into new technologies will demonstrate the power of multiplexing for forensic analysis. This chapter describes our efforts in this regard and our hope, in conjunction with our commercial partners, to develop an assay that could be routinely employed in a forensic laboratory.

## MATERIALS AND METHODS

### Sample Preparation

Blood, seminal fluid, saliva and urine samples were collected by pipetting known amounts of fresh fluid onto swatches of cotton cloth and allowing the spots to dry at room temperature. Vaginal swabs were collected on cotton swabs, whereas menstrual blood was collected on tampons and allowed to dry at room temperature. Each sample was stored in a glassine envelope, which was kept at room temperature in a box designated for the particular fluid at the Vermont Forensic Laboratory. Human tissues (kidney, colon, adipose, skin) were collected from the Surgical Pathology Suite at Fletcher Allen Health Care (Burlington, VT) and frozen at -20°C until use.

Human control RNAs (brain, heart, liver, kidney, intestine) were purchased from Ambion (Austin, TX). Additional human control RNAs (submaxillary gland, salivary gland, skin, blood) were purchased from BioChain (Hayward, CA). These RNAs were supplied as 1 µg/µl and diluted as noted for experiments.

## Serology Tests

### *Acid Phosphatase Presumptive Test (Brentamine Reaction)*
This presumptive test for seminal fluid involves the detection of the enzyme acid phosphatase (AP). The reaction is a result of the liberation of napthol from sodium α-naphthyl phosphate by the enzyme acid phosphatase and the subsequent formation of a purple azo dye by the coupling of napthol with buffered fast blue B. The visible result of this reaction is the development of a deep magenta-purple color.

### *Amylase Diffusion*
Amylase diffusion is a test to indicate whether amylase is present in a sample or stain at levels indicative of the presence of saliva. Amylase in vaginal swabs, semen stains, or other body fluid stains may also show activity, although usually at lower levels. Amylase breaks down starch into a variety of sugar products, and it is this reaction that allows for the detection of amylase. An agarose gel containing starch is prepared and the samples are placed into wells in the gel. If amylase is present, it will migrate away from the point of introduction and break down the starch into sugars. An iodine solution added to the plate will stain blue any areas still containing starch and any areas that were broken down into sugars by the present of amylase will remain clear.

## RNA/DNA Extraction

### *Organic DNA Extraction*
The organic extraction method (Forensic Science Research Training Center, 1989) as modified in Akane et al. (1993) was used in this chapter. Samples were lysed in Stain Extraction Buffer with Proteinase K overnight at 56°C. Phenol:chloroform:isoamyl alcohol (25:24:1, v/v) from Invitrogen (Carlsbad, CA) was added to the lysed samples. Samples were mixed into a milky emulsion and centrifuged to separate the DNA aqueous phase from the organic solvent. Tris-EDTA (TE) was added to a Microcon® 100 Concentrator (Millipore Corporation, Bedford, MA) to wet the membrane. The aqueous phase was added to the Microcon® 100 and centrifuged. A volume of TE was added to the Microcon® 100 and centrifuged. The filtrate cup was removed from the concentrator and placed in a new retentate cup. TE was added to the concentrator and the concentrator was inverted onto the retentate cup to allow for release of the DNA from the concentrator during centrifugation.

## *Tris-Buffered Phenol Method (Stain ID Extraction)*

This protocol is optimized for the simultaneous extraction of both DNA and RNA from a sample. To the sample, RNagents denaturation solution (Promega, Madison, WI), 1X PBS and 20 mg/ml proteinase K is added. The sample is vortexed and incubated for 10 minutes at 56°C. The sample is transferred to a spin basket and centrifuged at max speed for 2 minutes. To the retentate, 2M sodium acetate is added and mixed followed by the addition and mixing of 1M Tris (pH 9.0). A volume of phenol:chloroform:isoamyl alcohol is added and the sample vortexed and centrifuged at max speed for 5 minutes. The aqueous phase is removed into a new tube and chloroform:isoamyl alcohol is added and vortexed. The sample is centrifuged at max speed for 5 minutes and the aqueous phase is removed into a new 1.5 mL tube. Glycogen (5 µg/µl) and isopropanol is added and vortexed. The sample is centrifuged at max speed for 10 minutes and following removal of the supernatant, the sample is washed with ice-cold 95% ethanol. Centrifuge at max speed for 5 minutes and remove supernatant and wash the pellet with 75% ethanol. Centrifuge at max speed for 5 minutes and remove supernatant and allow pellet to air dry for 1 minute. The pellet is resuspended in TE$^{-4}$ and stored at -20°C.

## *TRIzol® Extraction*

Samples were combined with TRIzol® Reagent (Invitrogen) and incubated at 56°C for 20 minutes. To the samples, chloroform was added and the tube was shaken vigorously for 15 seconds. The sample was incubated at 56°C for 10-15 minutes and vortexed every few minutes. The tube was centrifuged for 15 minutes at 11,000 x g causing the sample to separate into a lower, red phenol-chloroform phase, an interphase, and a colorless upper aqueous phase. The aqueous phase containing the RNA was removed into a new tube and combined with isopropanol. The sample was incubated at room temperature for 10 minutes and centrifuged for 15 minutes at 11,000 x g. The supernatant was removed and the pellet was washed with 75% ethanol and then centrifuged for 5 minutes at 7,500 x g. The supernatant was removed and the pellet allowed to air dry prior to resuspension in sterile water. Samples were stored at -20°C.

## Reverse Transcription

Reverse transcription was performed on isolated RNA using the MessageSensor™ RT Kit (Ambion) with minor modifications. RNA extracts were combined with random decamer primers (Ambion) and nuclease-free water. The reaction mixture was heated at 80°C for 3 minutes. To the sample, 10X RT buffer, dNTPs, RNase inhibitor, and reverse transcriptase were added. The sample was mixed gently and incubated at 43°C for 1 hour followed by 92°C for 10 minutes. cDNAs were stored at -20°C.

## Real-Time PCR

### *TaqMan®*

Singleplex assays using real-time PCR on cDNAs were performed using Assays-on-Demand™ Gene Expression Products (Applied Biosystems, Foster City, CA). These are a comprehensive collection of pre-designed and tested primer and probe sets that allow researchers to perform quantitative gene expression studies on any human gene. They are designed against GenBank transcripts, transcripts from the Mammalian Gene Collection, and human Celera transcripts. Each assay is built on 5' nuclease chemistry and consists of two unlabeled PCR primers and a FAM™ dye-labeled TaqMan® minor groove binder (MGB) probe. The components are formulated into a single 20X mix and designed to run under universal conditions for reverse transcription and PCR.

For the real-time PCR reactions, TaqMan® Universal PCR Master Mix, No AmpErase UNG (Applied Biosystems), cDNA, Assay-on-Demand™ primer/probe mix and nuclease-free water were combined. Cycling was performed in a RotorGene 3000 or 6000 (Corbett Research, Sydney, Australia) according to the following temperature profile: hold at 95°C for 10 minutes, 50 cycles of 95°C for 15 seconds and 60°C for 60 seconds. Data were analyzed using RotorGene software from Corbett Research.

### *Plexor®*

The Plexor® technology (Promega) takes advantage of the specific interaction between two modified nucleotides to achieve quantitative PCR analysis. One of the primers contains a modified nucleotide (iso-dC) linked to a fluorescent label at the 5' end. The second PCR primer is unlabeled. The reaction mix includes deoxynucelotides and iso-dGTP modified with the quencher dabcyl. Dabcyl-iso-dGTP is incorporated opposite the iso-dC residue in the primer. The incorporation of the dabcyl-iso-dGTP at this position results in quenching of the fluorescent dye on the complementary strand and a reduction in fluorescence, which allows quantitation during amplification. Therefore, with the Plexor® technology, accumulation of product is accompanied by a decrease in fluorescence. As a quality check, the Plexor® System allows you to measure the melting temperature of the PCR products as homogeneous products create a well defined melting curve.

A single Plexor® reaction can contain multiple Plexor® primer sets; each primer pair is specific to a different target sequence, and labeled with different fluorophores. The dabcyl-iso-dGTP in the Plexor® master mix will quench the fluorescence of all the dyes present in the reaction. Plexor® primers were designed by Promega using the Plexor® Primer Design Software (Promega).

For the Plexor® Stain ID reactions, 2X Master Mix, RNasin® RNase Inhibitor, ImProm-II™ Reverse Transcriptase, Primer Mix and water were combined with unknown sample RNA. Cycling was performed in a RotorGene 6000 according to the following temperature profile: hold at 45°C for 5 minutes, hold at 95°C for 2 minutes, 38 cycles of 95°C for 5 seconds and 60°C for 35 seconds. This program was followed by a dissociation protocol of 95°C for 5 seconds, 50°C-95°C (2.5 acquisitions per °C), and 50°C for 30 seconds. Data were analyzed using Plexor® Analysis Software from Promega.

## Quantitation of DNA Extracts

The Plexor® HY System is a real-time PCR assay specifically designed to determine the concentration of total human DNA and male human DNA simultaneously in one reaction. The kit contains an internal PCR control (IPC) to test for false-negative results that may occur in the presence of PCR inhibitors, and a melt curve function to confirm the correct product was amplified. Plexor® HY is a sensitive multiplex kit, with routine detection of approximately 6.4 pg total DNA. PCR amplification setup is performed at room temperature and is compatible with automated platforms. After PCR, a melt analysis can be performed to provide an internal control for the final assay design or to expedite troubleshooting.

# RESULTS

## Determining the Half-life of mRNA in Different Types of Stains

In order for a candidate to be implemented into a stain identification assay, it needs to be detectable for years following deposition of the sample. The amount of RNA present was determined by real-time PCR TaqMan® assays using HBB (blood), PRM2 (seminal fluid) or the housekeeping gene B2M. Applied Biosystems has created TaqMan® primer/probe sets for many human genes (Assay-on-Demand™ products). These have been carefully designed and thoroughly tested for specificity. Most of these sets are mRNA specific (cross exon-exon boundaries and have no cross-reaction with pseudogenes) although some do react with genomic DNA. Since these sets are available, optimized and cost only $150 each, we decided to use these pre-designed sets for our initial studies rather than expend the time and resources necessary to design our own. Table 1 lists the Assay-on-Demand™ numbers for each of the genes of interest. The mRNA specific assays (probe spans an exon/exon junction) end in "_m1". Those ending in "_g1" are not guaranteed to be mRNA specific. We checked the results when using two of the _g1 probes (HBB and PSA) by amplifying with DNA. Figure 1 shows the result of amplification of cDNA and genomic DNA (256 ng in a 10 ul reaction) with five TaqMan® assays; only the cDNA was amplified.

One of the earliest experiments we performed was to determine if amplifiable RNA could be detected from an aged blood sample. From preliminary studies, we had 20 μl and 40 μl blood stains on cotton cloth which had been stored at room temperature in the dark for 13 and 26 months, respectively. Following amplification with the TaqMan® HBB assay, it was apparent that this candidate gene was very stable over time (Figure 2). Similar results were seen for detection of the candidate gene PRM2 in seminal fluid. Twenty μl seminal fluid stains aged for 16 or 24 months were easily detected using this assay (Figure 3).

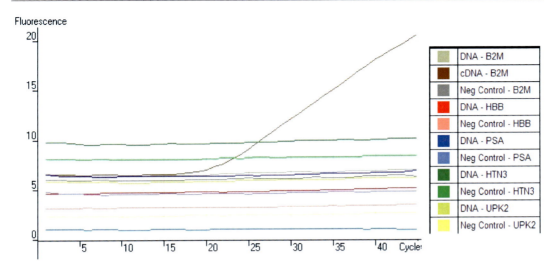

Figure 1. DNA and cDNA amplified with five cDNA-specific assays. After room temperature storage for 18 hours, a 20 μl blood stain was extracted using the TRIzol® reagent. Six μl of RNA was reverse transcribed using the MessageSensor™ RT Kit. Two μl of the resulting cDNA was used with the B2M Assays-on-Demand™ Gene Expression Product. Water as a negative control or control DNA (Promega; 256 ng in a 10 ul reaction) was used with the B2M, HBB, PSA, HTN3 and UPK2 Assays-on-Demand™ Gene Expression Products. Real-time PCR reactions were performed on a Corbett Rotor-Gene 6000 and data analyzed using the Rotor-Gene Software.

Now that we had determined the HBB and PRM2 genes were amplifiable in samples aged for two years, we performed time course studies to look at the stabilities over time. For blood, we used two sample volumes, 1 μl and 10 μl that had been aging at room temperature in the dark for 3 days to 510 days (1 μl) or 864 days (10 μl). As depicted in Table 2, there is a slight decrease in expression over time, but samples aged well over a year (or more) maintained a high HBB expression level.

In a similar experiment, we looked at two different sized seminal fluid stains, 1 μl and 20 μl that had been aging at room temperature in the dark for 16 days to 807 days (1 μl) or 791 days (20 μl). Table 3 shows that PRM2 expression is maintained in samples aged over 2 years. In fact, it appears as though the expression may even increase over time, perhaps due to the loss of an inhibitor.

### Table 1. Assays-on-Demand™ Gene Expression products used in the project

| TISSUE | Assays on Demand (ABI) | | |
|---|---|---|---|
| Blood | hemoglobin, beta [HBB] (Hs00747223_g1) | CD3G antigen, gamma polypeptide [CD3G] (Hs00173941_m1) | spectrin, beta, erythrocytic [SPTB] (Hs00165820_m1) |
| Semen | semenogelin I [SEMG1] (Hs00268141_m1) | kallikrein 3 [PSA] (Hs00426859_g1) | acid phosphatase, prostate [ACPP] (Hs00173475_m1) |
| | cysteine-rich secretory protein 1[CRISP1] (Hs00538261_m1) | microseminoprotein, beta- [MSMB] (Hs00159303_m1) | transglutaminase 4 [TGM4] (Hs00162710_m1) |
| Sperm | protamine 2 [PRM2] (Hs00172518_m1) | | |
| Saliva | statherin [STATH] (Hs00162389_m1) | histatin 3 [HTN3] (Hs00264790_m1) | |

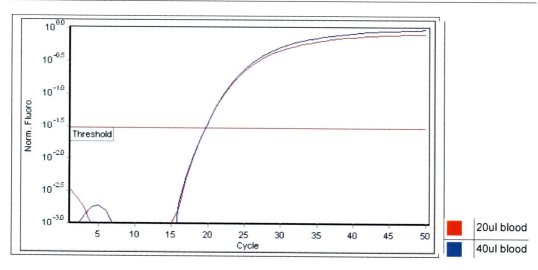

Figure 2. Amplification of aged blood with the HBB TaqMan® assay. After room temperature storage for 13 or 26 months, dried blood stains (20 and 40 μl, respectively) were extracted using the TRIzol® reagent. Six μl of RNA was reverse transcribed using the MessageSensor™ RT Kit. Two μl of the resulting cDNA was used with the HBB Assays-on-Demand™ Gene Expression Product. Real-time PCR reactions were performed on a Corbett Rotor-Gene 6000 and data analyzed using the Rotor-Gene Software.

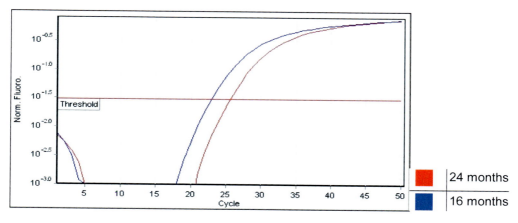

Figure 3. Amplification of aged semen with the PRM2 TaqMan® assay. After room temperature storage for 16 or 24 months, dried semen stains (20 μl) were extracted using the TRIzol® reagent. Six μl of RNA was reverse transcribed using the MessageSensor™ RT Kit. Two μl of the resulting cDNA was used with the PRM2 Assays-on-Demand™ Gene Expression Product. Real-time PCR reactions were performed on a Corbett Rotor-Gene 6000 and data analyzed using the Rotor-Gene Software.

Forensic samples are often exposed to a variety of environmental insults therefore, we stored parallel samples under ideal conditions (room temperature, dark) as well as in a sub-optimal condition (37°C). By comparing gene amplification between the samples, we hoped to determine whether RNA profiling would be feasible for weathered forensic stains. In the first experiment, between 0.25 μl and 20 μl of blood was spotted onto cloth and dried at either room temperature in the dark, or in a 37°C incubator. The samples were stored for 503 days prior to extraction with TRIzol®. cDNA was amplified using the HBB TaqMan® assay. Figure

4 shows that amplification of HBB is possible following storage at 37°C for 503 days. In fact, there does not appear to be a considerable decrease in the degree of amplification after prolonged exposure to elevated temperatures.

**Table 2. Time course of HBB expression in blood stains**

| BLOOD | AGE (DAYS) | HBB Ct |
|---|---|---|
| 1 µl | 3 | 19.94 |
| 1 µl | 23 | 19.99 |
| 1 µl | 461 | 23.30 |
| 1 µl | 496 | 23.52 |
| 1 µl | 510 | 23.15 |
| 10 µl | 3 | 17.68 |
| 10 µl | 420 | 19.94 |
| 10 µl | 490 | 20.27 |
| 10 µl | 855 | 20.15 |
| 10 µl | 864 | 20.51 |

Ct for the NTC was 35.15

**Table 3. Time course of PRM2 expression in seminal fluid stains**

| SEMEN | AGE (DAYS) | PRM2 Ct |
|---|---|---|
| 1 µl | 16 | 34.61 |
| 1 µl | 461 | 30.35 |
| 1 µl | 507 | 27.41 |
| 1 µl | 699 | 30.95 |
| 1 µl | 807 | 36.90 |
| 20 µl | 16 | 27.92 |
| 20 µl | 507 | 20.10 |
| 20 µl | 607 | 22.19 |
| 20 µl | 777 | 21.34 |
| 20 µl | 791 | 22.94 |

Ct for NTC was not observed during the 50 cycles

One experiment we performed was to evaluate blood samples which had been stored under both conditions (room temp/dark, 37°C) for an extended period of time with a relatively new sample. One µl blood stains were stored for 544 days at room temperature (dark) or in a 37°C incubator and extracted with TRIzol®. For comparison purposes, a 1 µl blood stain was stored for 3 days at room temperature (dark) in order to see how much amplification of HBB decreases with prolonged storage at either of the two conditions. Regardless of the storage length or conditions, the resulting Cts were essentially the same with a difference of less than 1 Ct between all 3 samples (Figure 5). This result further demonstrates how stable HBB RNA is over time.

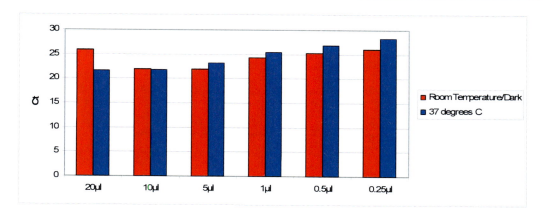

Figure 4. Effect of storage conditions on HBB amplification from blood stains. After room temperature or 37°C storage for 503 days, dried blood stains (0.25 – 20 µl) were extracted using the TRIzol® reagent. Six µl of RNA was reverse transcribed using the MessageSensor™ RT Kit. Two µl of the resulting cDNA was used with the HBB Assays-on-Demand™ Gene Expression Product. Real-time PCR reactions were performed on a Corbett Rotor-Gene 6000 and data analyzed using the Rotor-Gene Software.

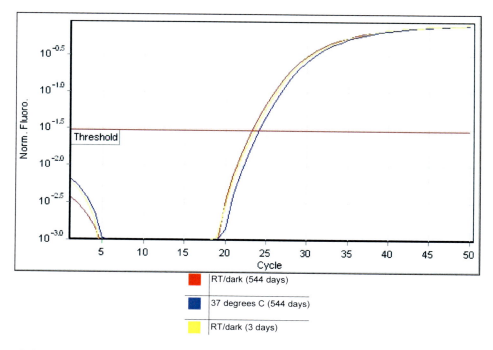

Figure 5. HBB expression in aged blood stains stored at various conditions. After room temperature or 37°C storage for 3 or 544 days, dried blood stains (1 µl) were extracted using the TRIzol® reagent. Six µl of RNA was reverse transcribed using the MessageSensor™ RT Kit. Two µl of the resulting cDNA was used with the HBB Assays-on-Demand™ Gene Expression Product. Real-time PCR reactions were performed on a Corbett Rotor-Gene 6000 and data analyzed using the Rotor-Gene Software.

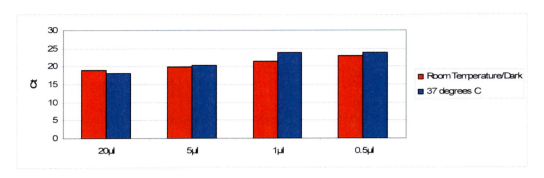

Figure 6. Effect of storage conditions on PRM2 amplification from seminal fluid stains. After room temperature or 37°C storage for 518 days, dried semen stains (0.5 - 20 μl) were extracted using the TRIzol® reagent. Six μl of RNA was reverse transcribed using the MessageSensor™ RT Kit. Two μl of the resulting cDNA were used with the PRM2 Assays-on-Demand™ Gene Expression Product. Real-time PCR reactions were performed on a Corbett Rotor-Gene 6000 and data analyzed using the Rotor-Gene Software.

In a similar experiment, between 0.5 μl and 20 μl of semen was spotted onto cloth and dried at either room temperature in the dark, or in a 37°C incubator. The samples were stored for 518 days prior to extraction with TRIzol®. cDNA was amplified using the PRM2 TaqMan® assay. Figure 6 shows that amplification of PRM2 is possible following storage at 37°C for 518 days. Similar to what was shown for blood and HBB expression, there does not appear to be a considerable decrease in the degree of amplification after prolonged exposure to elevated temperatures.

## Finding Genes Specific for Each Stain Type

Survey of literature including PubMed, Gene and other databases have allowed for the selection of several genes that appear to be specific for a number of different tissues (Table 1). The following alphabetical list is a brief description of each gene target utilized in this chapter:

*ACPP (acid phosphatase, prostate)* - enzyme which catalyzes the conversion of orthophosphoric monoester to alcohol and orthophosphate; secreted by the epithelial cells of the prostate gland;

*B2M (beta 2 microglobulin)* - serum protein found in association with the major histocompatibility complex class I heavy chain on the surface of nearly all nucleated cells;

*CD3G (CD3G antigen, gamma polypeptide)* - component of the T-cell receptor-CD3 complex;

*CRISP1 (cysteine-rich secretory protein 1)* - expressed in the epididymis and plays a role at fertilization in sperm-egg fusion;

*GAPDH (glyceraldehyde-3-phosphate dehydrogenase)* - catalyzes an important energy-yielding step in carbohydrate metabolism, the reversible oxidative phosphorylation of glyceraldehyde-3-phosphate in the presence of inorganic phosphate and nicotinamide adenine dinucleotide;

*HBB (hemoglobin, beta)* - iron containing oxygen-transport metalloprotein in red blood cells;

*HTN3 (histatin 3)* - non-immunological, anti-microbial role in the oral cavity;

*MSMB (microseminoprotein, beta)* - synthesized by the epithelial cells of the prostate gland and secreted into the seminal plasma;

*PRM2 (protamine 2)* - major DNA-binding protein in the nucleus of sperm and packages DNA;

*PSA (kallikrein 3)* - protease present in seminal plasma involved in liquefaction of seminal coagulum;

*SEMG1 (semenogelin 1)* - involved in formation of gel matrix that encases ejaculated spermatozoa;

*SPTB (spectrin, beta, erythrocytic)* - major component of red blood cell membrane;

*STAT (statherin)* - peptide that inhibits precipitation from calcium phosphate solutions, stabilizes saliva;

*TGM4 (transglutaminase 4)* - catalyzes the cross linking of proteins and the conjugation of polyamines to specific proteins in the seminal tract.

We tested the specificity, robustness and sensitivity of each assay by analysis of mRNA isolated from the body fluid of interest. Once the assay was been shown to be robust, we tested it on mRNA isolated from other fluids and tissues to demonstrate that the assay is specific. Additional fluids and tissues to those discussed previously included vaginal secretions and menstrual blood. For semen, we are interested in mRNAs specific for the sperm as well as for the prostatic components. In a number of cases, it is important to determine if semen is present even if the male is sterile or has had a vasectomy. In other cases, it is important to know if sperm are likely to be present. We obtained anonymous samples of a variety of tissues (kidney, colon, adipose, skin) from the Surgical Pathology Suite at Fletcher Allen Health Care. Lastly, control RNAs (liver, kidney, brain, heart, intestine) were purchased from Ambion to ensure that our assays are specific only for the intended tissue.

The sensitivity of the three candidate blood assays (HBB, CD3G, SPTB) was evaluated using a range of blood volumes spotted onto cotton cloth. Between 0.0001 µl and 20 µl of blood was allowed to air dry at room temperature for 18 hours prior to extraction using TRIzol®. cDNA was amplified using the three TaqMan® assays. The sensitivity of HBB was far superior to the other assays with amplification resulting from 0.0001 µl of blood, compared to a limit of 1 µl for the CD3G and SPTB assays (Table 4).

The sensitivity of the four candidate semen assays (SEMG1, PSA, MSMB, TGM4) and one sperm assay (PRM2) was evaluated using a range of semen volumes spotted onto cotton cloth. In one experiment (SEMG1, PSA, PRM2), between 0.01 µl and 20 µl of semen was allowed to air dry at room temperature for 8 days prior to extraction using TRIzol®. In a subsequent experiment (MSMB, TGM4), between 1 µl and 20 µl of semen was allowed to air dry at room temperature for 41 days prior to extraction using TRIzol®. cDNA was amplified using the five TaqMan® assays. The sensitivities of PSA and PRM2 were slightly higher than SEMG1 since both were able to amplify from 0.01 µl of semen (Table 5). However, since the Cts for PRM2 were significantly lower than those for PSA (and SEMG1) for most volumes, PRM2 appears to have a higher expression level, or is a more robust assay. Furthermore, the second experiment with MSMB and TGM4 suggests that those two candidates are expressed more than the other semen markers (SEMG1 and PSA) since the Cts are lower. But, since the two lowest volumes, namely 0.01 µl and 0.1 µl, were not analyzed with these two assays, the lower limits are unknown, but assumed to be lower than 1 µl based on the Cts.

### Table 4. Sensitivities of TaqMan® blood assays

| BLOOD VOLUME | HBB | CD3G | SPTB |
|---|---|---|---|
| NTC | 37.21 | ND | ND |
| 0.0001 µl | 33.13 | ND | ND |
| 0.001 µl | 29.92 | ND | ND |
| 0.01 µl | 26.28 | ND | ND |
| 0.1 µl | 24.31 | ND | ND |
| 1 µl | 21.60 | 33.41 | 35.00 |
| 5 µl | 19.08 | 29.63 | 34.35 |
| 10 µl | 16.67 | 28.69 | 31.56 |
| 20 µl | 15.84 | 28.62 | 31.24 |

ND = not detected

### Table 5. Sensitivities of TaqMan® semen and sperm assays

| SEMEN VOLUME | SEMG1 | PSA | MSMB | TGM4 | PRM2 |
|---|---|---|---|---|---|
| NTC | ND | ND | ND | ND | ND |
| 0.01 µl | ND | 37.20 | N/A | N/A | 35.67 |
| 0.1 µl | 33.79 | 34.15 | N/A | N/A | 32.26 |
| 1 µl | 30.80 | 31.39 | 25.42 | 28.33 | 28.93 |
| 5 µl | 31.43 | 32.48 | 28.90 | 30.69 | 27.57 |
| 10 µl | 31.55 | 35.13 | 29.74 | 31.15 | 24.80 |
| 20 µl | 31.86 | 34.02 | 28.35 | 30.79 | 27.24 |

ND = not detected
N/A = not determined

### Table 6. Sensitivities of TaqMan® saliva assays

| SALIVA VOLUME | STAT | HTN3 |
|---|---|---|
| NTC | ND | ND |
| 0.1 µl | ND | ND |
| 1 µl | 34.14 | ND |
| 5 µl | 33.93 | 39.45 |
| 10 µl | 37.80 | 37.93 |
| 20 µl | 34.68 | 36.25 |

ND = not detected

The sensitivities for saliva candidate markers (STAT, HTN3) were evaluated using a range of saliva volumes spotted onto cotton cloth. Between 0.01 µl and 20 µl of saliva was allowed to air dry at room temperature for 18 hours prior to extraction using TRIzol®. cDNA was amplified using the two TaqMan® assays. As shown in Table 6, only the STAT assay was able to detect 1 µl of freshly dried saliva, whereas the HTN3 assay had a 5 µl limit of detection. The Cts were not as low as seen in the blood and semen/sperm assays, but were different than the absence of Cts observed for the negative controls.

**Table 7. Specificity of blood, semen, sperm and saliva TaqMan® assays (grey = not tested)**

|  | BLOOD ||| SEMEN ||||||  SPERM | SALIVA | CONTROL |
|---|---|---|---|---|---|---|---|---|---|---|---|---|
|  | HBB | SPTB | CD3G | PSA | SEMG1 | ACPP | CRISP1 | MSMB | TGM4 | PRM2 | STAT | B2M |
| Blood | + | + | + | - | - | + | - | - | - | - | - | + |
| Semen | - | - | - | + | + | + | - | + | + | + | - | + |
| Saliva | - | - | - | - | - | - | - | - | - | - | + | + |
| Menstrual Blood |  |  |  |  | - | - | - | - | - |  |  | + |
| Vaginal Secretions |  |  |  | + | + | - | - | - | - |  |  | + |
| Kidney | - |  |  | - | - |  |  | - | - | - |  | + |
| Colon |  |  |  | - |  |  |  | - | - | - |  | + |
| Adipose |  |  |  | - |  |  |  | - | - | - |  | + |
| Skin |  |  |  | - |  |  |  | - | - | - |  | + |
| Ambion Brain |  |  |  | - |  |  |  | - | - | - |  | + |
| Ambion Heart |  |  |  | - |  |  |  | - | - | - |  | + |
| Ambion Liver |  |  |  | - |  |  |  | - | - | - |  | + |
| Ambion Kidney |  |  |  | - |  |  |  | - | - | - |  | + |
| Ambion Intestine |  |  |  | - |  |  |  | + | - | - |  | + |

The specificity of the chosen genes for the tissue of interest was also examined. To test the TaqMan® sets (only the control B2M and tissue-specific sets should give amplification), mRNA was isolated from dried blood, semen, saliva, menstrual blood or vaginal secretions using TRIzol®. Human tissues (kidney, colon, adipose, skin) were extracted using the Absolutely RNA® Kit. Control human RNAs from Ambion (brain, heart, liver, kidney, intestine) were diluted to 100 ng/µl. The RNA samples were then reverse transcribed and PCR performed with each of the TaqMan® sets. The amplification results for the blood, semen, sperm, and saliva assays are depicted in Table 7.

For the three blood assays, amplification only occurred in the blood sample as expected. For the 6 semen assays there were mixed results. PSA, SEMG1, MSMB and TGM4 all appeared to be specific for semen when tested against blood, semen and saliva. However, SEMG1 cross-reacted with vaginal secretions, albeit at a much lower level (Ct of 29.40 for semen vs. Ct of 33.67 for vaginal secretions). Interestingly, MSMB amplified from a control intestine sample, but not with human colon tissues. ACPP and CRISP1, although ideal candidates based on literature searches, were not suitable assays for the specific detection of semen. The sperm marker PRM2 amplified from a seminal fluid sample, but nothing else that was tested. For saliva, amplification only occurred with the STAT assay as expected. The control B2M was detected in each of the fluids and tissues. Based on these results, several of these TaqMan® assays appear to be specific (HBB, SPTB, CD3G, PSA, STAT), however, screening against an expanded sample set would strengthen that claim. Alternatively, TGM4 and PRM2 have demonstrated their specificity for semen/sperm through the course of these studies.

Table 8. Detection of semen and saliva using a Plexor®-based Stain ID assay

| SAMPLE | HTN3 (FAM) | SEMG1 (HEX) | GAPDH (ROX) |
|---|---|---|---|
| NTC | ND | ND | ND |
| NTC | ND | ND | ND |
| DNA | ND | 34.3 | ND |
| DNA | ND | 33.5 | ND |
| vaginal secretion | ND | ND | 22.1 |
| vaginal secretion | ND | ND | 22.3 |
| vagina | ND | ND | 21.4 |
| vagina | ND | ND | 21.1 |
| submaxillary gland | 8.8 | ND | 24.7 |
| submaxillary gland | 8.2 | ND | 24.8 |
| salivary gland | 14.8 | ND | 26.0 |
| salivary gland | 14.8 | ND | 25.8 |
| saliva | 27.0 | ND | 28.0 |
| saliva | 26.9 | ND | 27.2 |
| skin | ND | ND | 23.0 |
| skin | ND | ND | 23.0 |
| semen | ND | 19.7 | 25.1 |
| semen | ND | 19.8 | 25.5 |
| blood | ND | ND | 24.9 |
| blood | ND | ND | 25.5 |

ND = Not Detected

## Developing Multiplex Assays for the Detection of Stain Types

A major aim of stain identification using mRNA expression profiling is working towards multiplexing the real-time PCR assays once mRNAs are identified that clearly define specific types of stains. Since these assays are designed to function more qualitatively than quantitatively, a test of a single stain should typically give amplification with only one candidate. It is possible that a mixture could give several amplifications. However, it is of greater concern to know that a mixture does exist, than to know the exact amount of each fluid present.

One methodology to achieve this goal is the Plexor® system from Promega. Depending on the dye-capability of the real-time instrument that is utilized, this system allows multiple mRNAs to be combined in one assay, thus reducing the amount of sample needed and time of analysis. For example, using a 4-dye channel instrument, eight mRNA targets could be analyzed; two per dye-channel, each of which has a distinctive melt curve. The Plexor® qRT-PCR system takes advantage of the specific interaction between two modified nucleotides to achieve quantitative PCR analysis. Promega's Plexor® design software allows the generation of primers which span an intron by designating a certain base to include in the primer design.

During the course of our work, we were contacted by Promega with an offer to collaborate on the development of stain identification assays. The combination of Promega's extensive knowledge of the Plexor® platform with our sample inventory and insight into the needs of the forensic laboratory, it was a strong partnership. The goal was to generate Plexor® Tissue Typing Systems; multiplexed qRT-PCR systems for determining the source and quantity of a variety of human stains and/or tissues. The systems would include Plexor® primers for the detection of tissue-specific mRNA transcripts associated with semen, sperm, blood, menstrual blood, saliva, etc. By limiting the initial system to two-color detection (i.e. FAM and HEX detection), it would be compatible with the majority of real-time thermal cyclers in forensic laboratories. We sought to explore the potential to include controls (e.g. a housekeeping gene) or multiple, tissue-specific targets using the ability of the Plexor® Data Analysis Software to distinguish two different amplicons in the same dye channel, based upon thermal melt properties.

The Stain ID assay which we decided to first focus on was for detection of semen and saliva. Plexor® primers were designed to amplify the targets SEMG1 (semen), HTN3 (saliva) and GAPDH (housekeeper). Table 8 shows amplification of a variety of RNA samples using the triplex. The saliva primers (HTN3) show specific reactivity with saliva RNA (isolated in-house), and also with submaxillary gland RNA and salivary gland RNA that was purchased from a commercial vendor (BioChain). They show no cross-reactivity with other RNA samples tested, or with genomic DNA. The semen primers (SEMG1) show specific reactivity with semen RNA that was isolated in-house, and did not amplify any of the other RNA samples tested. However, they do show some minor reactivity with genomic DNA. This is likely due to some weak amplification across the intron in the genomic sequence. Therefore, new SEMG1 primers were designed that would hopefully address the genomic DNA amplification.

The modified SEMG1 primers were screened for the possibility of amplifying genomic DNA. The new primers did indeed eliminate cross-reactivity with genomic DNA, however the primers now yielded a product with RNA isolated from blood. The initial blood sample isolated showed no reactivity with the SEMG1 primers (old or new), but a commercial blood sample did show amplification with the SEMG1 primers. To confirm this, two additional RNA samples from blood were generated in-house and tested. Both of those showed amplification with the SEMG1 primers (Figure 7) with melt curves specific to the RNA product and not the product expected with genomic DNA. This indicates that the modified primers eliminated the amplification from genomic DNA, but not from RNA isolated from blood. Therefore, we assume that SEMG1 is expressed at low levels in blood. Although the article doesn't mention blood specifically, Lundwall et al. (2002) reported SEMG1 to be expressed in a number of non-genital tissues. As a result of these findings, we decided to replace SEMG1 with a different semen-specific target.

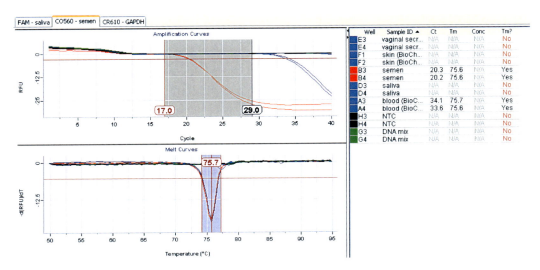

Figure 7. Cross-reactivity of SEMG1 Plexor® primers with blood. After room temperature storage for 18 hours, dried vaginal secretions, semen and saliva stains were extracted using phenol-chloroform or the Promega PureYield RNA midiprep kit (vaginal secretions). The RNA was quantitated and 100 ng of RNA was used in the Plexor® Stain ID assay. Control skin and blood RNA (BioChain) was also analyzed. Reactions were performed in duplicate on a RotorGene 6000 and data analyzed using the Plexor® analysis software.

Protamine 2 was identified as a potential target in early experiments, so primers were designed and screened for PRM1 and PRM2 transcripts. The PRM1 primers were designed so that one primer sits on the junction of the two exons, however some amplification of genomic DNA was detected. Three different sets of PRM2 primers were designed. The first set was designed so that one primer sits on the junction of two exons, but some amplification of genomic DNA was detected, as well as amplification from other RNA transcripts. The second set was designed so that one primer is on either side of the intron. Some amplification of genomic DNA was detected; however, the DNA melt curve was distinct from the RNA melt (84°C for RNA vs. 88°C for DNA). The third set of PRM2 primers was also designed so that one primer is on either side of the intron. Some amplification of genomic DNA was detected, however, the DNA melt curve was distinct from the RNA melt curve. Unfortunately, minor amplification of skin and blood also occurred with these primers. The second set of PRM2 primers looked the most promising although in theory, PRM2 is a sperm-specific marker and therefore, may not be expressed in vaseoctomized males. We isolated RNA from a semen sample donated by a vasectomized male and not surprisingly, PRM2 was not detected (Figure 8). At this point, because the screening assay only includes one semen/sperm marker, it was decided that PRM2 would not be a viable candidate since the presence of semen would go undetected in samples from vasectomized males or donors with low-sperm counts.

The next semen-specific candidate which was assessed was PSA. Initial studies with PSA primers showed non-specific amplification with all other RNAs that were tested, as well as genomic DNA and the no template control. Since all nonspecific amplification (including the no template control) was identical in the amplification and melt curves the cause was thought to be primer dimerization. However, additional experiments with variations in the PSA primer sequences yielded little improvement in the target specificity. Based on studies we had performed using the Gene Expression TaqMan® assays from Applied Biosystems, we switched our focus to MSMB and TGM4. Expression of MSMB occurred in both vasectomized and non-vasectomized semen samples, however, nonspecific amplification was observed with all the other RNAs as well as genomic DNA. Changing the fluorescent label to the opposite primer showed no improvement in target specificity. On the other hand, TGM4 was detected in both vasectomized and non-vasectomized semen samples without nonspecific amplification (Figure 9).

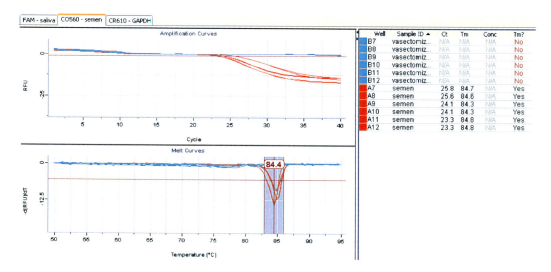

Figure 8. Absence of PRM2 expression in vasectomized males. After room temperature storage for 18 hours, dried semen stains from 6 individuals were extracted using phenol-chloroform. The RNA was quantitated and 100 ng of RNA was used in the Plexor® Stain ID assay. Reactions were performed in duplicate on a RotorGene 6000 and data analyzed using the Plexor® analysis software.

The preliminary experiments were not performed using sample types and sizes which are reflective of forensic-type samples. The RNA samples which were extracted in-house included vaginal secretions, whole blood, semen and saliva. In all cases, RNA was extracted from extremely large sample sizes (i.e. 2 mL of semen, 10 mL of saliva, 5 mL of whole blood) and the samples were all fresh. These were obviously not typical casework samples, but intended to isolate a large pool of RNA that experiments could be performed with. The semen, saliva and whole blood RNA samples were extracted with phenol-chloroform and the vaginal secretion was extracted using Promega's PureYield RNA midiprep kit. After extraction, the RNA was quantitated and 100 ng of RNA was used per reaction. Titration experiments were performed and indicated that semen had a detection threshold of approximately 10 pg of RNA whereas the threshold for saliva was approximately 1 ng of RNA. Although these studies gave an idea as to the relative sensitivities of the assay, it was important to assess how the assay would perform with typical forensic samples (i.e. various volumes of unknown RNA yields).

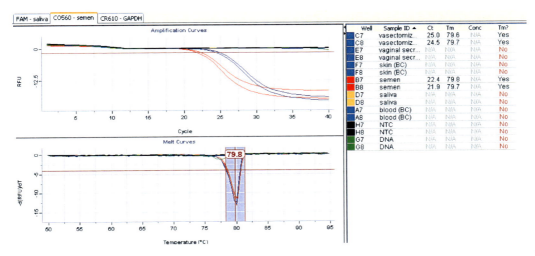

Figure 9. Specific expression of TGM4 in semen samples. After room temperature storage for 18 hours, dried vaginal secretions, semen and saliva stains were extracted using phenol-chloroform or the Promega PureYield RNA midiprep kit (vaginal secretions). The RNA was quantitated and 100ng of RNA was used in the Plexor® Stain ID assay. Control skin and blood RNA (BioChain) was also analyzed. Reactions were performed in duplicate on a RotorGene 6000 and data analyzed using the Plexor® analysis software.

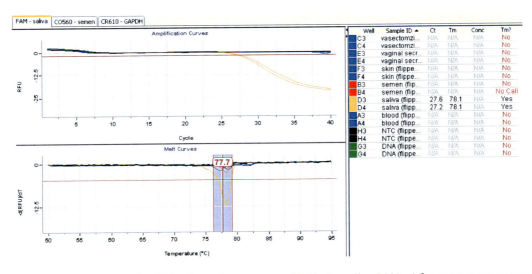

Figure 10. Modification of HTN3 primers increases specificity for saliva RNA. After room temperature storage for 18 hours, dried vaginal secretions, semen and saliva stains were extracted using phenol-chloroform or the Promega PureYield RNA midiprep kit (vaginal secretions). The RNA was quantitated and 100 ng of RNA was used in the Plexor® Stain ID assay. Control skin and blood RNA (BioChain) were also analyzed. Reactions were performed in duplicate on a RotorGene 6000 and data analyzed using the Plexor® analysis software.

A panel of samples was screened using the Stain ID assay which now consisted of HTN3, TGM4, and GAPDH. Samples included dried blood (20 µl aged 70 days), semen (1-20 µl aged 76 days), saliva (1-20 µl aged 4 days), menstrual blood (5x5 mm cutting aged 700 days) and vaginal secretions (1/2 swab aged 54 days) extracted with TRIzol®. Positive control samples of known RNA quantities were run along with the Plexor® Stain ID assay: semen (1 ng/reaction) and saliva (10 ng/reaction). The results are shown in Table 9. The HTN3 primers amplified from all four saliva samples ranging from 1-20 µl of dried saliva as well as the positive control sample. However, there was some nonspecific amplification in the vaginal secretions sample. The TGM4 primers only amplified extracts from the semen samples and positive control. Interestingly, GAPDH was not amplified in the four saliva samples even though HTN3 was clearly detected which suggests that the expression of the housekeeper in saliva is not as prevalent as the tissue-specific marker. Based on the HTN3 results, the primers were modified by moving the fluorescent label from one oligo to the other. The modified HTN3 primers no longer detect vaginal secretions (Figure 10).

**Table 9. Detection of semen and saliva with the Plexor® Stain ID assay**

| SAMPLE | HTN3 (FAM) | TGM4 (HEX) | GAPDH (ROX) |
|---|---|---|---|
| NTC | ND | ND | ND |
| Blood (20ul) | ND | ND | 30.1 |
| Semen (20ul) | ND | **27.5** | 34.9 |
| Semen (10ul) | ND | **27.0** | 35.9 |
| Semen (5ul) | ND | **25.6** | 33.5 |
| Semen (1ul) | ND | **25.0** | 35.3 |
| Saliva (20ul) | **20.9** | ND | ND |
| Saliva (10ul) | **22.3** | ND | ND |
| Saliva (5ul) | **22.6** | ND | ND |
| Saliva (1ul) | **25.4** | ND | ND |
| Menstrual Blood | ND | ND | 38.8 |
| Vaginal Secretions | 24.4 | ND | 24.4 |
| Semen (+) Control | ND | **24.4** | 36.5 |
| Saliva (+) Control | **21.6** | ND | 37.5 |

ND = Not Detected

**Table 10. DNA yield comparison of Tris-buffered phenol and RNagents extractions**

| | Pre-Processing Step | | No Pre-Processing Step | |
|---|---|---|---|---|
| SAMPLE | Tris (ng) | RNagents (ng) | Tris (ng) | RNagents (ng) |
| 10ul semen | 2851.25 | 21.07 | 361.88 | 0.53 |
| 1ul semen | 190.78 | 3.65 | 63.58 | 0.27 |
| 10ul saliva | 166.45 | 0.56 | 89.38 | 0.94 |
| 1ul saliva | 3.49 | 0.01 | 6.66 | 0.04 |

A major selling point of the Stain ID assay was the development of a co-isolation method for RNA and DNA extraction. By utilizing one extraction step, a DNA sample would be ready and waiting for STR profiling if the RNA screening assay deemed it worthy of such analysis. In addition, obtaining RNA and DNA from a single stain would prevent the possibility of conclusions being drawn regarding the identity of one stain which may not hold true for a nearby stain. Therefore, a significant amount of time was spent optimizing a procedure which would co-extract the two nucleic acids so that they were of sufficient quality and quantity for downstream analyses.

Table 11. RNA yield comparison of Tris-buffered phenol and RNagents extractions

| SAMPLE | Pre-Processing Step | | No Pre-Processing Step | |
|---|---|---|---|---|
| | Tris (Ct) | RNagents (Ct) | Tris (Ct) | RNagents (Ct) |
| 10ul semen | 35.1 | 39.2 | 22.9 | 22.1 |
| 1ul semen | 38.1 | 37.6 | 25.2 | 24.8 |
| 10ul saliva | ND | ND | 29.6 | 30.3 |
| 1ul saliva | ND | ND | 34.6 | 34.8 |

ND = not detected

Table 12. DNA yields and RNA expression of semen and saliva samples extracted with the Tris-buffered phenol procedure

| SAMPLE | DNA (ng/ul) | HTN3 RNA (Ct) | TGM4 RNA (Ct) | GAPDH RNA (Ct) |
|---|---|---|---|---|
| 10ul semen | 17.3 | ND | 21.9 | 23.7 |
| 1ul semen | 2.0 | ND | 25.0 | 25.0 |
| 10ul saliva | 13.8 | 29.0 | ND | 29.0 |
| 1ul saliva | 1.3 | 32.9 | ND | 32.4 |

An initial comparison of DNA yields using two different extraction techniques was made. One and ten μl of semen and saliva were extracted via the RNagents Total RNA Isolation System (Promega) or an organic method which used Tris-buffered phenol. Prior to extraction with these methods a pre-processing step consisting of incubation with 1.8 mg/mL proteinase K and 100 mM DTT at 56°C for 2 hours was performed. In parallel samples, this step was omitted and the samples went immediately into lysis with the guanidine denaturation solution. DNA yields were determined using the Plexor® HY quantitation assay. RNA yields were assessed using the saliva-semen screening assay. The Tris-buffered phenol extraction provided the best results since the DNA yield was better than for the RNagents extraction while the RNA yields were equivalent (Table 10). The DNA yields were significantly higher when the pre-processing step was included in the protocol, however the RNA was virtually destroyed and undetectable in the Stain ID assay (Table 11).

Experiments were undertaken to improve the sample lysis without compromising RNA integrity. Reducing agents were added to the guanidine-HCl denaturation solution which itself should protect the RNA. A protocol was optimized which yielded sufficient quality and quantity DNA and RNA for downstream analyses. The final optimized extraction method was used to extract 1 and 10 μl of semen and saliva. The resulting DNA was quantitated using the Plexor® HY assay with yields shown in Table 12. This extraction procedure yielded sufficient quantities of DNA to perform STR analysis. The RNA was used in the Stain ID assay to detect the presence of HTN3, TGM4 and GAPDH. The only amplification of HTN3 was in the saliva samples, whereas amplification of TGM4 only occurred with the semen samples. Alternatively, GAPDH was detected in both sample types. This experiment supports the use of Tris-buffered phenol extraction as a method to isolate sufficient quantities of quality nucleic acids for downstream analyses.

Promega generated a draft Technical Manual to accompany the Stain ID kit and subsequently distributed the prototype kits to several forensic laboratories for alpha-testing of the assay. As one of the testing sites, we extracted samples including blood, menstrual blood, saliva, semen, urine, vaginal secretions, buccal swabs on FTA®, kidney, adipose, colon and skin. In addition, mixtures of blood/saliva, blood/semen, and saliva/semen were tested. The samples ranged in age and size and were extracted using the Tris-buffered phenol protocol. In the multiplex Stain ID reaction we demonstrated that amplification of each fluid only occurred with the tissue-specific genes as expected; semen was amplified with TGM4 primers, whereas only saliva was amplified with the HTN3 primers (Table 13). Additionally, the artificial mixtures containing semen and saliva RNA extracts show that these primer sets are able to discriminate their target RNA in a heterogeneous sample. This experiment shows that the Stain ID assay can detect down to 1 μ of aged seminal fluid and saliva – the lowest volumes tested to date. Furthermore, there was no cross-reactivity with other commonly encountered bodily fluids such as blood, menstrual blood, vaginal secretions or urine. In order to compare the Stain ID assay with presumptive tests currently performed in forensic laboratories, we analyzed this set of samples using the acid phosphatase and amylase diffusion tests. As shown in Table 13, the acid phosphatase results mirrored the Stain ID results, however the amylase diffusion results were far inferior compared to the Stain ID assay. All of the samples containing saliva amplified with the HTN3 primers, but went undetected when subjected to the amylase diffusion test for the presence of saliva. These results suggest that the Stain ID assay is more sensitive and robust than at least one of the presumptive tests routinely used in the forensic laboratory.

**Table 13. Analysis of forensic samples using the Plexor® Stain ID assay**

| Sample | Size | Age (months) | HTN3 (FAM) | TGM4 (HEX) | GAPDH (ROX) | AP | Amylase |
|---|---|---|---|---|---|---|---|
| NTC | N/A | N/A | - | - | - | ND | ND |
| Positive Control | N/A | N/A | Yes | Yes | Yes | ND | ND |
| Blood | 1ul | 23 | - | - | Yes | - | - |
| Blood | 10ul | 21 | - | - | Yes | - | - |
| Blood/Saliva | 5ul each | 31 | Yes | - | Yes | - | - |
| Blood/Semen | 5ul each | 28 | - | Yes | Yes | Yes | - |
| Buccal (FTA) | 5mm punch | 27 | - | - | Yes | - | - |
| Menstrual Blood | 5x5mm cutting | 27 | - | - | Yes | - | - |
| Saliva | 1ul | 31 | Yes | - | Yes | - | - |
| Saliva | 10ul | 29 | Yes | - | Yes | - | - |
| Saliva/Semen | 5ul each | 31 | Yes | Yes | Yes | Yes | - |
| Semen | 1ul | 7 | - | Yes | Yes | Yes | - |
| Semen | 10ul | 7 | - | Yes | Yes | Yes | - |
| Urine | 1ul | 31 | - | - | No Call | - | - |
| Urine | 10ul | 31 | - | - | Yes | - | - |
| Vaginal Secretions | 1/4 swab | 29 | - | - | Yes | - | - |
| Kidney | 10mg | 17 | - | - | Yes | ND | ND |
| Adipose | 10mg | 17 | - | - | Yes | ND | ND |
| Colon | 10mg | 17 | - | - | Yes | ND | ND |
| Skin | 10mg | 17 | - | - | Yes | ND | ND |
| Neg Control | N/A | N/A | - | - | - | ND | ND |

ND - not determined

In addition to the in-house mock forensic samples which were tested using the prototype kit from Promega, we also extracted and analyzed four swabs of unknown origin as a blind test of the assay's performance (Table 14). For swabs A-C, the results were as expected; swab A (10 μl semen) amplified from the TGM4 primers, swab B (10 μl saliva) amplified from the HTN3 primers, swab C (1 μl blood) did not amplify from either HTN3 or TGM4. Swab D was a vaginal swab to which 10 μl of semen was added. Each of these swabs was sent in duplicate and for swab D, one of the samples amplified from the TGM4 primers, but the other did not based on calls made by the software examining the melt curves. However, the raw data (Cts) indicates a positive reaction with the TGM4 primers for both swab D samples (Cts of ~25 for TGM4; equivalent to swab A). These results indicate the potential for false negatives if the melt curves are the only criteria used for making calls since samples containing a large amount of biological material (i.e. vaginal swabs) can lead to drift out of the melting temp range set based on the positive control samples. Therefore, both the raw data and calls made by the Stain ID software must be taken into account when analyzing data.

Table 14. Blind analysis of mock forensic samples using the Plexor® Stain ID assay (Key: Swab A – 10 μl semen, Swab B – 10 μl saliva, Swab C – 1 μl blood, Swab D – vaginal swab with 10 μl semen)

| Sample | HTN3 (FAM) | TGM4 (HEX) | GAPDH (ROX) |
|---|---|---|---|
| NTC | - | - | - |
| Positive Control | Yes | Yes | Yes |
| Swab A | - | Yes | Yes |
| Swab B | Yes | - | Yes |
| Swab C | - | - | Yes |
| Swab D | - | -/Yes | - |
| Negative Control | - | - | - |

## CONCLUSION

The classical biochemical analysis of evidence involved the determination of the nature of a biological stain. Through the use of simple enzymatic color reactions, crystal tests or microscopy, forensic examiners could probe a stain to determine if it contained blood, semen, saliva or some other tissue. The characterization of a stain was the basic question a forensic scientist was technically able to answer when presented with evidence from a homicide, sexual assault or other crimes where body fluid stains may be found. Through the years, researchers developed methods to permit some level of individualization of the evidence and knowledge of the material detected permitted the examiner to determine which typing tests were appropriate for the stain in question. For example, saliva stains contain a limited number of biological markers that could be typed, whereas semen allowed a better discrimination and blood even more so. Understanding the nature of the biological stain permitted the forensic scientist to select those appropriate stain specific typing methods. The identification of semen on clothing from a sexual assault victim or human blood on a suspect involved in a homicide, coupled with some limited typing information was seen in its day as useful information.

Today DNA analysis can essentially pin point the donor of a stain and discussions within the forensic community debate the need to identify the tissue of origin of the stain when individual identity is assumed.

These discussions have merit since limiting the number of tests performed on an item would save time and resources especially given the backlogs existing in today's crime laboratories along with the need to meet judicial deadlines with limited resources. However, one could think of a number of crimes where stain identification may be crucial to a case. Finding a low level male DNA profile on a child's underwear from a father accused of sexual assault may not be truly meaningful given the sensitivity of DNA typing. In a court of law, a semen stain containing suspect DNA can have far more serious consequences than DNA deposited from shed epithelial cells due to incidental contact. In this case and similar cases, tissue identification would be important in the evaluation of the evidence. Prosecutors are seeking an answer to the CSI effect where juries expect forensic science to play a major role in solving cases. It is not unusual for a prosecutor to parade a number of experts in front of the jury to showplace forensics even if only limited or no useful forensic information was gleamed from the evidence. A forensic expert who offers court testimony about a DNA profile but says she didn't bother to identify a stain as seminal fluid in origin may not be appreciated by the members of a jury well versed in "CSI". The analysis of biological evidence without tissue identification is probably a procedural step backwards and should be viewed as a short term fix until technology catches up in the front-end analysis of crime scene evidence.

The work conducted in our laboratory and others concerning mRNA is an attempt to make improvements in tissue identification technology. Molecular biological testing has revolutionized the individualization of stains and research hopes to show these same improvements can be achieved with tissue identification. The first goal was to evaluate the stability of RNA in different types of stains. For over 5 years we have been collecting samples for the sole purpose of determining the stability of candidate mRNAs for stain identification. In order for a candidate to be implemented into a stain identification assay, it needs to be detectable for years following deposition of the sample. It was long believed that RNA was very unstable and difficult to work with, requiring dedicated equipment and laboratory space. However, due to the development of new techniques and the recent increase in knowledge concerning RNA, it has been shown to be relatively stable. Various groups have demonstrated the stability of RNA in forensic stains by traditional RT-PCR and more recently, RT reactions coupled with real-time PCR (Juusola and Ballantyne, 2003; Alvarez et al., 2004; Bauer et al., 2003; Nussbaumer et al., 2006). Furthermore, Setzer et al. (2008) recently addressed concerns on the stability, and hence recoverability, of RNA in forensic samples (blood, saliva, semen, and vaginal secretions) exposed to a range of environmental conditions from 1 to 547 days.

In support of these findings, we used amplification of HBB and PRM2 genes as an indicator of mRNA stability in blood and semen samples, respectively. Regardless of the sample size (i.e. down to 1 µl), we were able to detect these genes in samples aged well over 3 years. In fact, PRM2 was amplified from RNA extracted from the first sample collected for this project, a seminal fluid stain aged for 1666 days at room temperature in the dark. In fact, it appears as though PRM2 expression may even increase over time, perhaps due to the loss of an inhibitor.

Since forensic samples are often exposed to a variety of environmental insults, we stored parallel blood and semen samples under ideal conditions (room temperature, dark) as well as in a sub-optimal condition (37°C). By comparing gene amplification between the samples, we hoped to determine whether RNA profiling would be feasible for weathered forensic stains. There was no considerable decrease in the degree of amplification after prolonged exposure (>500 days) to elevated temperatures. These results further demonstrate how stable HBB and PRM2 RNA are over time. In conclusion, our results together with work published by other groups (Juusola and Ballantyne, 2003; Alvarez et al., 2004; Bauer et al., 2003; Nussbaumer et al., 2006; Setzer et al., 2008) prove that RNA can be recovered from forensically relevant biological stains in sufficient quantity and quality for mRNA analysis.

A major goal of ours was to identify 2-3 gene candidates which were specific for each tissue of interest. The gene candidates utilized through the course of this chapter were identified through surveys of the literature including PubMed, Gene and other databases. Initially we identified 2-3 genes that appeared to be specific for each tissue. These screening studies were performed using TaqMan® primer/probe sets from Applied Biosystems because they were pre-designed, inexpensive and already optimized for their intended target. For each target, the sensitivity and specificity for the body fluid of interest were assessed. Once the assay was shown to be robust, we tested it on mRNA isolated from other fluids and tissues to demonstrate that the assay was specific.

A sensitivity study of the three candidate blood assays (HBB, CD3G, SPTB) demonstrated how minute volumes of blood could be detected using mRNA profiling. Amplification with the HBB probe/primers occurred with as little as 0.0001 µl of blood. Although the seminal fluid genes were not as sensitive as the HBB assay, amplification using the PSA and PRM2 TaqMan® sets occurred with 0.01 µl of semen. The lower detection limit for TGM4 was not determined, but assumed to be lower than the 1 µl tested based on the Ct since it was far from nearing Cts typically observed in negative samples.

The sensitivities for saliva candidate markers (STAT, HTN3) were not as low as found for the blood and semen assays; 1 µl for STAT and 5 µl for HTN3. However, the result is significant because there are no Cts observed for the negative controls.

Our diverse sample bank was used to assess the specificity of the candidate tissue-specific genes. These samples included blood, semen, saliva, menstrual blood, vaginal secretions, kidney, colon, adipose, skin, and control RNAs (brain, heart, liver, kidney, intestine). The fluid results were fairly straight-forward. HBB, SPTB and CD3G (blood markers) only amplified in blood samples, whereas STAT (saliva marker) only amplified in saliva samples. There was some cross-reactivity with the semen candidates. Some minor amplification occurred with vaginal secretions (SEMG1 and ACPP) and blood (ACPP). But, for the most part, the assays only amplified from semen stains. Based on these studies PSA, TGM4 and PRM2 were the most specific.

A major aim of stain identification using mRNA expression profiling is working towards multiplexing the real-time PCR assays once mRNAs are identified that clearly define specific types of stains. Since these assays are designed to function more qualitatively than quantitatively, a test of a single stain should typically give amplification with only one candidate. It is possible that a mixture could give several amplifications. However, it is of greater concern to know that a mixture does exist, than to know the exact amount of each fluid present.

Work from Juusola and Ballantyne (2005) identified tissue-specific genes for the more common forensic casework samples: blood, saliva, semen and vaginal secretions. They developed a multiplex RT-PCR assay composed of eight genes (SPTB, prophobilinogen deaminase [PBGD], STAT, HTN3, PRM1, PRM2, human beta-defensin 1 [HBD1] and mucin 4 [MUC4]) which could be analyzed on a standard capillary electrophoresis platform. However, we sought to develop multiplex assays which could be performed more efficiently using real-time PCR; a technology currently used in most forensic laboratories.

A Plexor®-based multiplex assay arose out of collaboration with Promega to develop stain identification assays. The long-term goal of the collaboration is to generate a panel of Plexor® Tissue Typing Systems; multiplexed qRT-PCR systems for determining the source and quantity of a variety of human stains and/or tissues. The systems would include Plexor® primers for the detection of tissue-specific mRNA transcripts associated with semen, sperm, blood, menstrual blood, saliva, etc. By limiting the system to two-color detection (i.e. FAM and HEX detection), it is compatible with the majority of real-time thermal cyclers currently in place in forensic laboratories. We sought to include controls (e.g. a housekeeping gene) or multiple, tissue-specific targets using the ability of the Plexor® Data Analysis Software to distinguish two different amplicons in the same dye channel, based upon thermal melt properties.

The Stain ID assay which we have developed detects semen and saliva. Plexor® primers were designed to amplify the targets TGM4 (semen), HTN3 (saliva) and GAPDH (housekeeper). Through numerous optimization studies, we generated saliva primers that show specific reactivity with saliva RNA and no cross-reactivity with other RNA samples or with genomic DNA. The semen primers (TGM4) show specific reactivity with semen RNA and no cross-reactivity with other RNA samples or with genomic DNA. Although initial studies were performed using RNA extracted from large sample volumes, unlike what's encountered in routine forensic work, titration experiments were performed and indicated that semen had a detection threshold of approximately 10 pg RNA whereas the threshold for saliva was approximately 1 ng of RNA. Furthermore, we assessed how the Stain ID assay would perform with typical forensic samples (i.e. various volumes of unknown RNA yields). The only non-specific amplification that occurred was from the HTN3 primers and the vaginal secretions sample. Since this experiment was performed, the HTN3 primers have been modified and no longer detect vaginal secretions.

A major outcome of the Stain ID assay development was the generation of a co-isolation method for RNA and DNA extraction. A combination of the RNagents Total RNA Isolation System (Promega) with a Tris-buffered phenol protocol was optimized for simultaneous extraction of the nucleic acids. The final extraction method was shown to extract sufficient quantities of quality RNA and DNA from 1 and 10 μl of semen and saliva demonstrating its utility as a dual extraction technique. Although this method involves numerous hands-on steps, it is faster than the TRIzol® method, and produces significantly better DNA yields. To date, it's the best co-isolation method we've tested in terms of yields and amplifiability.

The research indicates that mRNA may have a significant impact in forensic analysis in the years to come. This change in the way we identify stain types may be ushered into forensics via mRNA analysis or perhaps other methods will become available and more appropriate for use. The National Institute of Justice (NIJ) has funded a number of projects that look at streamlining the screening of biological materials (http://www.dna.gov/audiences/researchers/r_funding/). Our laboratory has been involved with a project to automate the microscopic search of sperm on slides from evidence retrieved from a sexual assault. An automated approach to scan and record the locations of sperm on a slide would reduce the time it takes an examiner to process a sexual assault case. Other NIJ projects include one from Towson University whose researchers will attempt to use DNA as the tissue determent for tissue identification with their project "Development of a DNA-Based Real-Time PCR Assay for Identification of Semen, Blood and Saliva". Additional NIJ grants are looking at proteomics as a means to provide a new way forward. The New York Medical Examiner's office has a project to evaluate proteomics as a method to determine body fluid cell type and researchers at the University of Denver have NIJ funding to identify proteins as markers for biological stains. A private company (MicroBioSystems, North Logan, UT) has performed research that has produced a hand held instrument with the qualities similar to that of the Star Trek "Tricorder". This device uses a variety of wavelengths of light to identify stains from crime scene materials and was developed under the NIJ funded project "Development of an Optical Handheld Biological Evidence Detection System".

The switch from a conventional to an mRNA or other non-traditional approach will not be an easy transition. Current testing methods are available for the majority of routinely encountered forensically important tissues. These tests are relatively fast and require limited resources and examiner training to perform. Each test does require a separate sampling consuming a portion of the specimen for each subsequent test. In addition, some of these tests have limited specificity and sensitivity. mRNA may be able to overcome these difficulties and with enough research one could imagine a streamlined extraction technology that would allow a simplified co-extraction of RNA and DNA. The extract could be used to identify a number of tissues in one test and then permit DNA analysis of that same extract, avoiding sampling question issues. More information could be derived from a single sample undergoing one test. This assay could be substituted for the numerous tests now required to identify semen, blood, saliva and others tissues with a single unified approach to the problem. Research and development of solutions for tissue identification is but one hurdle the forensic community must overcome to use mRNA in tissue typing. Training for non-DNA analysts currently performing only biological screening could be extensive. In the United States, those involved with DNA analysis must attain a certain level of training and experience as determined by the DNA Advisory Board which could be an obstacle for some laboratories. Identifying appropriate space to do the testing with concerns about contamination issues and resources to do the testing with high tech equipment would also need to be addressed. These are issues that the forensic community encountered when DNA typing was first introduced. The community was able to meet those challenges and in the years to come, as mRNA analysis matures, the community will once again need to face these concerns to see if the community will embrace a new technology to revolutionize how biological material is identified.

## COMPETING INTEREST

This project was supported by Award number 2004-DN-BX-K002 and 2007-DN-BX-K149 awarded by the National Institute of Justice, Office of Justice Programs, US Department of Justice. The opinions, findings, and conclusions or recommendations expressed in this publication are those of the authors and do not necessarily reflect those of the Department of Justice.

## ACKNOWLEDGMENTS

The authors would like to thank Doug Storts, Nadine Nassif and Len Goren at Promega Corporation for help in development of the Stain ID assay.

## REFERENCES

Akane, A; Shiono, H; Matsubara, K; Nakamura, H; Hasegawa, M; Kagawa M. Purification of forensic specimens for the polymerase chain reaction (PCR) analysis. *Journal of Forensic Science*, 1993 38, 691-701.

Alvarez, M; Juusola, J; Ballantyne, J. An mRNA and DNA co-isolation method for forensic casework samples. *Analytical Biochemistry*, 2004 335(2), 289-298.

Bauer, M. RNA in forensic science. *Forensic Science International: Genetics*, 2007 1, 69-74.

Bauer, M; Kraus, A; Patzelt, D. Detection of epithelial cells in dried blood stains by reverse transcriptase-polymerase chain reaction. *Journal of Forensic Science*, 1999 44, 1232-1236.

Bauer, M; Patzelt, D. Evaluation of mRNA markers for the identification of menstrual blood. *Journal of Forensic Science*, 2002 47, 1278-1282.

Bauer, M; Patzelt, D. A method for simultaneous RNA and DNA isolation from dried blood and semen stains. *Forensic Science International*, 2003 136, 76-78.

Bauer, M; Patzelt, D. Identification of menstrual blood by real time RT-PCR: technical improvements and the practical value of negative test results. *Forensic Science International*, 2008 174, 55-9.

Bauer, M; Polzin, S; Patzelt, D. Quantification of RNA degradation by semi-quantitative duplex and competitive RT-PCR: a possible indicator of the age of bloodstains? *Forensic Science International*, 2003 138, 94-103.

Bourlet, T; Berthelot, P; Grattard, F; Genin, C; Lucht, F; Pozzetto, B. Detection of GB virus C/hepatitis G virus in semen and saliva of HIV type-1 infected men. *Clinical Microbiology and Infection*, 2002 8, 352-357.

Cao, J; Cousins, R. Metallothionein mRNA in monocytes and peripheral blood on nuclear cells and in cells from dried blood spots increases after zinc supplementation of men. *Journal of Nutrition*, 2000 130, 2180-2187.

Chomczynski, P. A reagent for the single-step simultaneous isolation of RNA, DNA, and proteins from cell and tissue samples. *Biotechniques*, 1993 15(3), 532-537.

Daja, M; Aghmesheh, M; Ow, K; Rohde, P; Barrow, K; Russell, P. Beta-human chorionic gonadotropin in semen: a marker for early detection of prostate cancer? *Molecular Urology*, 2000 4, 421-427.

Dulioust, E; Tachet, A; De Almeida, M; Finkielsztejn, L; Rivalland, S; Salmon, D; Sicard, D; Rouzioux, C; Jouannet, P. Detection of HIV-1 in seminal plasma and seminal cells of

HIV-1 seropositive men. *American Journal of Reproductive Immunology*, 1998 41, 27-40.

Forensic Science Research Training Center. Procedure for the detection of restriction length polymorphisms in Human DNA. Quantico VA: FBI Laboratory, 1989.

Fourney, R; DesRoches, A; Buckle, J. Recent Progress in Processing Biological Evidence and Forensic DNA Profiling. A Review: 2004 to 2007. 15th International Interpol Forensic Science Symposium. Lyon, France. October 23-26, 2007.

Goodwin, L; Karabinus, D; Pergolizzi, R; Benoff, S. L-type voltage-dependent calcium channel alpha-1C subunit mRNA is present in ejaculated human spermatozoa. *Molecular Human Reproduction*, 2000 6, 127-136.

Jin, L; Vyse, A; Brown, D. The role of RT-PCR assay of oral fluid for diagnosis and surveillance of measles, mumps and rubella. *Bulletin of the World Health Organization*, 2002 80, 76-77.

Juusola, J; Ballantyne, J. Messenger RNA profiling: a prototype method to supplant conventional methods for body fluid identification. *Forensic Science International*, 2003 135, 85-96.

Juusola, J; Ballantyne, J. Multiplex mRNA profiling for the identification of body fluids. *Forensic Science International*, 2005 152, 1-12.

Juusola, J; Ballantyne, J. mRNA profiling for body fluid identification by multiplex quantitative RT-PCR. *Journal of Forensic Science*, 2007 52, 1252-1262.

Li, J; Wirtz, R; McCutchan, T. Analysis of malaria parasite RNA from decade-old Giemsa-stained blood smears and dried mosquitoes. *American Journal of Tropical Medicine and Hygiene*, 1997 57, 727-731.

Lundwell, A; Bjartell, A; Olsson, A; Malm, J. Semenogelin I and II, the predominant human seminal plasma proteins, are also expressed in non-genital tissues. *Molecular Human Reproduction*, 2002 8, 805-810.

Matsubara, Y; Ikeda, H; Endo, H; Narisawa, K. Dried blood spot on filter paper as a source of mRNA. *Nucleic Acids Research*, 1992 20(8), 1998.

Miller, D. Analysis and significance of messenger RNA in human ejaculated spermatozoa. *Molecular Reproduction and Development*, 2000 56, 259-264.

Nicklas, J; Buel, E. Simultaneous determination of total human and male DNA using a duplex real-time PCR assay. *Journal of Forensic Science*, 2006 51(5), 1005-1015.

Noreault-Conti, T; Buel, E. The use of real-time PCR for forensic stain identification. *Profiles in DNA*, 2007 10, 3-5.

Nussbaumer, C; Gharehbaghi-Schnell, E; Korschineck, I. Messenger RNA profiling: a novel method for body fluid identification by real-time PCR. *Forensic Science International*, 2006 157, 181-186.

Richter, W; Dettmer, D; Glander, H. Detection of mRNA transcripts of cyclic nucleotide phosphodiesterase subtypes in ejaculated human spermatozoa. *Molecular Human Reproduction*, 1999 5, 732-736.

Setzer, M; Juusola, J; Ballantyne, J. Recovery and stability of RNA in vaginal swabs and blood, semen, and saliva stains. *Journal of Forensic Science*, 2008 53, 296-305.

Watanapokasin, Y; Winichagoon, P; Fuchareon, S; Wilairat, P. Relative quantitation of mRNA in beta-thalassemia/Hb E using real-time polymerase chain reaction. *Hemoglobin*, 2000 24, 105-116.

Zhang, Y; McCabe, E. RNA analysis from newborn screening dried blood specimens. *Human Genetics*, 1992 89, 311-314.

Zubakov, D; Hanekamp, E; Kokshoorn, M; van, I; Kayser, M. Stable RNA markers for identification of blood and saliva stains revealed from whole genome expression analysis of time-wise degraded samples. *International Journal of Legal Medicine*, 2008 122, 135-42.

In: Forensic Genetics Research Progress
Editor: F. Gonzalez-Andrade

ISBN: 978-1-60876-198-2
© 2010 Nova Science Publishers, Inc.

*Chapter 2*

# TRACE DNA ANALYSIS

## Kaye N. Ballantyne[*]

Department of Forensic Molecular Biology, Erasmus University Medical Center,
Rotterdam, The Netherlands

## ABSTRACT

Trace DNA has become a large part of the average forensic laboratories' workload. Remarkably low DNA amounts (<100pg) have been successfully analysed to obtain profiles from a wide range of sample types. Touched objects constitute the most common source of trace DNA, but any type of biological material present in low amounts may be considered as trace, including minute blood deposits, saliva residue on partially consumed food, or even epithelial cells from the interior surface of condoms. In addition to supplementing existing analysis techniques in serious crime cases, trace DNA can allow investigation of volume crime cases such as burglary or vehicle theft, where DNA evidence had not previously been considered usable. However, despite the widespread use of trace DNA, at present there are very few specific validated methods. This has led to controversy in the use of trace DNA, and particularly the low copy number amplification technique. It has been established that the use of existing methodology (developed for high-copy number samples) leads to significant levels of artefacts with trace DNA, including allele drop-out and drop-in, stutter, and allelic/locus imbalance. To minimize these, there are numerous modifications that can be made to existing methods to increase the success of trace DNA analysis. These include reduced extraction volumes, increased cycle number, reduced PCR volume, and increased injection time for capillary electrophoresis. In addition, new research shows that the introduction of techniques such as whole genome amplification, molecular crowding, and post-PCR purification can significantly increase success rates with trace DNA. It is clear that each step of the analysis procedure (including collection, extraction, amplification and fragment detection) can, and should, be optimized with regards to trace DNA. However, the use of increasingly sensitive trace DNA analysis techniques must bring an increasing awareness

---

[*] E-mail: k.ballantyne@erasmusmc.nl

of the potential for contamination, both within the laboratory and at crime scenes. In particular, this has implications for the analysis of trace DNA from cold cases, which were not collected or stored with highly sensitive DNA detection techniques in mind. Although it is certain that trace DNA will continue to be used within forensic biology, there may need to be modifications to a wide range of practices to ensure accuracy and reliability.

## INTRODUCTION

Trace (n): 1. a sign or evidence of some past thing. 2. A minute and often barely detectable amount or indication. 3. An amount of a chemical constituent not always quantitatively determinable because of minuteness. (Merriam-Webster Dictionary, 2009)

The use of trace amounts of evidentiary material for DNA profiling is now common within forensic science, ever since the first description in 1997 of the production of DNA profiles from fingerprints (van Oorschot and Jones 1997). Following this, it has been demonstrated that trace DNA can be obtained from a wide variety of substrates, including touched objects (van Oorschot and Jones 1997), drinking containers (Abaz et al 2002), bedding (Petricevic et al 2006), shoes (Bright and Petricevic 2004), documents (Sewell et al 2008) and ropes (Wickenheiser 2002), amongst many other items. As profiling techniques become more sensitive, the number and type of cases that can now be considered for DNA profiling has been considerably expanded, particularly when considering volume crime such as auto theft or burglary. Trace DNA has now become both a large research field within forensic genetics, and an important issue for many laboratories and courts. As increasing numbers of trace DNA samples are analysed as part of routine casework, and more challenges are raised to its theory and use, it has become apparent that there is still a considerable amount to be learnt, researched and validated within this field. This chapter will provide an overview of the current state of trace DNA knowledge and usage within forensic biology, and describe some of the newer methods that can be used to increase success rates from these minute samples.

Before beginning, it will be useful to define exactly what is meant by the term trace DNA. There has come to be a large number of terms associated with minute quantities of DNA within the realm of forensic molecular biology. Trace DNA is sometimes used to refer to *any* small quantity of biological material, regardless of cellular origin (such as this chapter, or Wickenheiser 2002). In other instances, trace DNA may refer to only epithelial cells transferred by skin contact with items. This may also be referred to as 'contact DNA', or 'touch DNA'. Further terms often seen are 'Low Copy Number', and also 'Low Template DNA typing' (Gill et al 2001, Caddy et al 2008), which are commonly used to refer to the specialised analysis procedures (see below), rather than the nature of the sample itself. This terminology refers to any DNA sample containing less than 100pg of amplifiable DNA, regardless of its source (epithelial, salvia, blood, semen etc). For the purposes of this chapter, the term 'trace DNA' shall refer to any minute quantity of cellular material from any source, which yields less than 100pg of amplifiable DNA for analysis. The 100pg limit, although somewhat arbitrary and laboratory/analyst dependant, is commonly regarded as the lower threshold to which the current commercial STR amplification kits (such as Identifiler, SGM Plus and PowerPlex 16) can be reliably used. However, any user familiar with these kits will have experienced that incomplete profiles may occur from 500pg and less, and conversely that 50pg may result in complete profiles. As such, it may not always be a simple matter to interpret trace DNA results within the casework framework, or in researching effective strategies for the analysis of trace DNA.

## ORIGIN AND DEPOSITION OF TRACE DNA

While trace DNA can be from any biological material, it is most commonly seen originating from epithelial cells on touched objects. Any skin contact, be it with hands, ears, legs etc can result in cellular transfer from the donor to the object. The process of deposition of epithelial cells is essentially a transfer process, where sloughed epithelial cells, oils and sweat are transferred to the surface contacted. In addition to the transfer of nucleated and non-nucleated cells, it has been demonstrated that small amounts of fragmented DNA from apoptotic cells are carried within the sweat and sebaceous oils that are transferred (Kita et al 2008), thus suggesting that STR profiles may be retrievable from touched objects even when no cells are transferred. Crucially, the length of contact is of little consequence to the amount of material deposited – a short contact will deposit similar amounts of material to prolonged contact (Wickenheiser 2002).

There are several factors important in the level of DNA transferred. It has been suggested by several authors that there are 'good' and 'bad' shedders – certain individuals deposit more cells/DNA than others (Lowe et al 2002). However, the effect does not appear to be consistent, with variation occurring within the same individual over time, and also between different hands on the same individual at the same time (Phipps and Petricevic 2007). While it may be true that some individuals are consistently good shedders, it would appear that their percentage in the population is considerably lower than first estimated (45%, Rutty et al 2003), and that the same individual may be both a good and bad shedder at different time points. In addition to variation between (and within) individuals, the substrate onto which the cells are deposited plays a large role. Porous substrates such as paper or wood show in considerably higher transfer rates than non-porous glass or plastic (Alessandrini et al 2003). However, the substrate may also have a considerable effect on the recovery of the deposited DNA, rather than the actual amount deposited.

While the presence of trace DNA on an object is usually indicative of the last person to touch an object, this may not always be the case. There is very little knowledge of the persistence of trace DNA – whether it lasts days, weeks, or months, and the extent to which environmental conditions play a role in persistence. It is conceivable that under the correct conditions, cellular deposits may adhere to surfaces for weeks or months, although empirical research testing persistence is still lacking. In preliminary research, Raymond et al (2008) suggested that the retrieval of DNA from deposits declines rapidly, with the majority not detectable after 1 day, and completely gone after 2 weeks outside

The dearth of knowledge regarding primary transfer rates and persistence of DNA leads to an important issue that is currently facing the trace DNA field. The occurrence of secondary transfer has been a much debated issue for around a decade. While primary transfer (person-person or person-object) is accepted without exception, secondary transfers (person-person-object, person-object-person etc), and the rate at which they occur, are yet to be exhaustively examined. Early papers gave conflicting results, with some demonstrating the phenomenon (van Oorschot and Jones 1997, Petricevic et al 2006, and Polley et al 2006), and others failing to find evidence it occurred frequently enough to be a concern (Ladd et al 1999). However, subsequent studies have shown secondary transfer can occur relatively easily, although estimates of frequency differ widely. Phipps and Petricevic (2007) found only 2% of alleles did not match the primary donor (and were theorised to be transferred from another, secondary donor), while Lowe et al (2002) found transfer rates between 11% and 75%, depending on the 'shedder' status of each individual in the transfer. The occurrence of secondary transfer, and the variation in its occurrence, raises considerable issues for forensic biology and criminology, as discussed below.

## CURRENT METHODOLOGY FOR TRACE DNA ANALYSIS

At present, there are no globally recognised, validated procedures for the analysis of trace DNA. The vast majority of laboratories use standard methodologies for all samples, regardless of quantity – all of which have been developed, optimised and validated for use on higher quantities (generally 1ng) of DNA. Despite considerable research, it can be argued that there are no completely new methods specifically developed for trace DNA. However, there have been many modifications developed to existing methods, which can increase success rates. Within this section, current methodologies for each stage of the analysis procedure (collection, extraction, quantification, amplification, detection and profile interpretation/genotyping) will be described briefly, with a summary of potential improvements for trace DNA.

### DNA Collection

The detection and collection of trace DNA at the crime scene could be argued to be one of the most significant factors affecting the success rate of subsequent DNA profiling. Unfortunately, at present there are no defined guidelines on the best methods to use. Fingerprint enhancement methodology is commonly used to detect the presence of epithelial deposits, although dusting powders and ninhydrin may negatively affect subsequent PCR amplifications (Sewell et al 2008, Grubwieser et al 2003). However, there do not appear to be any new methods developed specifically for detecting trace epithelial cells at crime scenes. Additionally, there is no clear consensus on the best methods to collect trace DNA deposits. Different collection matrices, such as cotton cloths, nylon, foam and cotton swabs, adhesive tape, and vacuuming have all been trialed with no clear consensus on the best method for trace DNA. All methods leave considerable amounts of material on the surface of the object, or that which is collected is not able to be retrieved from the matrix for extraction. However, the double wet-dry swabbing method has been shown to be the most efficient of the current methods (Sweet et al 1997, Pang and Cheung 2007), while the use of solvents such as dilute ethanol has also been shown to retrieve more material than sterile water, yet the vast majority of crime scene examiners still use the single swab method with water (Franke et al 2008).

Certainly, one of the best methods to increase the collection of trace DNA from crime scenes and exhibits would be improved education of crime scene examiners and laboratory staff. Knowledge is one of the most powerful tools to increase the collection rate. Further research into the best method to collect, and then recover, the maximal amount of sample would also be beneficial. However, teaching crime scene personnel to use the double swab method, whilst rotating the swab around the stain/contact trace would increase collection rates above those currently seen (Raymond et al 2008).

## DNA Extraction

It has previously been demonstrated that two commonly used extraction methods, Chelex and phenol chloroform, result in the loss of significant amounts of DNA (van Oorschot et al 2003). Chelex extraction commonly loses 20-76% of the DNA present on a substrate, while phenol-chloroform extractions have 37-75% losses. Although the percentage loss decreases as lower amounts of DNA are extracted, it is for these trace amounts where the loss of any material is the most critical for success. There are conflicting reports on the effectiveness of the newer extraction kits, including silica columns (such as Qiagen's QiaAmp) or silica-coated magnetic bead extraction (such as Promega's DNA IQ). Some reports suggest that they are not as effective with trace DNA samples as simpler Chelex or lysis methods (Schiffner et al 2005), while others suggest that they produce better results (Greenspoon et al 2004).

For most extraction methods, there have been modifications to standard methods developed to attempt to increase the success rate, and particularly the final concentration, of trace DNA extracts. Commonly, this involves reducing the volume of extraction reagents used (for example from 200µl to 50µl in the case of Chelex extractions, Walsh et al 1991). While this effectively concentrates the DNA, it may also result in lower yields due to incomplete recovery of cells from the substrate, or only partial elution of the DNA from silica columns. Alternatively, the introduction of carriers such as salmon sperm DNA or Poly A RNA (see Schiffner et al 2005), can increase the yield from silica-based extractions of very low template amounts (Kishore et al 2006). Carriers in DNA extractions are thought to increase efficiency and recovery rates either by preventing the sample binding to the plastic tube or filters, or by increasing the DNA-silica binding rate by binding to free water molecules, thus preventing them binding to the silica. This may aid in recovering the maximum amount of DNA possible.

With the increasing use of laser-microdissection (LMD) techniques in forensic biology, the use of the direct lysis technique is becoming more possible. Direct lysis, using either proteinase K/SDS or alkaline solutions, has the distinct advantage of having no tube transfers during extraction. For this reason, it is commonly used in reproductive genetics, to avoid the loss of precious cells. Previously, lysis has not been considered a viable option for forensic samples, as the sample is not purified in any way, potentially leaving PCR inhibitors in the sample. However, if cells are microdissected away from the substrate they were deposited on, direct lysis methods can then be used without concern of substantial inhibition. For example, LMD has been successfully used to isolate buccal cells from soil mixtures (Anoruo et al 2008). Direct lysis of the sample within the PCR tube has been shown to minimise allelic dropout, through the removal/reduction of stochastic sampling effects (Thornhill et al 2001, Thornhill & Snow 2002).

## Quantitation of Trace DNA

Quantitation of trace DNA samples is not always regarded as necessary, as if the sample is assumed to have very low template amounts it is customary to simply add the maximum amount possible to the amplification reaction. However, in practice, it may be advisable to quantitate all samples, to prevent over-amplification of samples containing more DNA than expected. Real-time PCR multiplexes such as Quantifiler and Quantifiler Duo (Applied Biosystems), now in common use in forensic laboratories; allow accurate quantitation and an indication of potential PCR inhibitors present in the sample. It is often possible to quantitate as little as 6pg/µl with these kits, offering much greater sensitivity than previous methods. As recommended in the Caddy report (2008), quantitation of trace DNA samples prior to amplification offers much greater control over the amplification, improved results, and can prevent the loss of precious samples through the need for re-amplifications.

## Amplification of Trace DNA

At present, most laboratories use standard amplification methodology with trace DNA samples. Most commercially available and widely used STR multiplex kits are optimised for use with between 0.5 and 2ng of DNA. While these kits all work exceptionally well with 1ng of high quality DNA, when the template amounts are reduced below 100-200pg, a range of artefacts are commonly seen. Allelic and locus dropouts are commonly seen, allele drop-in (contamination) may be seen, and stutter percentages are often increased (Kloosterman and Kersbergen 2003, Gill et al 2000). Dropout and stutter are both usually the result of stochastic processes, which may occur at any point in the reaction set-up and analysis. At such low template levels, random fluctuations in the representation of each template molecule in the DNA sample added to the PCR will have a large influence on the resultant STR profile. Some alleles/loci may be over-represented within the aliquot of sample taken for amplification, while others will be under-represented. To compound this, imbalanced amplification between alleles or loci within the reaction itself can add to the bias seen in the final profile. Navidi et al (1992) give a comprehensive mathematical simulation of stochastic fluctuations, while Taberlet et al (1996) give a practical demonstration of the effects of low template amounts. Both papers demonstrate the need for replicate reactions to give statistical accuracy of low template amplifications – at least 10 are recommended for very low template amounts (such as trace DNA amounts).

There is also a certain level of stochastic variation in the sampling of the PCR product for electrophoresis. Certainly, different aliquots of the same PCR product will produce slight variations in peak heights and allele balance. Additionally, when the products are near the baseline detection limit of the capillary electrophoresis instrument, this can result in profiles differing between replicate injections of the same aliquot of PCR product (even when separated by only 45 minutes in time, data not shown). Different machines will have different baseline thresholds, and the correct limits for each machine need to be determined empirically.

Unfortunately, there is little that can be done to reduce the stochasticity of trace DNA amplifications. Most strategies have revolved around increasing the generation of PCR product, or subsequently increasing the concentration/purity of the product following amplification. There are several strategies currently in use and some contention over the best methods to use. The longest standing method is the Low Copy Number (LCN) technique, pioneered by the Forensic Science Service in the UK. This involves increasing the number of PCR cycles used to amplify the STRs from 28 to 34. With the increased levels of amplification, it is possible to obtain STR profiles from as little as 30-60pg, compared to 300-600pg with the standard 28 cycles. This strategy results in large increases in peak height, with higher percentages of alleles observed (from 0% at 28 cycles to 100% at 34, Gill et al 2000). While this technique has proved very effective for profiling trace DNA samples, there are a number of factors to be aware of when applying this protocol. Increases in artefacts are observed, with peak imbalance and stutter commonly seen (Whitaker et al 2001). Additionally, there is increased mixture and contamination detection, due to the greater sensitivity. Due to allele drop-in and dropout, it is strongly recommended to perform a minimum of two independent amplifications for each sample, allowing the production of a consensus profile without the artefacts. Because there are a number of limitations with this technique, it has not been widely adopted. At present, only the Forensic Science Service in the UK, the Netherlands Forensic Institute, the Switzerland and New York Chief Medical Offices and New Zealand's Environmental Science Research (ESR) routinely use the LCN technique.

Several alternatives to the 34 cycle LCN method have been proposed, including the use of 30 instead of 28 or 34 cycles (Roeder et al 2009) and a 28+6 approach, where additional Taq polymerase is added after 28 cycles, and thermal cycling is continued for a further 6 cycles (Kloosterman and Kersbergen 2003). One advantage to this 28+6 approach is the ability to stop the PCR after 28 cycles, analyse the results, and only perform the additional cycles if required. However, like the standard 34 cycle approach, artefacts are often observed.

There are also many other options to increase the amplification success of trace DNA. Reducing the reaction volume from 50μl to 5 or 10μl can substantially increase the amount of product generated, with a four-fold increase in sensitivity (Gaines et al 2002). When the volume is reduced to 10 or 25μl, there is no significant increase in the level of artefacts, and relative peak height information is retained, allowing accurate mixture interpretation (Fregeau et al 2003, Leclair et al 2003). The DNA sample may also be dried directly in the PCR tube, further increasing the amplification through the addition of large amounts of DNA. The development of chemically structured glass chips such as Advalytix's AmpliGrid slides allow the amplification of single or few cells in a total volume of 1μl. Successful amplification of 15 STRs was achieved from only 32pg (6 cells), and partial STR profiles from 4pg (Schmidt et al 2006). As well as having increased sensitivity, the use of chip-PCRs dramatically reduces the volume of sample needed; allowing either concentration of extracts, or increased numbers of replicate reactions to be performed.

It is also possible to alter the chemical components of the PCR to maximise amplification efficiency and success. Altering the concentrations of certain components can substantially change the way a PCR assay responds to various sample types or template amounts. Increasing the amount of Taq polymerase (from 1 unit to 3-5 units) can give higher amplification success, while the use of hot-start polymerases (such as Ampli-Taq Gold from Applied Biosystems) increases specificity (Moretti et al 1998). The addition of bovine serum albumin can aid in overcoming inhibition of the polymerase.

New research has shown that the use of molecular crowders can substantially increase PCR efficiency (Ballantyne et al, manuscript in preparation). For many enzymatic reactions, it can be beneficial to 'crowd' the reaction by adding a large inert polymer. This has the effect of reducing the space available to reactants, and increases the probability of diffusion-constrained reactions between template, primers, dNTPs and polymerase occurring. Previously, crowders such as polyethylene glycol (PEG) have been used to increase the amplification success of whole genome amplification methods (see below, and Ballantyne et al 2008). Therefore, three common crowders, PEG, Ficoll and Dextran were all trialed as potential crowders for commonly used STR multiplexes. As molecular crowding has a complex effect on the biochemistry of reactions, different crowders, and levels of crowding, may have very different effects on different amplification systems.

Following extensive empirical testing of each crowder, it was found that a 1% v/v solution of Dextran crowded amplifications most effectively. Multiple STR multiplexes were tested for amplification success of trace amounts of DNA both with and without crowding with Dextran 70. PowerPlex (Promega), Identifiler, SGM Plus, Yfiler (Applied Biosystems) and the miniSTR multiplex NC01 (Coble and Butler 2005) all showed increased numbers of alleles amplified, and increased peak heights, when the reaction was crowded. Across all multiplexes, there was an average increase of ~2 fold in peak height in amplifications containing less than 100pg. The number of alleles and loci called were also substantially increased, with 2.5 fold increases in the number of alleles seen from 6pg amplifications. The greatest effect was seen with PowerPlex, where up to 9-fold increases were seen in the number of alleles. No increases in artefacts were seen – no instances of allele drop-in were observed, peak balance was retained compared to non-crowded samples, and stutter was not significantly increased. A substantial advantage of this technique is that it does not require any additional steps, or sample manipulations – the dextran can simply be added to, and thoroughly mixed with the PCR master mix. The dextran does not affect capillary electrophoresis, and interpretation of the resultant profiles is simplified due to the increased peak height.

## Whole Genome Amplification

All of the previous modifications mentioned work by increasing the efficiency of the amplification, or detection of the product. However, in some cases this may not be enough to generate a usable product. Whole genome amplification (WGA) is a useful technique to increase the amount of DNA available prior to the STR genotyping PCR. A subtype of WGA, multiple displacement amplification (MDA) has been shown to be the most effective for small sample amounts (Ballantyne et al 2007a). This method uses a highly processive enzyme, Phi29, to replicate long (up to 70kb) sequences, with random hexamer primers ensuring coverage across the majority of the genome. Commercial MDA kits, such as GenomiPhi (GE Biosciences), are able to amplify trace DNA quantities to produce increased material for STR profiling, although not with complete success. Although more complete profiles (up to 70% increases in numbers of alleles) were produced from the WGA material, compared to standard protocols, there was also a large increase in the level of artefacts observed. Although allele drop-in was not commonly observed, allele dropouts were still common, and there was greatly increased peak height imbalance seen (Ballantyne et al 2007a).

A series of optimisation tests were undertaken, both to further increase the amplification success, and to decrease the level of amplification bias seen. Initially, to increase the level of amplification, molecular crowding with PEG400 was used during the WGA reaction. Amplification success (in terms of the numbers of STR alleles observed) nearly doubled with crowding the solution, particularly for amplifications containing 50-100pg (Ballantyne et al 2006). As with standard PCR, it is theorised that crowding the amplification reaction increases the chance of diffusion-limited reactions between components occurring. However, the amplification bias between alleles and loci is still frequently observed with crowded WGA products, as it is an inherent feature of the Phi29 polymerase. Therefore, an altered denaturation strategy was applied, where the initial denaturation phase (prior to WGA) was omitted for half of the DNA template, and performed for the other half. By combining the two reactions, it was possible to drastically reduce the amount of bias seen (Ballantyne et al 2007b). With standard WGA, the average peak height ratio was a very low 39%, indicating substantial bias. When the modified denaturation strategy was used, the bias was substantially reduced, with an average PHR of 68%.

Combining both molecular crowding, and the denaturation strategy, resulted in more complete and even WGA amplifications, with an average 34% increase in STR profile success compared to standard PCR alone (Ballantyne et al 2007c). Although the improved MDA method developed does require additional sample manipulations, it can be used to generate substantial amounts of material from limited samples, allowing repeated testing for STRs, or the use of greater numbers of loci (such as testing autosomal, Y-, X- and mitochondrial markers) on precious crime scene or archived samples.

## Post-PCR Detection/Genotyping

In addition to manipulating/optimising all the sample collection, extraction and amplification steps, it is also possible to improve trace DNA genotyping success by optimising the detection of the PCR product. Rather than performing increased cycle numbers, it is also possible to use post-PCR purification to maximise trace DNA amplification success. Silica gel membrane columns such as the MinElute kit (Qiagen) are most commonly used, for their ease of use and effectiveness. In addition to removing excess primers, dNTPs and salts, purification can be used to concentrate the sample to 5-10µl, allowing more product to be injected into the capillary. This procedure gives greater success than the standard, non-purified 28 cycle method, increasing peak heights 3-67 fold, depending on the method of purification used (Smith and Ballantyne, 2007, Forster et al 2008). Although artefacts such as allele drop-in, dropout, peak imbalance and increased stutter are still observed, they are commonly less severe when the product is purified, compared to 34-cycle products.

Increased injection times for capillary electrophoresis may also be used to increase genotyping success. This effectively introduces more product into the capillary, allowing increased detection and thus greater success. However, this may also increase the artefact level, particularly in terms of stutter allele heights and spectral pull-up. It may be advisable to purify the product prior to increasing the injection time, to prevent excess salts and ions interfering with the electrokinetic injection (Forster et al 2008).

The concentration of PCR product can also be increased prior to injection, either by concentrating the product during purification, or by drying the product completely and reconstituting with formamide. While this provides improved peak heights and genotyping success, it must be balanced against the increased levels of artefacts and inhibition of injection by excess salts and ions.

## Interpretation of Trace DNA Profiles

When low amounts of DNA are used for amplification, and high levels of artefacts are present, it is necessary to apply strict interpretation guidelines for genotyping and profile use. Peak height imbalance between alleles and loci can reduce genotyping accuracy, and particularly increase the likelihood of false homozygote calls. Inadvertent contamination (either within the laboratory or at the crime-scene) is more likely to be detected when low levels of DNA and methodological enhancements are used. Mixture genotyping can be extremely difficult when very low levels of DNA are used, due to peak imbalance and increased stutter allele heights. As such, replicate reactions for any trace DNA should be performed to enable elimination of spurious alleles. The use of consensus profiles generated from replicates can aid in determining the 'correct' alleles – only when alleles are duplicated can they be reported (Gill et al 2000). In addition, a new statistical method for determining the stochastic threshold for allele dropout has been described, allowing the calculation of the risk of false inclusions and exclusions when very low template levels are used. This may allow the use of the most conservative likelihood ratio for potential matches, and the determination of a conservative peak height threshold for homozygote calls that reduces the chance of false inclusions (Gill et al 2009).

Past the genotyping and profile interpretation stages, the trace DNA evidence must be placed into the context of the case. There is a level of concern within the forensic biology community that trace DNA evidence may at times be over-stated in terms of its evidentiary value. A crucial feature of trace DNA is that the origin of the biological material cannot be determined. Unlike visible saliva, semen or bloodstains, there is no presumptive test for epithelial cells, and at times the level of biological material may be so low that current tissue origin tests will not provide a result. Therefore, any speculation on the origin of the cells is scientifically invalid, and may unfairly bias the DNA results against the defendant.

## COMING ISSUES FOR TRACE DNA

Although there has already been considerable research and discussion within the community regarding trace DNA analysis and interpretation, there are a number of unresolved issues, which may impact its future use in criminal cases. The lack of validated techniques for trace DNA analysis was criticised in the recent Omagh bombing trial (the Queen v Sean Hoey, Northern Ireland, 341/05), leading to a review of the science of low template DNA analysis in the United Kingdom (Caddy et al 2008). This report highlighted the need for training of personnel involved, the need for stricter contamination control and interpretation guidelines, and the need for considerably more research and validation into specific areas of trace DNA (low-template DNA) analysis. The 21 recommendations of the investigating committee, and the newly established Forensic Science Regulator's responses, all appear to be a positive step towards adopting a 'best-practice' approach to trace DNA analysis. However, while implementing stricter controls and procedures into the laboratory will assist in resolving some of the current issues with trace DNA, there are several remaining. These include secondary transfer and persistence, contamination and the over-reliance on trace DNA as probative evidence.

The occurrence of secondary transfer has been a much-debated issue for around a decade. While primary transfer (person-person or person-object) is accepted without exception, secondary transfers (person-person-object, person-object-person etc), and the rate at which they occur, are yet to be exhaustively examined. Early papers gave conflicting results, with some demonstrating the phenomenon (van Oorschot and Jones 1997), and others failing to find evidence it occurred frequently enough to be a concern (Ladd et al 1999). However, subsequent studies have shown secondary transfer can occur relatively easily, although estimates of frequency differ widely. Phipps and Petricevic (2007) found only 2% of alleles did not match the donor (and were theorised to be transferred from another donor), while Lowe et al (2002) found transfer rates between 11% and 75%, depending on the 'shedder' status of each individual in the transfer.

This large variation in results obtained creates considerable debate over the potential effects of secondary transfer. If it does occur with high or moderate frequencies, there are large implications for trace DNA use as probative evidence. In some scenarios, it raises the possibility that an individual's DNA may be found at a crime scene, *without that person ever being at the scene*. This scenario, although unlikely, is possible, particularly if the first individual is a 'good' shedder, while the second (transfer) individual is a poor shedder, and the time between contacts is short. It has been reasonably well demonstrated that the last person to touch an object is usually the major profile donor, but with the increasingly sensitive analysis techniques described in this chapter, it is becoming more likely that the minor profile of the 'non-present' individual could be detected in its entirety, despite being present in very small amounts. Whether or not this is demonstrated conclusively, the possibility of it occurring may be enough to raise doubt about the ability to match an individual to a scene using only trace amounts of DNA. At the moment, the presence of an individual's DNA on an object is generally considered enough to imply their use/contact with the object. However, as research into secondary transfer grows, there is a distinct possibility that this will no longer be possible. As such, it will be imperative to have an understanding of the rate of secondary transfer, situations where it is likely or unlikely to occur, and how length of time since contact affects transfer.

The persistence of trace DNA in different environments is also an area where further research is required. No large-scale studies have been conducted, particularly with long time periods. While it could be reasonably theorised that trace DNA would degrade at a standard rate, and would therefore become undetectable with relative speed, there has been no research confirming this. Therefore, the possibility that trace DNA could be detected after months, or conversely, not detected after a week, remain open, and sources of uncertainty for interpretation and attribution of profiles.

The rate of contamination of trace DNA samples is also a growing concern. Any addition of DNA to an object after a crime is contamination, whether it occurs at the crime scene by investigators or the public, or in the laboratory. Within the laboratory, it is necessary to take specific precautions when working with trace DNA exhibits. Simply speaking may introduce detectable amounts of DNA to an exhibit as far away as 120cm (Finnebraaten et al 2008). Simulations of crime scene examinations showed that individuals might contaminate exhibits simply by moving or talking near exhibits (Rutty et al 2003). More worryingly, cross-exhibit contamination within the laboratory is entirely possible, with tertiary transfer occurring from exhibits, onto the gloved hands of the examiner, then onto examination equipment (Poy and van Oorschot, 2006). While quaternary transfer back to other exhibits was not detected, it remains a possibility. Thus, stringent cleaning and decontamination procedures must be in place following each examination. Manufacturer contamination of 'sterile' plasticware has also been demonstrated (Howitt et al 2003). Other forensic scientists must also be aware of the possibility of contamination – if an exhibit is sent for fingerprint enhancement or handwriting analysis prior to swabbing for DNA, the analyst may introduce their DNA inadvertently to the exhibit, or transfer DNA between two exhibits, due to incomplete knowledge of the risks involved, and incorrect procedure. Thus, it is not only biologists that need to be educated about contamination prevention, but all members of forensic investigation team.

While it is (relatively) easy to control for contamination within laboratories, the events prior to and during sample collection are considerably harder to control. The use of and frequent changing of gloves, cover-alls and masks for crime-scene personnel considerably reduce contamination (Rutty et al 2003). The addition of police and crime-scene personnel to DNA exclusion databases would also aid in detecting contamination at the scene, and has been recommended in the United Kingdom (Caddy et al 2008). The occurrence of contamination at the scene raises considerable issues regarding the analysis of cold cases for DNA. If exhibits were collected by personnel not wearing protective equipment, there is a strong possibility that contamination occurred. Prior to knowledge about trace DNA, there were few precautions taken during scene examinations. Gloves were changed infrequently (if worn at all), thus introducing the possibility for cross-exhibit contamination, or even cross-scene contamination. Exhibits may have been packaged together for transport or storage, resulting in transfer of DNA between exhibits. As such, placing significance on the finding of DNA on particular objects in such cases could be considered doubtful, and, in light of the current knowledge of transfer and trace DNA, unscientific. Such factors were key in the dismissal of the previously mentioned Omagh bombing case (the Queen v Sean Hoey, Northern Ireland 341/05), and should be kept firmly in mind when any cold cases are considered for DNA analysis.

## CONCLUSION

Trace DNA is an expanding and important area within forensic molecular biology. The increasing sensitivity of methods allows profiles to be generated from smaller and smaller traces of biological material, and the limit of detection is now approaching single cell level.

Although not yet applied in most laboratories, there are numerous improvements to existing methods, which can be used to further increase success rates with trace samples.

However, simply because we are capable of obtaining profiles from single cells, it does not mean we necessarily should. At the present time, there are large gaps in our knowledge of many areas of trace DNA. Without having the entire picture, there is a question over relying on trace DNA as probative evidence. At best, trace DNA should be considered as circumstantial evidence, where it *may* imply presence at a crime-scene, or involvement in a crime, rather than definite proof of guilt. Over-reliance on trace evidence can be prejudicial against suspects, and should be avoided until the remaining questions on trace DNA can be answered.

There is no question that trace DNA is extremely useful, and very common, in forensic cases. Considering the evidence with an eye on the limitations of our current knowledge is far more conservative to the defendant, and beneficial to the entire forensic biology community, than blindly applying trace DNA analysis to every case that comes in.

## ACKNOWLEDGMENTS

Kaye Ballantyne is supported by the Erasmus University Medical Center Rotterdam and the Netherlands Forensic Institute. Research described in this chapter was supported by the Department of Forensic Molecular Biology, Erasmus University, the Victorian Police Forensic Services Department in Melbourne, Australia, and La Trobe University in Melbourne, Australia. Roland van Oorschot and R. John Mitchell are thanked for their considerable assistance with research into trace DNA amplification.

## COMPETING INTERESTS

The authors declare that they have no competing interests. The authors alone are responsible for the content and writing of the paper.

## REFERENCES

Abaz J, Walsh SJ, Curran JM, Moss DS, Cullen J, Bright J, Crowe GA, Cockerton SL, Power EB. (2002). Comparison of the variables affecting the recovery of DNA from common drinking containers. *Forensic Science International,* 126 233-240.

Alessandrini F, Cecati M, Pesaresi M, Turchi C, Carle F, Tagliabracci A. (2003). Fingerprints as evidence for a genetic profile: Morphological study on fingerprints and analysis of exogenous and individual factors affecting DNA typing. *Journal of Forensic Science* 48, 586 – 592.

Anoruo B, van Oorschot R, Mitchell J, Howells D. (2007). Isolating cells from non-sperm cellular mixtures using the PALM microlaser micro dissection system. *Forensic Science International* 173, 93 – 96.

Ballantyne KN, van Oorschot RA, Mitchell RJ, Koukoulas I. (2006). Molecular crowding increases the amplification success of multiple displacement amplification and short tandem repeat genotyping. *Analytical Biochemistry* 355, 298 – 303.

Ballantyne KN, van Oorschot RA, Mitchell RJ. (2007a). Comparison of two whole genome amplification methods for STR genotyping of LCN and degraded DNA samples. *Forensic Science International* 166, 35 – 41.

Ballantyne KN, van Oorschot RA, Muharam I, van Daal A, Mitchell RJ. (2007b). Decreasing amplification bias associated with multiple displacement amplification and short tandem repeat genotyping. *Analytical Biochemistry* 368, 222 – 229.

Ballantyne KN, van Oorschot RAH, Mitchell RJ. (2007c). Increasing amplification success of forensic DNA samples using multiple displacement amplification. *Forensic Science, Medicine and Pathology* 3, 182 – 187.

Bright JA, Petricevic SF. (2004). Recovery of trace DNA and its application to DNA profiling of shoe insoles. *Forensic Science International* 145, 7 – 12.

Caddy B, Taylor GR, Linacre AMT (2008). A review of the science of low template DNA analysis; Executive Summary. Available from http://police.homeoffice.gov.uk/publications/operational-policing/Review_of_Low_Template_DNA_1.pdf?view=Binary

Coble MD, Butler JM. (2005). Characterisation of new miniSTR loci to aid analysis of degraded DNA. *Journal of Forensic Science* 50, 43-53.

Finnebraaten M, Graner T, Hoff-Olsen P. (2008). May a speaking individual contaminate the routine DNA laboratory? *Forensic Science International: Genetics Supplement Series* 1, 421 – 422.

Forster L, Thomson J, Kutranov S. (2008). Direct comparison of post-28-cycle PCR purification and modified capillary electrophoresis methods with the 34-cycle "low copy number" (LCN) method for analysis of trace forensic DNA samples. *Forensic Science International: Genetics* 2, 318-328.

Franke N, Augustin C, Puschel K. (2008). Optimisation of DNA-extraction and typing from contact stains. *Forensic Science International: Genetics Supplement Series* 1, 423-425.

Fregeau CJ, Bowen KL, Leclair B, Trudel I, Bishop L, Fourney RM. (2003). AmpFlSTR Profiler Plus short tandem repeat DNA analysis of casework samples, mixture samples, and nonhuman DNA samples amplified under reduced PCR volume conditions (25μl). *Journal of Forensic Science* 48, 1014 – 1034.

Gaines ML, Wojtkiewicz PW, Valentine JA, Brown CL. (2002). Reduced volume PCR amplification reactions using the AmpFlSTR Profiler Plus kit. *Journal of Forensic Science* 47, 1224 – 1237.

Gill P, Whitaker J, Flaxman C, Brown N, Buckleton J. (2000). An investigation of the rigor of interpretation rules for STRs derived from less than 100 pg of DNA. *Forensic Science International* 112, 17 – 40.

Gill P, Puch-Solis R, Curran J. (2009). The *low-template DNA* (stochastic) threshold – its determination relative to risk analysis for national DNA databases. *Forensic Science International: Genetics* 3, 104-111.

Greenspoon SA, Ban JD, Sykes K, Ballard EJ, Edler SS, Baisden M, Covington BL. (2004). Application of the BioMek 2000 laboratory automation workstation and the DNA IQ system to the extraction of forensic casework samples. *Journal of Forensic Science* 49, 29 – 39.

Grubweiser P, Thaler A, Kochl S, Teissl R, Rabl W, Parson W. (2003). Systematic study on STR profiling on blood and saliva traces after visualization on fingerprint marks. *Journal of Forensic Science* 48, 733-741.

Howitt T, Johnson P, Cotton L, Rowlands D, Sullivan K. (2003). Ensuring the integrity of results: A continuing challenge in forensic DNA analysis. *Proceedings of the 14th International Symposium on Human Identification*. Madison, Wisconsin. Available at http://www.promega.com/geneticicproc/ussymp14proc/oralpresentations/Howitt.pdf.

Kita T, Yamaguchi H, Yokoyama M, Tanaka T, Tanaka N. (2008). Morphological study of fragmented DNA on touched objects. *Forensic Science International: Genetics* 3, 32-36

Kishore R, Reef Hardy W, Anderson VJ, Sanchez NA, Buoncristiani MR. (2006). Optimisation of DNA extraction from low-yield and degraded samples using the BioRobot EZ1 and BioRobotM48. *Journal of Forensic Science* 51, 1055-1061.

Kloosterman AD, Kersbergen P. (2003). Efficacy and limits of genotyping low copy number (LCN) DNA samples by multiplex PCR of STR loci. *Journal de la Societe de biologie* 197: 351 – 359.

Ladd C, Adamowicz MS, Bourke MT, Scherczinger CA, Lee HC. (1999). A systematic analysis of secondary DNA transfer. *Journal of Forensic Science* 44, 1270 – 1272.

Leclair B, Sgueglia JB, Wojtowicz PC, Juston AC, Fregeau CJ, Fourney RM. (2003). STR DNA typing: increased sensitivity and efficient sample consumption using reduced PCR reaction volumes. *Journal of Forensic Science* 48, 1001 – 1013.

Lowe A, Murray C, Whitaker J, Tully G, Gill P. (2002). The propensity of individuals to deposit DNA and secondary transfer of low level DNA from individuals to inert surfaces. *Forensic Science International* 129, 25 – 34.

Moretti T, Koons B, Budowle B. (1998). Enhancement of PCR amplification yield and specificity using AmpliTaq Gold DNA polymerase. *BioTechniques* 25, 716 – 722.

Navidi W, Arnheim N, Waterman MS. (1992). A multiple tubes approach for accurate genotyping of very small DNA samples by using PCR: statistical considerations. *American Journal of Human Genetics* 50, 347 – 359.

Pang BC, Cheung BK. (2007). Double swab technique for collecting touched evidence. *Legal Medicine (Tokyo).* 9, 181 – 184.

Petricevic SF, Bright JA, Cockerton SL. (2006). DNA profiling of trace DNA recovered from bedding. *Forensic Science International.* 159, 21 – 26.

Phipps M, Petricevic S. (2007). The tendency of individuals to transfer DNA to handled items. *Forensic Science International* 168, 162 – 168.

Polley D, Mickiewicz P, Vaughn M, Miller T, Warburton R, Komonski D, Kantautas C, Reid B, Frappier R, Newman J. (2006). An investigation of DNA recovery from firearms and cartridge cases. *Canadian Society of Forensic Science* 39, 217 – 228.

Poy A, van Oorschot RAH. (2006). Beware; gloves and equipment used during the examination of exhibits are potential vectors for transfer of DNA-containing material. *International Congress Series* 1288. 556-558

Raymond JJ, van Oorschot RAH, Walsh SJ, Roux C. (2008). Trace DNA analysis: Do you know what your neighbour is doing? A multi-jurisdictional survey. *Forensic Science International: Genetics* 2, 19 – 28.

Raymond JJ, Walsh SJ, van Oorschot RAH, Gunn PR, Evans L, Roux C. (2008). Assessing trace DNA evidence from a residential burglary: Abundance, transfer and persistence. *Forensic Science International: Genetics Supplement Series* 1, 442 – 423.

Roeder AD, Elsmore P, Greenhalgh M, McDonald A. (2009). Maximising DNA profiling success from sub-optimal quantities of DNA: A staged approach. *Forensic Science International: Genetics* 3, 128-137.

Rutty GN, Hopwood A, Tucker V. (2003). The effectiveness of protective clothing in the reduction of potential DNA contamination of the scene of the crime. *International Journal of Legal Medicine* 117, 170 – 174.

Schmidt U, Lutz-Bonengel S, Weisser HJ, Sanger T, Pollak S, Schon U, Zacher T, Mann W. (2006). Low volume amplification on chemically structured chips using the PowerPlex 16 DNA amplification kit. *International Journal of Legal Medicine* 120, 42 – 48.

Schniffer LA, Bajda EJ, Prinz M, Sebestyen J, Shaler R, Caragine TA. (2005). Optimisation of a simple, automatable extraction method to recover sufficient DNA from low copy number DNA samples for generation of short tandem repeat profiles. *Croatian Medical Journal* 46, 578 – 586.

Sewell J, Quinones I, Ames C, Multaney B, Curtis S, Seeboruth, Moore S, Daniel B. (2008). Recovery of DNA and fingerprints from touched documents. *Forensic Science International:Genetics* 2, 281-285.

Smith PJ, Ballantyne J. (2007). Simplified low copy number DNA analysis by post-PCR purification. *Journal of Forensic Science* 52, 820 – 829.

Sweet D, Lorente M, Lorente J, Valenzuela A, Villaneuva E. (1997). An improved method to recover saliva from human skin: the double swab technique. *Journal of Forensic Science.* 42, 320 – 322.

Taberlet P, Griffin S, Goossens B, Questiau S, Manceau V, Escaravage N, Waits LP, Bouvet J. (1996). Reliable genotyping of samples with very low DNA quantities using PCR. *Nucleic Acids Research* 24, 3189 – 3194.

Thornhill AR, McGrath JA, Eady RA, Braude PR, Handyside AH. (2001). A comparison of different lysis buffers to assess allele dropout from single cells for preimplantation genetic diagnosis. *Prenatal Diagnostics* 21, 490 – 497.

Thornhill AR, Snow K. (2002). Molecular diagnostics in preimplantation genetic diagnosis. *Journal of Molecular Diagnostics* 4, 11 – 29.

van Oorschot RA, Jones MK. (1997). DNA fingerprints from fingerprints. *Nature* 387, 767.

van Oorschot RAH, Phelan DG, Furlong S, Scarfo GM, Holding NL, Cummins MJ. (2003). Are you collecting all the available DNA from touched objects? *International Congress Series* 1239, 803 – 807.

Walsh PS, Metzger DA, Higuichi R. (1991). Chelex 100 as a medium for simple extraction of DNA for PCR-based typing from forensic material. *BioTechniques* 10, 506-513.

Wickenheiser RA. (2002). Trace DNA: a review, discussion of theory, and application of the transfer of trace quantities of DNA through skin contact. *Journal of Forensic Science* 47, 442 – 450.

Whitaker JP, Cotton EA, Gill P. (2001). A comparison of the characteristics of profiles produced with the AmpFlSTR SGM Plus multiplex system for both standard and low copy number (LCN) STR DNA analysis. *Forensic Science International* 123, 215 – 223.

In: Forensic Genetics Research Progress
Editor: F. Gonzalez-Andrade

ISBN: 978-1-60876-198-2
© 2010 Nova Science Publishers, Inc.

Chapter 3

# THE CONTINUING EVOLUTION OF FORENSIC DNA DATABASES

## *Simon J. Walsh[1,\*], John S. Buckleton[2,†], and Olivier Ribaux[3,‡]*

[1]Forensic & Data Centres, Australian Federal Police, Canberra, ACT, Australia
[2]ESR Ltd., Auckland, New Zealand
[3]Institut de police scientifique, Universite de Lausanne, Switzerland

### ABSTRACT

In terms of forensic-specific applications of DNA technology, few have had a more profound effect on the field than the launching of databases around the world. The expansion of this phenomenon has not only required an appropriate level of scientific sophistication, but also unprecedented legislative, political and financial backing. In practical terms DNA database implementation and operation has brought massive increases in case submissions and a demonstrable change in case and evidence profiles. Forensic DNA databases also remain high profile and retain some element of controversy, typically in relation to socio-legal issues. Despite this impressive impact, it is important to acknowledge that forensic DNA database applications are still young, still only partially developed and understood and still requiring of our attention, monitoring and effort to ensure an ongoing positive contribution.

Fresh complexities are emerging in the management and development of DNA databases. Some of these problems have been examined in detail in this chapter, and, new solutions that allow cross-comparison of database performance are discussed. These methods should assist, not only in identifying present strengths and weaknesses but also in enhancing future database performance and effectiveness. Effective and creative database management has to be seen as a key priority for the forensic community. Achieving it will require a concerted effort of oversight that scientists themselves must be prepared to participate in as it is crucial to maximising the benefits of their work.

---

[\*] E-mail: simonjoseph.walsh@afp.gov.au
[†] E-mail: john.buckleton@esr.cri.nz
[‡] E-mail: Olivier.Ribaux@unil.ch

Forensic science has traditionally focussed on the production of evidentiary outcomes – retrospectively, and with a view to confirming or refuting an already-held belief. DNA databases also offer, however, the potential for proactive forensic contributions to investigations. Delivering these requires functional and philosophical adjustments to the process by which forensic outcomes are produced. This chapter also outlines specific steps that need to be taken to progress beyond the traditional operational framework to one that is also conducive to effective policing and crime resolution.

## INTRODUCTION

Typically forensic DNA databases consist of two separate collections of profiles. A database of the profiles of individuals who have either volunteered or been compelled to submit samples, and a database of profiles obtained from samples from crime scenes, or exhibits associated with an alleged offence (Figure 1). The administrator of a database typically has capacity to compare profiles from; (a) individuals to individuals, (b) crime samples to individuals (and individuals to crime samples) and (c) crime samples to other crime samples.

The overall database is comprised of (at least) two separate indices. One contains the DNA profiles from individuals whilst the other stores DNA profiles from crimes. The separate databases are matched either internally (as depicted by arrows (a) and (c) in Figure 1). These matches seek to locate duplicate entries on the "offender database" or crimes with a common DNA profile, respectively. The databases are also matched against each other (as depicted by arrow (b) in Figure 1). This is often regarded as the most informative match process as it links individuals with profiles associated with crimes.

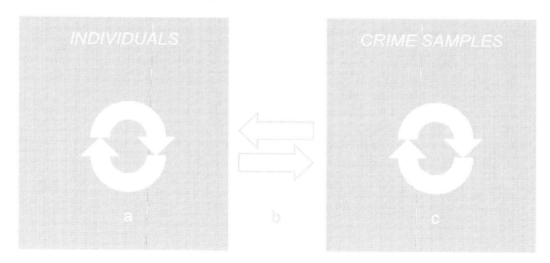

Figure 1. Summary of functionality of a standard DNA database system.

In a relatively short period, the growth of DNA databases internationally has been rapid with tens of millions of short tandem repeat (STR) profiles now held from convicted offenders, suspects and unsolved crimes. Links provided through DNA database searches have contributed valuable intelligence to literally millions of criminal investigations. Often links are provided for crimes which are notoriously difficult to resolve, such as property crime (for example burglary and vehicle theft) and historic unsolved crimes (commonly referred to as "cold cases"). The global scale of DNA database use, its relative infancy, the complexity of addressing requisite socio-legal concerns and the expanding capability of forensic DNA profiling combine to create a challenging law enforcement tool that demands careful assessment and management. In this chapter we introduce the emergence of forensic DNA databases in more detail and isolate aspects of their recent, and future development for more detailed consideration.

## A BRIEF SUMMARY OF NATIONAL DNA DATABASE PROGRAMS

Over the past 10-15 years the establishment of a forensic DNA database has been a focal point of development for police and forensic agencies. There has been a wide uptake of the concept and large-scale DNA database operations now exist in most developed countries.

As the initial National DNA Database, the UK has benefited from a broad legislative regime and consistent funding and has grown remarkably since 1995. The UK National DNA Database (UK NDNAD) contains over 4,400,000 person profiles, over 330,000 crime profiles and has contributed investigative links in over 900,000 cases. National DNA databases also exist in at least 24 EU countries Austria, Belgium, Bulgaria, Croatia, Czech Republic, Denmark, Estonia, Finland, France, Germany, Hungary, Lithuania, Luxembourg, The Netherlands, Norway, Poland, Portugal, Romania, Scotland, Slovakia, Spain, Sweden, Switzerland and Ukraine (data provided by ENFSI, see www.enfsi.eu ). By late 2008 there were over 2,400,000 person profiles and 385,000 crime profiles on European databases. These had led to over 288,000 links involving previously unsolved crimes.

In 1989 the FBI launched the Combined Offender DNA Index System (or CODIS) as a pilot program. This was fortified in 1994 with the creation of the *DNA Identification Act*. The technology was standardised to a panel of 13 STR loci (known colloquially as the CODIS loci). All 50 states have enacted legislation to establish a State index and once uploaded at the State level the data are combined at the National level through CODIS. At March 2009 there were over 6,830,000 individual profiles and 259,000 crime profiles on CODIS. There have been more than 86,000 investigations aided through CODIS over its history. The information management system that operates CODIS is made freely available by the FBI and has been adopted in at least 27 countries.

The Canadian Government committed to DNA databasing by introducing the *DNA Identification Act in 1998*, and implementing the national database in June 2000. The National DNA Database of Canada has shown consistent growth over its 9-year history. Currently (May 2009) the National DNA Database holds over 162,000 person profiles and 49,000 crime profiles and has contributed links to over 11,700 previously unsolved crimes.

China recently established a National DNA Database program that grew from 28,000 in 2005 to over 1,600,000 by 2008. Profiles are contributed by over 200 laboratories including Hong Kong which itself has over 20,000 profiles on a database that was established in 2001. Japan began DNA DB operations in December 2004 and each province is equipped for standardised DNA analysis. Singapore has over 100,000 profiles on a successful National system. Smaller more restrictive national DB programs exists in Korea and Taiwan but other major Asian countries such as Malaysia, Thailand and Indonesia currently have no National DNA database system. There is no National DNA database in India although mechanisms to develop one are underway with a draft Bill released in 2006 advocating the sharing of State data at the national level.

Australia is a federation of six States and two Territories. Each has implemented a DNA database with the first (Victoria) beginning in 1997. Due to difficulties harmonising laws data were only combined onto a National system in 2007. The National Criminal identification DNA Database (NCIDD) is managed by the Federal agency CrimTrac and now holds over 315,000 person profiles and 110,000 crime profiles. Since linking the databases there have been over 9,000 interstate links. The New Zealand (NZ) National DNA DB began in 1995 as the 2nd national DB in the world. In global terms it remains small with over 95,900 person samples and 22,000 crime profiles but it contains profiles from 2.2 % of the NZ population which is a higher proportion than countries such as the USA (2.0%) and Canada (0.5%) but lower than the UK (7.0%). The NZ DNA database has a high crime-to-person hit rate (63 % of crimes loaded) and has contributed over 13,900 links to unsolved investigations.

An appealing aspect of forensic DNA technology has always been the potential for the standardised STR outputs to be shared widely by police and/or forensic agencies. Whilst this potential has not yet reached the point of widespread international exchange, the recent heightened awareness around the threat of trans-national crime and terrorism has precipitated significant early steps towards the formation of international DNA exchange capabilities. In Europe, the Council of the European Union released the first Resolution covering the exchange of DNA analysis results in 1997. The Resolution called on Member States to consider establishing their own national DNA databases and to agree common standards for DNA profiling to facilitate the exchange of data. This approach was acknowledged as an important tool for investigating and combating cross border crime. Work on agreeing common standards for DNA profiling was being advanced under the umbrella of the European Network of Forensic Science Institutes (ENFSI). The Prüm Treaty, signed by Belgium, Germany, France, Luxembourg, the Netherlands, Austria and Spain in May 2005 provides for enhanced cross-border cooperation of the police and judicial authorities. The signatories agreed to give one another access to their DNA and fingerprint files using a *"hit/no hit"* system.[1] This approach creates a necessary distinction between databasing and speculative searching of DNA profiles between states and the preferred process of exchanging specific profiles during serious international investigations.

An example of *bona fide* international databasing is the Interpol DNA Database, set up by the Interpol General Secretariat in 2003 following a resolution by the 67th General Secretariat in 1998. The database (or Gateway) provides a resource through which Interpol's member countries can exchange and compare DNA profile data. Access to the Interpol database (by what are termed "beneficiaries" or "users") is allowable only following a written undertaking. Existing users can also object to any new beneficiary being granted access. The submitting countries retain ownership of the profiles and have direct control of submission, access and deletion, in accordance with (their own) national legislation. Once a match occurs

---

[1] The "hit/no hit" system describes a process by which a country can query the database of another signatory. The result of the query is an advice that the search has resulted in a "hit", or "no hit". In the event of a hit contact information is provided to allow official follow-up to reveal the particulars of the hit.

and the submitting country has been notified, then that country can communicate or request additional material to or from another country, subject to restrictions imposed by that country. This framework is aimed at meeting understandable concerns about privacy of, and control of, profiles once they leave national borders. By 2009 Interpol's DNA database held just over 83,500 profiles from 50 countries and had produced over 180 hits. Several of the successes have involved multiple crimes, some of them most serious, over multiple countries. Given in all cases the act of searching involved only adding a profile already collected and analysed, each of these instances of success must be seen as adding quite significant value towards achieving an otherwise improbable identification.

The National DNA database systems of the selected countries mentioned herein hold over 16,000,000 profiles and collectively they have contributed links to over 1,310,000 unsolved crimes. This represents the product of considerable investment from national governments and the police and forensic agencies responsible for law enforcement. Although, whilst this progress is impressive, DNA database operations are still relatively recent additions to the criminal justice system (CJS) and the principal focus to date has been on their establishment and growth. It is important to acknowledge that forensic DNA database applications are still requiring of our attention, monitoring and effort to ensure an ongoing positive contribution is not only maintained, but maximised.

## OPERATIONAL IMPACT OF FORENSIC DNA DATABASES

As the technology that forms the basis for DNA intelligence databases is specialised, the operational components have remained the responsibility of forensic biology laboratories. In general, the database and its products are the property of law enforcement agencies with the analytical and matching processes administered on their behalf by forensic institutions. All aspects of the process whether handled by police or scientists are subject to governing legislation. Often this legislation contains clauses that facilitate external review of operations by delegated parliamentary authorities. From a forensic scientist's perspective the legal basis for the administration of DNA databases represents an additional level of governance over their work and that prescribe the appropriate conditions under which a DNA sample can be collected, analysed and stored, and the criminal sanctions that are enforceable for individuals in breach of these requirements.

In a practical context the impact of the operational management of forensic DNA databases has had a much more profound effect on police and forensic organisations than the need to adjust processes to adhere to the governing legislation. The snapshot of global database models provided above illustrates that a unifying trend in major jurisdictions has been an increase in the scale of database operations. Whilst this has occurred in concert with increasingly broad legislative regimes it is more likely to have been a critical impetus for iterative legislative expansion. The workload generated through DNA database operations has been a major burden on forensic DNA providers and has compelled forensic laboratories to find efficiency gains in the analytical process. Many have simply not coped with the volume of submissions and have experienced considerable backlogs and case processing delays.

This circumstance has resulted in a vastly different model of case management. Historically, police and forensic scientists have had a focus on clearing one crime at a time.

Cases were submitted to the forensic laboratory after considerable investigation had occurred and in most cases, a suspect had been identified. The role of the scientist was to process these cases and determine whether there was evidence that could assist either the prosecution or defence of that specific crime. Occasionally there were cases where the forensic analysis contributed vital investigative information that assisted the location and arrest of a suspect. The broad utilisation of DNA databasing has seen this paradigm change. Essentially the analysis of evidence items occurs earlier in the investigative process with the hope that the scientist can produce intelligence information (such as a database link) in crimes for which no suspect has been identified through other means. The increased volume of submissions has also seen a trend away from individual case management and towards batch processing. It has also led to a greater prevalence of automated laboratory techniques that seek to achieve high-throughput analysis without extensive human involvement at all. The drastic increase in the size of databases and volume of information provided from them, has, in turn, imposed a dramatic change on the capacity of the CJS to absorb and utilise this information. For instance, the volume of hits now cannot be fully handled by the police due to sheer lack of resources. This then leads to the event where police work is driven by hits coming from manifold databases, and not by a response to or analysis of the situation (intelligence).

Another trend associated with the emergence of DNA database operations has been the broadening range of crimes submitted to forensic biology laboratories for analysis. In the 1980's DNA profiling was primarily used to solve serious crimes. It now contributes to the investigation of a broad spectrum of crimes, including property offences such as burglary. The variation in jurisdictional legislative and operational frameworks can impact the case submission profile, for example, certain countries in Europe initially focused on the investigation of serious violent and sexual offences (Schneider and Martin, 2001). In general there has been a clear pattern of increase in the proportion of cases submitted from volume crime categories (Walsh, 2007). A unifying factor is that the profile of casework received by the laboratory has changed since the beginning of DNA database operations.

The changing nature of case submissions, represented above, has also been accompanied by an associated change in the type of exhibit located, and hence the type of sample(s) presented for DNA analysis. For example, serious violent crimes would be expected to result in injuries and bleeding from those associated and therefore a higher likelihood of receiving blood as the principle evidence type. Likewise crimes of a sexual nature predominantly involve a male offender and hence will typically be associated with semen evidence. Property crimes and drug crimes are less simple to classify in this way and are not thought to be strongly associated with a characteristic evidence (or sample) type. A general trend however is that these types of incidents often result in the submission of more discrete evidence types, such as cigarette butts, drinking containers, food remnants, tools or swabs from surfaces or objects that the offenders are believed to have touched or handled (commonly referred to as "trace DNA") (Raymond et al., 2004).

As the contribution of forensic DNA evidence has increased in the past 5-10 years, so too has the profile of the field and its effect and impact in terms of positive outcomes of the CJS. However, the increased volume of casework and the alteration in the nature of core evidence types can each be seen as associated with a series of accompanying pressures. In summary, forensic biology practitioners must cope with greater personal expectations in terms of their casework output. This is in the context of more complex technical and interpretative challenges that are associated with the analysis of discrete, low template evidence types (such as touched surfaces, bottles and cans). Frequently, laboratories have been simply unable to cope with the rising volume of casework. Many jurisdictional centres in Australia and overseas have accrued casework backlogs that have in turn brought delays in the presentation of DNA evidence in court, or in some circumstances, trials having to proceed without any DNA evidence at all. At the same time, there is a recurrent demand from the CJS to obtain rapid results in relation to solving specific crimes or so as to decide how a suspect should be handled (detention, surveillance, arrest, etc). Backlogs are in conflict with these new demands and expectations of the CJS and can act as an additional source of pressure on forensic professionals.

From a scientist's perspective this operational environment can obviously cause pressure. This in turn can heighten the potential for error and exacerbate feelings of disempowerment, a lack of ability to adequately prepare personally for court testimony, insufficient time for research, training and professional development, or a diminished emphasis on best-practice models that may incur unmanageable commitments of staff time. In a review of laboratory backlogs in US State Crime Laboratories staff training was ranked 6$^{th}$ out of the top 10 spending priorities behind salaries, equipment, construction, consumables and outsourcing (Lovrich, *et al.*, 2003). This emphasises the importance placed on meeting current demand ahead of future development of staff or capabilities. This problem translates to fewer options for staff progression and monetary reward and these have been documented as affecting staff retention rates in forensic laboratories (Dale and Becker, 2004).

The changing nature of the submitted DNA evidence from traditional sources such as blood and semen to more discrete evidence types such as trace DNA and discarded items has an associated effect on the probative value of such evidence. This can indirectly place the scientist in a difficult position, particularly in interpreting questions focused on the link between any recovered DNA evidence and the actions or activities alleged to have taken place in a criminal event. These are of course the areas that are the primary concern of the courts – as they often contribute directly to resolving pivotal legal points such as culpability or intent. In evaluating these sorts of ambiguities, a forensic witness would routinely turn to a body of experimental data and interpret the current findings in the context of this empirical information. The dual challenge of working with discrete evidence sources is that 1) ambiguities relating to the source of the deposit, the duration it has been in the location it was recovered from and the mechanism by which it was deposited remain unanswerable; and 2) where experimental data exists it is as yet inconclusive and may never adequately address the myriad of potential propositions that could be advanced to explain the origins of trace DNA evidence. When these limitations of the DNA evidence are brought before a court they are often met with concern and/or alarm by members of the judiciary or the jury.

The increasing use of forensic DNA databases also has the effect of incorporating DNA evidence in cases where there is a lack of other supporting evidence. This is particularly true for historic cases which are submitted for DNA analysis as *"cold cases"* in the hope of re-invigorating unresolved investigations (*Using DNA to Solve Cold Cases*, 2002). In many circumstances the probative value of the DNA link may be unequivocal. However in others it will be more tenuous (*R v Hoey*, 2008). This also may present a source of pressure for a forensic scientist. It is important, given the often high profile nature of this kind of testing, to reinforce once more that DNA remains an item of physical evidence only and is not in itself proof of guilt or innocence. In this regard it is scientists who must ensure that the wrong impression of the potential strength of the evidence is not propagated by those wishing to inflate or denigrate its potential. A failure to engender this understanding will only increase pressure on witnesses and foster unreasonable expectations on the part of police, prosecutors and the public.

A final point that forensic scientists must consider in relation to the use of forensic DNA databases is the increased need for awareness of relevant socio-legal issues brought about by an increased public awareness of forensic DNA as a field. This increases the pressure on practitioners but has also increased the level of legislative and policy influence over the field. In a practical context, DNA-based legislation represents an additional level of governance for forensic professionals and one of the first pieces of law that places direct requirements on the manner in which they undertake their professional work. In addition, it prescribes sanctions for individuals or institutions who contravene the administrative processes detailed in these laws. Fervent debate has continued on many of the issues associated with the use of forensic DNA profiling in the CJS, and this debate has now expanded to encompass applications of the scientific process that are primarily the responsibility of the forensic community. Unfortunately, the forensic community has remained largely mute in this discussion. As such it has been dominated by a generalist tone that is abstracted from the practical context. Notwithstanding this, forensic professionals (and particularly the administrators of forensic institutions) would do well to acquaint themselves with these issues and enter the existing debate. Failure to do so could mean that the direction for the application of our scientific tools will become the responsibility of people well removed from the forensic community itself.

There are different DNA database models in different jurisdictions. All can be seen as successful and based on a cursory analysis there is little ability to isolate obvious examples of good or poor practices. The variation in the operating models occurs both between and within countries (Australia and the USA are examples of the latter). There appears from a first-level analysis of database composition to be a distinction in whether a sampling regime focuses on collecting samples from people, or from crimes. Occasionally – but not commonly – there appears to be an equivalent focus on each. The growth of DNA databases seems to have been premised on a belief that *"more is better"*. An analysis of DNA database growth demonstrates that there is a common trend that legal changes occur in favour of increased sampling powers to authorities leading to greater population of the DNA database (Walsh *et al.*, 2008).

Undeniably the area of forensic DNA databasing remains reasonably high profile, and this appears to be a unifying characteristic of various national systems. They also seem to retain some element of controversy. Importantly, we must acknowledge that forensic DNA database applications are still young, still only partially developed and understood and still (in fact more so than ever, it could be argued) requiring of our attention, monitoring and effort to ensure a continued positive contribution.

## ASSESSING THE EFFECTIVENESS OF FORENSIC DNA DATABASES

Despite the rather spectacular effects of DNA databases and the considerable degree of notoriety and adulation they have generated, the truth is that constructing a forensic database to provide some links between crimes and suspects is relatively simple. Some truisms of the CJS make this so. DNA evidence is frequently found at crime scenes. Many criminals are recidivist – particularly in property crime offences where it is estimated that a large proportion of the total number of crimes (some say as high as 90%; Smith, 1999) are committed by a small proportion of the criminal population (some say as low as 10%; Smith, 1999). There is considerable evidence to suggest that most serious offenders will have offended previously (Broadhurst and Maller, 1991; Simon, 1997; Zamble and Quinsey, 1997; Heide, et al., 2001; Hunt, 2002) and convicted serious offenders are ubiquitously sampled for DNA database inclusion. The DNA profiles generated in all cases are in a form that greatly assists computerised comparison. The combination of these routine features of the CJS leads to a guarantee of success when the composite parts are united through a database search.

The first crucial question at the macro level is what defines success from a forensic DNA database (solving crimes, impact on certain criminal phenomena, deterrence) and how much success should we expect? In contrast with other forensic disciplines, the social, political, legal and fiscal investment in State or National DNA databases has been extreme. Some reward has clearly flowed from that investment, but does it justify the commitment, or are there ways that we could better ensure optimal efficiency and maximal return? It seems vital that the performance of forensic DNA databases be monitored and optimised. Tracking performance is bound to lead to improvements (Asplen and Lane, 2003).

The second crucial question is: how do we measure the success of forensic DNA databases in order to answer the first question? To do this effectively is a complex undertaking that requires the coalescence of a range of experimental methodologies across numerous spheres of society. Most jurisdictions do not monitor the performance of their databases beyond reporting a one-dimensional index of output relating to the number or proportion of hits. This is a major omission.

To date, there has been little attention to either question – due mainly to the fact that over the history of databases up to now, there has been minimal demand for the answers. Forensic DNA databases have always provided outcomes, many of which involve spectacular and unprecedented contributions to the most serious of cases. These results have taken little strategic thought to achieve, and to some degree this will always be the case. However, it is our view that the days of database models based on overly simplistic expectations and guaranteed success are diminishing. An era is arriving where more profound performance management and consideration of database effectiveness will be essential to ensure an ongoing contribution and to manage future challenges.

As a database ages a number of changes occur, some of which are detrimental. Consider the crime sample database. These are samples from crime scenes and may be from the true offender or may be from an irrelevant source – such as the home owner of a house that has been burgled. Scenes of crime officers (SOCOs) seek to keep the fraction of relevant samples high but certain types of sample, such as cigarette butts have a risk of irrelevancy as they may be discarded or transported randomly, and with little relevance to the scene or offence. Let us say that the fraction of relevant samples when submitted is □. As time passes crimes are solved which can result in the removal of relevant samples from the database. However, case resolution does nothing for irrelevant samples, and so those samples largely remain on the database. Therefore the fraction of irrelevant samples on the unsolved part of the crime database may slowly rise.

Even relevant samples that generate hits also gradually diminish in their overall value over time. This is based on an expectation that resolving old crimes is of lesser value (and is often harder) than resolving recent crimes. Whilst this is a general statement it is certainly true of property crimes, which make up the vast bulk of database cases and links. There is less justification in investigating old property crimes as there is a reduced chance of recovering property and/or finding associated probative evidence.

The database comprised of samples from people also ages. In a very coarse model this database is comprised of active offenders and non-offenders. In general, there is a movement of some active offenders towards non-offending. This occurs as active offenders retire from crime, die, or become imprisoned. Let us denote the fraction of active offenders on the suspect database ☐. This fraction has a tendency to decline over time. This decline can be exaggerated if selection criteria for inclusion on the database increases the fraction of non-offenders sampled. We acknowledge that this model is very simplistic and that the division of people into active offenders and non-offenders overlooks the large range of behaviours exhibited by people. However this thinking is very useful when considering the value of database sampling strategies and how they interrelate with performance.

An additional factor that further compromises the efficiency of the person database is that there is a small but almost unavoidable accrual of duplicate samples as people are sampled twice due to aliases, subterfuge (by deliberate repeat submission under similar names or aliases), or due to the existence of numerous legislative models feeding into the one national database (each requiring samples to be collected from locally apprehended suspects or offenders). This latter example exists in Australia.

Presently, assessment of the effectiveness of forensic DNA databases is almost exclusively limited to primary indexes such as profile inclusions and crime-to-person ($C \rightarrow P$) *"match rates"* or *"hit rates"*. These terms are interchangeable and generally are calculated by the total number of hits (or matches, $H$) divided by the total number of crime samples loaded to the Crime Sample Database ($C$) at the point in time at which the loading or comparison occurs ($t$).

$$HR_{C \rightarrow P} = \frac{H_{C \rightarrow P}}{C_t}$$

These indexes are limited in their informativeness, particularly in relation to using them to determine optimal strategies for database operation. They measure output rather than outcomes (Bieber, 2006) and are not corrected for influencing factors.

An inferential model for database performance has been developed and tested (Walsh *et al.*, 2009). The model itself is not data driven but is logic-based, however, the predictions of the model hold particularly well when assessed on the training set (in this case the SDIS data from the FBI's CODIS system). The model provides a mechanism to cross-compare the performance of database systems operating under different legislative and operational frameworks because it is data independent. This comparison was undertaken on publicly available data from four major National DNA Database programs (UK, NZ, Canada and USA).

The modelling of Walsh *et al.* (2009) suggests several key observations related to database performance management:

- Database performance can be assessed by a metric described as the return index (*RI*) which is estimated by $\frac{H}{NC}$ where *H* is the number of crime-to-person hits, *N* is the number of person samples on the database and *C* is the number of crime samples on the crime sample database.
- A high *RI* indicates a database with a high return; that is maximum hits per person and crime sample tested. In our opinion, given the financial and ethical costs of operating a forensic DNA database this is the objective that database operators, legislators and policy makers must strive for.
- The primary output from a database, hits (*H*) is modeled by $H = \frac{\alpha N}{M} \times \omega C$. This model suggests that $H \approx NC$ but is conditioned by two parameters $\alpha$ and $\omega$, quality factors for the selection of person and crime samples, respectively and *M* is the *active criminal population*. High $\alpha$ and $\omega$ maximise *H* and in turn *RI* and are therefore of critical importance in optimising database performance. This has important implications for continuing research into drivers of success across all stages of police, forensic and database operations.

## OPERATIONAL FRAMEWORK FOR THE USE OF FORENSIC DNA DATABASES

As mentioned earlier, the establishment of forensic DNA databases has been a contributor to a change in thinking within forensic science. Historically each case was processed as a unit or perhaps as a small series. The analyst adopted a *"cradle-to-grave"* approach and usually sought to refute or corroborate the version(s) of events suggested during either the investigation or trial. Typically a suspect had been identified through other means and the forensic analysis was comparative rather than suggestive.

This model has changed significantly. Forensic DNA databases have catalysed profound changes in the volume and profile of forensic case submissions meaning that with the exception of certain serious crimes, the focus has shifted to a batch-processing model within which the DNA database is an embedded component and where all cases and individual samples are viewed as potentially linked. At an organisational level the crucial objective is efficiency; maximising the processing capacity in the minimal time and with the minimal associated expense. These objectives have typically been set and driven by police users as they align best with their operational priorities.

The ability to link cases and identify a crime series has been an effective strategy in law enforcement for some time (Gotlieb, 1998). Incorporating DNA outcomes into the existing array of investigative data provides an additional mechanism to link cases committed by the same individual or organisation, adding also a highly discriminating mechanism for identification. Through the ability to provide technical information capable of directing police investigations (such as by identifying a suspect or a crime-to-crime link), DNA databases are able to operate as an investigative tool. Another important investigative feature of DNA databases is their ability to transcend jurisdictional boundaries which may have hampered abilities of law enforcement agencies to link crimes and offenders which transcend such boundaries. This is particularly true in large countries, for example the US, Canada and Australia, where states or provinces have responsibility for law enforcement within particular physical and legislative boundaries. This more proactive use of forensic DNA outcomes also presents opportunities for more integrated and intuitive use of the technology. Achieving this relies upon a complete understanding of the nature and scope of the investigative contribution that forensic DNA profiling can make; presently and in the future.

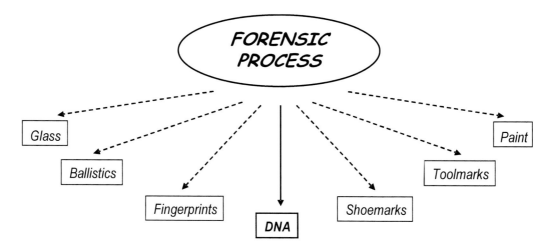

Figure 2. Common examples of discipline forensic databases.

It is the process of databasing which has provided the impetus for regarding forensic outputs as a potential source of investigative leads, rather than its traditional role as corroborative information, provided at the conclusion of an investigation. Champod & Ribaux (2000) correctly point out that *"databases must be seen as tools used in a process which begins with the crime scene investigation and ends with the criminal trial"*. To that end, although they deliver information, databases should not be mis-represented as a stand-alone intelligence cycle or as the sole and final arbiter. The benefits in terms of the CJS will be maximised if databases themselves are part of a broader framework of crime investigation that is capable of integrating forensic outcomes with other systems for qualitative linking based on crime analysis and investigative trends. This section will present a hierarchy of models for forensic database systems to work either independently in an intelligence-providing role or, ideally, as a component of a genuinely integrated investigative framework.

As illustrated in Figure 2 there are a number of examples across the forensic sciences where databases exist within disciplines. Despite the conceptual similarities of these systems there are significant operational barriers to effective integration within police systems or to exchange among disciplines or jurisdictions (notwithstanding legal impediments to such possibilities). A diagram describing the typical structure of a discipline database model (using DNA as the example discipline) is provided in Figure 3.

Under the DNA *Discipline Database Model* there are two repositories of information; the National DNA Database (NDD) and the Crime Sample Database (CSD). The NDD is populated by samples from persons who for some reason have been encountered by law enforcement agencies. As earlier discussed, the practicalities of who (and how many) is (are) sampled is constrained by a combination of policy, legislative and resource factors.

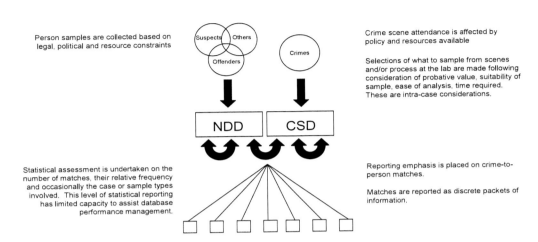

Figure 3. An example of a typical structure of a *Discipline Database Model*. This has been based on forensic DNA databases as this discipline is the focus of this chapter.

From the perspective of crime sample selection and inclusion onto the CSD there are a number of limiting factors. The list of factors and their key influences include:

1. Whether the crime scene is attended at all
   This is typically based on an assessment of the incident report to the police. A decision whether or not to attend is largely effected by resources, policy, and conflicting priorities at the time.
2. Whether the crime scene is attended by forensically trained personnel
   This is part of the initial police assessment of the incident report however it will be affected considerably by the jurisdictional framework and policy regarding crime scene response capability.
3. What evidence (if any) is recovered from the crime scene
   This will be affected by the decision of the forensic member attending, which in turn is a product of their training, professionalism and awareness and the timeliness with which the scene is attended. There are also practical limitations of resourcing, time and policy that will constrain what is recovered from the crime scene.
4. Whether the recovered evidence is submitted for laboratory analysis
   This is essentially a decision affected by the probative or investigative value of what is recovered, resources and likelihood of successful analysis. In a volume crime context, resources and likelihood of success are principal limiters.
5. Whether "sub-selection" occurs as part of the laboratory process
   As above, this is essentially a decision affected by the probative or investigative value of what is recovered, resources and likelihood of successful analysis. In a volume crime context, resources and likelihood of success are principal drivers.

Importantly, the laboratory may or may be not aware of the specific imperatives of the case, particularly, when the laboratory is remote from the police. This exacerbates the difficulty of making this assessment.

6. Whether analysis is successful.

This is affected by the laboratory capability, technology, the evidence type submitted for analysis. Internal policy (such as reporting or matching thresholds) may have a minor impact on this.

Matching occurs within each index of both the NDD and the CSD and between the NDD and CSD (refer to Figure 1). Typically the focus of result reporting is in relation to links between entries on the CSD and an entry on the NDD (crime-to-person links). Matches tend to be reported as discrete packets of information (i.e. links generated on a particular day or following the inclusion of a particular sample).

As earlier discussed, there is typically limited statistical analysis of the database holdings and database outputs. When it occurs it is focused only on the number of database entries and the number and frequency of links made. Occasionally the case or sample types involved in database entries and links is reported. This level of statistical reporting limits capacity to assist database performance management.

The contribution of this form of discipline database is mostly confined to low-end tactical level intelligence with outcomes provided in relation to particular cases or series. Occasionally in serial matters there is a potential for this simple discipline database model to contribute operational level intelligence and assist decisions regarding resourcing and investigative strategies in specific inquiries.

The next level of discipline database operation is what we have referred to as the *Managed Discipline Database Model* (Figure 4).

There are subtle but noteworthy changes at all levels of the *Managed Discipline Database Model*. Firstly, *all* outputs from the database comparison process are collated into a separate holding that is managed and overseen at a global level. Result reporting from this information is multi-layered and goes beyond the automated dissemination of links. The primary purpose of this additional level of analysis is to provide a more efficient capacity to review database outcomes holistically. The vast numbers of cases and crime information residing on forensic DNA databases (and indeed other forensic holdings) is not typically analysed holistically. This is an oversight and is dismissive of unique characteristics of these datasets. That is that they already contain numerous records of links made through highly informative scientific analyses and that they are an amalgamation of crime types and localities that often remain separate in police investigative and intelligence structures.

This additional level of analysis has a number of benefits. Firstly, the outcomes of database comparison are reported as clusters of information. Secondly, trend analysis is more easily undertaken to continuously monitor performance. And thirdly, it establishes an effective feedback mechanism to inform decision-making at the early stages of the forensic process to ensure the information entered into the NDD and CSD indices is of high relevance. Walsh *et al.* (2009) have shown that this is a crucial driver of maximised DNA database performance and one that is best led from within the forensic environment as police agencies notoriously have a limited understanding of the range and scope of forensic capabilities (Lambert, *et al.*, 2007) and cannot be expected to drive more effective uptake of relevant forensic evidence.

## MANAGED DISCIPLINE DATABASE MODEL

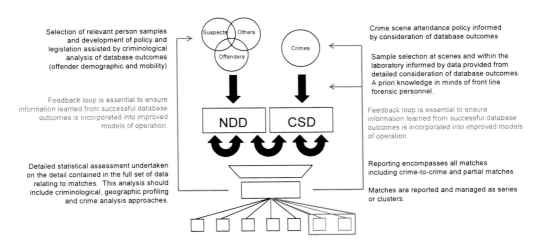

Figure 4. An example of a proposed structure of a *Managed Discipline Database Model*. Once again this model is based on forensic DNA databases.

This level of operation has been achieved by a number of jurisdictions and should be an accepted minimum operating standard for forensic DNA (or other discipline) databases. There is value in considering forensic DNA database outputs holisitically to identify tactical level intelligence that ultimately can be redirected back into the system to improve its operability. This model advances the application of forensic databases from a consideration of singular outputs (of cases or series) to the analysis of general trends from the totality of the data. Notwithstanding these examples, there has been limited exploration of practical mechanisms whereby the intelligence contribution of forensic DNA science or forensic DNA databases could be enhanced through purposeful analysis of database outcomes. Some examples of potential sources of information that could further enhance the *Managed Discipline Database Model* are provided below:

1. Criminological value of DNA database outcomes

    The expanding use of DNA databases offers significant value as a source of criminological awareness through greater analysis of trends in criminal behaviour. Such analysis could contribute to proactive policing strategies that are based on a contemporary understanding of criminality. It is foreseeable that by analysing outcomes (links) from a DNA Database from a criminological standpoint the operational success of the DNA Database can be capitalised on as a contemporary subset of data on crime, crime investigation and criminals. Analysis of this data could inform current understanding of the extent and nature of high-volume crime and the demographic and criminological profile of those who commit it. The net outcome would be a greater understanding of criminality and recommendations for strategic responses to it that could be implemented across the justice sector.

2. Criminal mobility

    There are limited studies that specifically investigate offender travel. Those that have tend to report a limited extent of travel by offenders, usually within the radius of neighbouring law enforcement jurisdictions (Leitner, et al., 2007). Analysis of the geographic distribution of offences linked through the DNA database and the evaluation of relationships between localities using geographical information systems could be highly profitable. Another way of "measuring" mobility is to globally study crime to person hits, mapping the collection point of the person specimen against the crime scene location (Walsh et al., 2002).

3. Systematic management of crime-to-crime (forensic) links

Importantly, the identifications of suspects through DNA Database (crime-to-person) links follow a process which is generally well formalised. By contrast, the results of comparisons between criminal events (crime-to-crime links) are not the subject of the same level of global or systematic management. These links however are capable of being promptly used in specific investigations or intra-jurisdictional series which can be pursued by a single police force. The extensive number of crime-to-crime links (for most database systems they are at least as common as crime-to-person links) shows the extent of this under-utilised potential. The practical value that could be realised through more comprehensive use of crime-to-crime link information includes a contribution at the tactical, operational and strategic levels. It is a serious oversight to not be analysing this information in closer detail.

4. Identifying the existence of a crime series

Good quality, timely knowledge of a crime series is likely to influence operational decisions by proactive tasking of investigatory or uniform police resources towards the series. Of course DNA outcomes are not the sole factor contributing to these decisions, but are often a fundamental contributor.

5. Assist decisions regarding sample submission

The analysis of DNA from biological traces is expensive and, in most jurisdictions, decisions as to which samples to submit to the database are important. The decision-making process surrounding database submissions requires the interpretation of several parameters including the available budget, the probative value of the sample, the quality of the sample (as it affects the likelihood of obtaining a complete profile), the probability of obtaining a hit (as much as this is predictable) and the importance of the case. All of these criteria are assisted by a more comprehensive awareness of the criminal situation in one's jurisdiction.

The next level of database operation involves the combination of a range of forensic disciplines in what I have referred to as the *Managed Multi-Discipline Database Model* (Figure 5).

Extending the *Managed Discipline Database Model* to incorporate multiple disciplines relies essentially on extending the capability of the results analysis unit to include other relevant forensic disciplines. The value of a multi-discipline approach is based on the assumption that the activity of serial offenders is specific and that this affects the evidence available and how and when it is deposited. As a consequence of this, some criminal signatures will be more easily visualised through certain data (for example modus operandi, shoemarks etc), whereas others will be visible through an entirely different set of data (for example DNA). The principal objective and advantage of this model is that it overcomes the silo-effect of the forensic discipline structure. The benefit of networking forensic outcomes is realised both in terms of efficiency gains by avoiding the duplication of analytical effort and in the value of outcomes and reports. As an example, fingerprints and DNA are both commonly sought in volume crime investigation and examination of the fingerprints at a scene that already has DNA link information has been useful at identifying associates of donor of the DNA link, who are potential co-offenders. By combining the outcomes of various discipline databases additional links will be observed that were not obvious previously. This augments the criminological analyses recommended under the *Managed Discipline Database Model*. In addition, reporting the full extent of these outcomes through the feedback mechanisms develops a high level of situational awareness amongst forensic crime scene and laboratory personnel. This should have a flow-on effect of improving the capacity to select relevant samples and further improve the effectiveness of the entire system. The contribution of this system extends across tactical, operational and strategic intelligence. This should be seen as a desirable end-point for forensic organisations responsible for multiple disciplines.

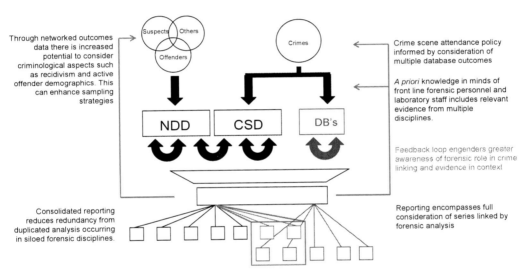

Figure 5. An example of a proposed structure of a *Managed Multi-Discipline Database Model*. Once again this model is based on forensic DNA databases.

To date progressing through the levels of models proposed could be achieved within the walls of a forensic agency and are more examples of effective information management rather than *"intelligence"*. The models above focused on forensic case data and its use and management in the context of an intelligence-based contribution. The ultimate value of this information will be realised when the comprehensive forensic outcomes are maximised and then incorporated into well-developed law enforcement crime analysis and intelligence systems.

The ultimate level of operation, however, proposes full integration of the *Managed Multi-Discipline Database Model* within a broader context of law enforcement crime analysis and intelligence systems (Figure 6). This is based on the assumption that any single evidence type (discipline) is only able to explain part of the story regarding criminal activity. Intelligence definitely requires the logical processing of all available information, whatever its type. The separation of forensic disciplines may be an organisational necessity, but compromises forensic sciences ability to explain singular criminal activities on the basis of the evidence types available. In this sense, it should not be expected that criminality will conform to these organizational constraints, but, in fact, the other way around!

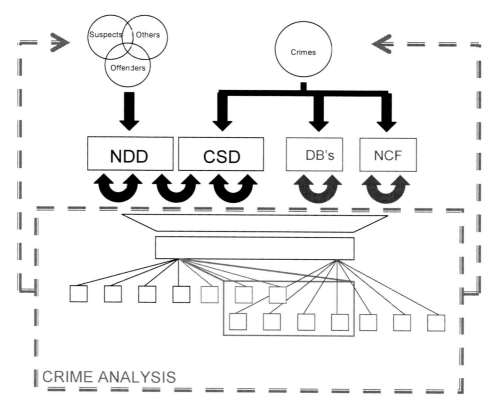

Figure 6. An example of an *Integrated Model*. This model embeds the Managed Multi-Discipline Model within existing crime analysis structures.

An additional component included in the *Integrated Model* is the use of *Non-Comparative Forensics* (NCF, in Figure 6). By this term we refer to forensic science tools that have the capacity to suggest intelligence links by virtue of their outcomes and do not rely on direct comparison with material from a known source. Their value in this context should not be underestimated. We have mentioned them as part of the *Integrated Model* as we believe that it is necessary to ensure there is a capacity to utilise the information they generate effectively in an intelligence context, prior to considering them for routine use. NCF techniques included in this category are familial searching, the use of partial (degraded) DNA and mixture and DNA phenotyping.

## SUMMARY

Through their ability to provide technical information capable of directing police investigations (such as by identifying a suspect or a crime-to-crime link), DNA databases can operate as a source of tactical and operational intelligence. As mentioned this proactive role is somewhat novel for forensic DNA evidence which is usually employed to corroborate or refute a previously held belief or version of events. In some respects the remnants of this retrospective, identification-driven use of DNA evidence provide a conceptual barrier to its exploitation under a truly intelligence-based model. These include:

- A lack of timeliness such as that identified above through the work of Blakey (2000, 2002) and in the discussion regarding the evidential versus investigative models;
- The lack of a framework to integrate DNA links with other forensic or investigative information. This can be accentuated by attempts to replicate the identification-based approach of DNA and AFIS databases with other forms of forensic evidence. This has proven to be complex and computationally laborious due to the fragmentary and visual nature of other trace evidence types and the complexity of the comparison process;
- An under-utilisation of the value of crime-to-crime DNA links due to a myopic emphasis on identifications. Scene-linking is a fundamental goal of crime analysis and DNA databases can complement and reinforce these efforts;
- An under-utilisation of the potential union between DNA links/outcomes and qualitative links generated through crime analysis and criminal and technical intelligence gathering. Some obvious advantages of this union include a lateral increase in the number of *"detections"* related to each DNA link and the recognition of serial-crimes and crime *"hot-spots"*;
- A tendency for the *"aura of certainty"* associated with DNA matches to supplant rather than complement other investigative strategies;
- A failure to systematically exploit information associated with DNA-based cases and links, such as characteristics of the crime and the evidence, criminal mobility or the offender demographic profile.

As yet, the forensic community has not determined the most effective manner in which to coordinate and exploit the intelligence potential of DNA (and other) evidence and have largely failed to develop systems capable of contributing higher-level operational and strategic intelligence. At the basic level forensic science needs to consider the intelligence cycle and whether we consider ourselves to be a contributor of information into an intelligence process that is abstract from our domain. This is a limited view of the role of forensic science in this area but it is realistic and possibly an accurate reflection of our role in jurisdictions operating under a *Discipline Database Model*. If this is the contribution that we seek then the onus is on us to produce the highest quality information for the purpose. That is, the best outcomes possible from the forensic process that in turn are best suited to use in this way.

At the next level it is possible for forensic science to operate our own (internal) intelligence cycle. If this is our desire then we must question how well we collect, collate, analyse and disseminate our information; and, whether or not the products of our work aide our understanding of the crime problem that we seek to resolve. At present it is not apparent that the forensic DNA field operates systematically at this level, however, this chapter has attempted to provide a blueprint via which forensic DNA database administrators and forensic administrators more generally, can progress towards achieving this objective. At the heart of this framework is effective information management and communication. These are implemented with the objective of improving the situational awareness of forensic and police personnel in order to have a positive influence on their ability to examine crimes and evidence holistically, selecting and processing relevant forensic samples, with the most appropriate forensic mechanism available. The models proposed also engender a greater understanding of criminality and the contribution forensic science can make to its management.

It is important that the forensic science community acknowledges that our focus with regard to forensic DNA database operations has not progressed markedly from the priorities established to support the implementation and growth phases. Undeniably there has been profound success in this area, but the future holds different challenges that will require from us further inventiveness and initiative to address. The true potential of this impressive forensic advance is still to be realised.

## COMPETING INTERESTS

The authors declare that they have no competing interests. The authors alone are responsible for the content and writing of the paper.

## REFERENCES

Asplen, C. H. and Lane, S. A. (2003) Considerations in the development of DNA databases. *Interfaces* 36: 1-2.

Bieber, F. R. (2006) Turning base hits into earned runs: improving the effectiveness of forensic DNA data bank programs. *Journal of Law and Medical Ethics* 34: 222-233.

Blakey, D. (2000) *Under the Microscope: Thematic Inspection Report on Scientific and Technical Support*. Report of the Her Majesty's Inspectorate of Constabulary, Ditching.

Blakey, D. (2002) *Under the Microscope - Refocused*. Report of the Her Majesty's Inspectorate of Constabulary, Ditching.

Broadhurst, R. G. and Maller, R. A. (1991) Estimating the numbers of prison terms in criminal careers from one-step probabilities of recidivism. *Journal of Quantitative Criminology* 7: 275-290.

Champod, C. and Ribaux, O. (2000) Forensic identification databases in criminal investigations and trials. In: Nijboer, J. F. and Spranger, W. J. J. M. (Ed). *Harmonisation in Forensic Expertise*. Thela Thesis: Amsterdam, pp. 463-484.

Dale, W. M. and Becker, W. S. (2004) A Case Study of Forensic Scientist Turnover. *Forensic Science Communications,* volume 6(3), available from http://www.fbi.gov/hq/lab/fsc/backissu/july2004/index.htm (accessed 12 January 2007).

Gotlieb, S. (1998) *Crime Analysis - From First Report to Final Arrest*. Alpha Publishing: Montclair, Ca.

Heide, K. M., Spencer, E., Thompson, A. and Solomon, E. P. (2001) Who's in, who's out, and who's back: follow-up data on 59 juveniles incarcerated in adult prison for murder or attempted murder in the early 1980's. *Behavioral Sciences and the Law* 19: 97-108.

Hunt, N. Crime and crime again: The offenders who will never learn. *The Advertiser* (Adelaide), 5 October 2002, pp. 1.

Lambert, E. G., Hogan, N. L., Nerbonne, T., Barton, S. M., Watson, P. L., Buss, J. and Lambert, J. (2007) Differences in forensic science views and needs in law enforcement: A survey of Michigan law enforcement agencies. *Police Practice and Research* 8: 415-430.

Leitner, M., Kent, J., Oldfield, I. and Swoope, E. (2007) Geoforensic analysis revisited - The application of Newton's geographic profiling method to serial burglaries in London, UK. *Police Practice and Research* 8: 359-370.

Lovrich, N. P., Gaffney, M. J., Pratt, T. C., Johnson, C. L., Asplen, C. H., Hurst, L. H. and Schellberg, T. M. (2003) *National Forensic DNA Study Report*. Report of the Division of Governmental Studies and Services, Washington State University and Smith Alling Lane, Professional Services, Available from http://www.dnaresource.com (accessed 13 September 2004).

Raymond, J. J., Walsh, S. J., van Oorschot, R. A., Gunn, P. R., Roux, C. Trace DNA: an underutilised resource or Pandora's Box? *Journal of Forensic Identification* 56(4) (2004) 668-686.

Schneider, P. M. and Martin, P. D. (2001) Criminal DNA databases: the European situation. *Forensic Science International* 119: 232-238.

Simon, L. M. J. (1997) Do criminal offenders specialize in crime types? *Applied and Preventative Psychology* 6: 35-53.

Smith, D. Cops and swabbers. *The Sydney Morning Herald* (Sydney), 1 December 1999, pp. 19.

The Queen v Sean Hoey, *Crown Court Northern Ireland*, Bill No: 341/05, 21 December 2007.

Walsh, S. J., Buckleton, J. S., Ribaux, O., Roux, C., Raymond, T. Comparing the Growth and Effectiveness of Forensic DNA Databases. *Forensic Science International: Genetics Supplement Series* 1 (2008) 667-668.

Walsh, S. J., Curran, J. M., Buckleton, J. S. Modelling forensic DNA database performance. In press *J. Forensic Sci.* (accepted May 2009).

Walsh, S. J. Current and future trends in forensic molecular biology. In Rapley R and Whitehouse D. *Molecular Forensics*. John Wiley & Sons: London, 2007, pp. 1-20.

Zamble, F. E. and Quinsey, G. (1997) *The Criminal Recidivism Process*. Chicago University Press: Chicago.

In: Forensic Genetics Research Progress
Editor: F. Gonzalez-Andrade

ISBN: 978-1-60876-198-2
© 2010 Nova Science Publishers, Inc.

*Chapter 4*

# HOMICIDE INVESTIGATION: ANTHROPOLOGY AND GENETIC ANALYSIS FOR THE CRIME SCENE

## I. Roca, M. Beaufils[*], A. Esponda, G. Said and C. Doutremepuich

Laboratoire d'Hématologie Médico-Légale, 41-43 Avenue de la République,
33019 Bordeaux Cedex, France

### ABSTRACT

Dr Watson has been replaced by Sir Jeffreys in 1985, day when a criminal case was elucidated thanks to genetic analysis; forensic laboratories have tried to decrease the DNA/cells quantity necessary to obtain a profile and to increase the analysis sensibility.

The DNA profile is put in evidence from each kind of tissue as epithelium, sperm, blood, bones and hairs. Two kinds of samples are realised: the samples of traces and those of comparison. The first step of the analysis is to investigate the stains or traces. Several techniques are used: chemical, cytological or visual. A specific organisation has been elaborated in the laboratory in order to eliminate the cross contamination and the contact between victim samples and suspect samples. This organization is present in the entire laboratory, for all the steps of the analysis. The second step is the extraction of the DNA from tissue. Since 2008, a new technique, the laser microdissection, is used in complement of classical method to analyse contact cells. This one is chosen as a function of the potential quantity of cells on the support. One to ten cells are sufficient to obtain a DNA profile. The laser microdissection permits to directly select and analyse the interest cells. The result is as efficient as it was with the classical one but on less than ten cells. With the reduction of the numbers of analysed cells, the number of DNA blend is reduced too. Since the use of the laser microdissection, the percentage of results has been significantly increased: results are obtained where no result was revealed with the classical technique of extraction.

The obtained profiles are compared either between them, or "trace" profiles with "comparison" profiles. A statistical analysis is realised for the "trace" profile corresponding to the "comparison" profile. Because of the importance of the results, quality assurance has to be present in the laboratory. One possibility is the accreditation ISO 17025 which permits to set the quality system and the methods after a checking and a control. All the used laboratory techniques are certified ISO 9001 and accredited ISO 17025 to assure the competency, the quality and the performance of the laboratory.

Nowadays, the analysis DNA becomes widespread and complementary to the other analysis for the investigators because of the numerous information it brings. To find one or several profiles thanks to a contact cells or sperm or blood permit to orient the investigation, to find a suspect and sometimes to understand the progress of the crime or the facts.

## 1. INTRODUCTION

The characterisation of a person from DNA began in ninety's thank to a new technology invented by Sir Alec Jeffreys from Leicester University in 1985. DNA analysis is based on the fact that two persons have a majority of their DNA in common and a part specific to the individual. The analysis consists in analysing the specific part or polymorph part of DNA present in the nucleus of cells (nuclear DNA - n-DNA) or in the mitochondria (mitochondrial DNA - m-DNA). The cells include one nucleus and much more than one hundred mitochondria. Each nucleus contains one molecule of n-DNA guise twenty three pairs of chromosomes (human genome), the half of chromosomes results from the mother and the other half from the father. Mitochondria contain about one hundred copies of m-DNA resulting only from the mother; m-DNA is specific of maternal lineage.

Cells are present in all tissues (blood, muscles, bones, epithelium etc…). Therefore, the identification of person is realised by analysing the DNA extracted from blood cells, bone cells or epithelial cells resulting from handled object. For one person, DNA is identical in all cells and specific to the person.

Nowadays, thanks to technical progress like PCR (Polymerase Chain Reaction) and Laser microdissection, one cell is sufficient to obtain a DNA profile.

The aim of a scene crime investigator is to well collect cells present on an object or to collect directly the object when it is possible to realise an exploitable and right DNA profile, that's mean without contamination.

## 2. IDENTIFICATION OF TRACES OR STAINS

Scene crime investigators collect different samples or evidences as a function of the case. For a mass crash and cadaver identification, bones are harvested. In case of paternity analysis, victims or suspects identification, buccal cells are taken on swabs and/or FTA. For a scene crime investigation, different samples as blood, cells, semen and/or hairs are collected depending on the case. For instance, cells and roots are taken for murder, sexual assault and robbery whereas blood is mainly collected for murder and semen for sexual assault.

[*] E-mail : adn.laboratoire@wanadoo.fr

Blood or semen evidences are present on a scene of crime under two forms. Some evidences are visible like blood stains or semen stains in opposition with traces which are not visible. For blood or semen traces, a chemical analysis is realised in order to reveal their presence.

The blood presence is tested chemically with Bluestar® Forensic (composed of luminol) on a scene crime and with Kastle Meyer method in laboratory. Bluestar® Forensic is more sensitive but a lot of false positive occurs. Moreover this chemical dilutes the stains or traces which complicate the analysis when there is little white blood cell (only cells with DNA presented in blood). These two techniques reveal the presence of blood by inducing a reaction of oxydo-reduction in presence of iron which is located in the heme of red blood cells.

A positive reaction with Kastle Meyer is recognizable by a pink color whereas Bluestar® Forensic produce a chemiluminescence in presence of blood.

Semen presence is revealed with a crimescope on a scene crime whereas in laboratory the presence of semen is tested with Brentamine and confirmed by a cytological investigation. This chemical reacts with acid phosphatase located in semen. Fresh semen stains give a fast, deep purple, color reaction.

The hairs are investigated visually, a presence of roots is determined on binocular magnifying glass.

For contact cells, it's more complicated because none chemicals allow enlightening the epithelial cells. Crime scene investigator has to imagine the contact zones in order to collect the interest samples. In the laboratory, the contact cells are investigated following the specification of the crime scene investigator or following the protocol benched by the laboratory. Aeras susceptible to be handled by the victim or the suspect are privileged.

During a contact, cells could be transferred in two ways. Te first one is from a person to an object which it is called primer transfer. The second one occurs less often, it corresponds to a transfer from the primary object to another object, it is named secondary transfer.

For each transfer, a loose of cells operated what returns the cells analysis more difficult.

This consideration allows us defining two work lines which will be based on the collect. First, the crime scene investigator has to collect cells deposited on an object or on another person and to collect unknown object in order to look for cells potentially present.

For instance, it's important to collect with swabs the contact area between the assailant and the victim and the objects handled by the aggressor.

## 3. SAMPLES REALISATION

As described previously, the aim of a sampling is to save cells, present on an object with a swab (whatever the kind of cells) or to take this object without contamination of the sampling.

Some rules have to be followed in order to collect the maximum of cells with meticulousness, to avoid the contamination and to conserve the sampling.

The first important point to realise a sample is the equipment of the investigator. Whatever the sampling, the technician has to wear a blouse (or overalls), a cap (or charlotte), a mask, overshoes and gloves. This set must be used for a unique purpose.

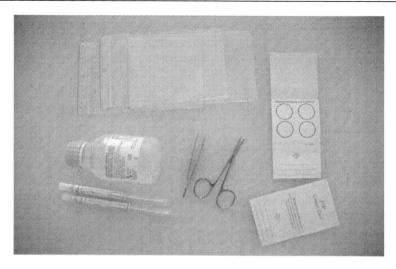

Photo 1. Material used for a sampling.

Gloves have two principal functions. The first one is to protect the investigator from bacteria and virus eventually presented on a stain and the second one is to protect samples from a contamination between samples or between the sample and the investigator. Gloves have to be worn only during the sampling and have to be changed between two samples.

All the materials and all the chemicals (Photo 1) have to be exempt from DNA. A cleaning with diluted bleach (10%) ensures a perfect decontamination or destruction of DNA.

Two kinds of samples are collected by the scene crime investigators, the mobile objects but also the non mobile objects which are susceptible to have been touched by the victim or the suspect. Theses samples can contain contact cells or cells from blood or sperm in the form of spot or traces.

For mobile supports, investigators collect objects with forceps when it's possible or take them by the area which probably no contains cells. Wet supports have to be dried before their conservation. Each collected support is identified, put under seal and stocked at room temperature for dried supports and at negative temperature (-20°C) for perishable supports like food or condom. Mobile samples are directly sent to the laboratory.

For non mobile samples, the scene crime investigator has to collect carefully the traces or stains (blood, cells sperm) with a swab in order to be sent to the laboratory quickly.

The swab case is identified; after the collect, the swab in its case is let opened in order to be dried. The swab is put under seals and conserved dried at room temperature. For wet swabs, the conservation has to be at negative temperature.

### a) Buccal Swabs

These samples are realised to compare an unknown DNA profile to a person, to discriminate victims or to identify suspects but also to analyse filiations.

This sample consists to take buccal cells (Photo 2) in the interior of the mouth by rubbing the cotton part on the intern face of the cheek. After drying the swab, and identification of the swab case, the sample is put under seals. In some cases, cells collected on swabs are transferred on a FTA paper (Fast Technology Analysis) by rubbing the cotton swabs on it. Put under seals, these samples are stocked dried at room temperature.

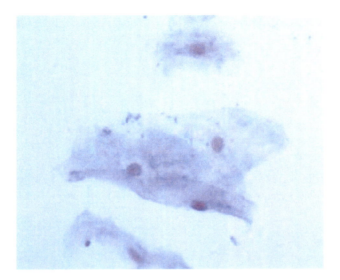

Photo 2. Buccal cells.

## b) Samples for Sexual Assault

Sampling are realised depending on the kind of sexual assault in order to find cells and spermatozoa (Photo 3). On the victims, vaginal swabs, buccal swabs, anal swabs and/or swabs on penis are made whereas on suspect only buccal swabs and sometimes swabs on penis are sampled. Clothes or bedding can be collected on the crime scene depending on victim's declaration.

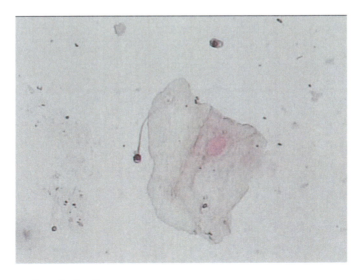

Photo 3. Spermatozoa and vaginal cell.

## c) Samples for Mass Crash and Cadaver Identification

Usually a bone is harvested like thighbone. The DNA profile obtained from the bone analysis is compared to DNA profile of the supposed mother and father or to supposed personal objects belonging to cadaver (teeth brush, brush). This comparison permits to establish the identification of the cadaver.

## d) Hair Samples

Hairs are collected on a crime scene or on clothes with forceps in order to avoid contamination.

Some root hairs do not contain root nuclear DNA (Photo 4) and others do (Photo 5). In this last case, root is composed of fat acid. But in all hairs, mitochondrial DNA is present in a stem from hairs.

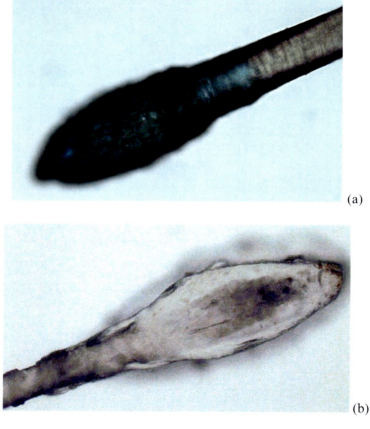

Photo 4. (A) stained Root hair without DNA. (B) Roots hair.

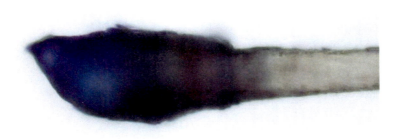

Photo 5. Root hairs with DNA.

## e) Teeth Samples, Muscles Samples, Blood Samples

To identify a dead body, sometimes it is not possible to collect bones. For these particular cases, an alternative is to collect teeth or muscles or blood. For teeth, it is preferable to analyse the DNA from cheek-teeth. For muscles and blood, it is recommended to freeze the samples.

## f) Nail Samples

After aggression or murder, cut nails of the victim is reasonable, that's allow collecting cells of the suspects eventually present. Swabs under the nails are dissuaded because cells of the victims are collected in the same time that induces mixed profiles after analysis.

## g) Contact Cells Samples

The epithelial cells are more or less protected by keratin (Photo 6) that's why its detachment from the skin and its transfer is difficult. Buccal cells present no keratin protection (Photos A1 and A2) whereas cells from skin (Photos B1 and B2) and particularly cells from hands skin or feet skin (Photos C1 and C2) are keratinised.

Some supports facilitate the cells transfer by its nature and/or the texture, for instance latex gloves or rough objects.

When it is possible, all the support is collected with forceps. But for the non mobile supports, a swab is realised on the area which is liable to be handled to contain cells of interest (Photo 7).

In conclusion, whatever the samples, in order to guarantee the quality of the samples, samples has to be adapted as a function of the case, non contaminated and preserved in adapted conditions (light, temperature, humidity).

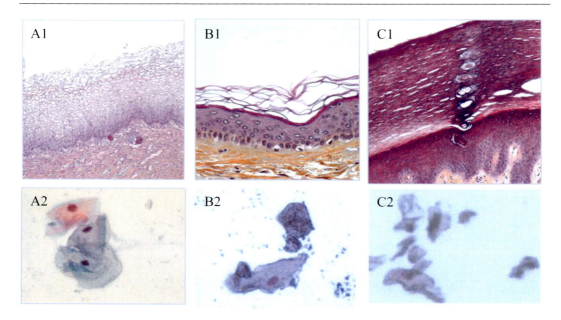

Photo 6. A1, B1 and C1: histological sections of 3 kinds of epithelium: A1 mucous epithelium, B1 classical epithelium, C1 epithelium of hands and feet. A2, B2 and C2: view on microscope of cells after a contact with a slide: A2 cells with nuclei of the mucous membrane, B2 cells of skin with few nuclei, C2 squama of hands and feet with not many nuclei.

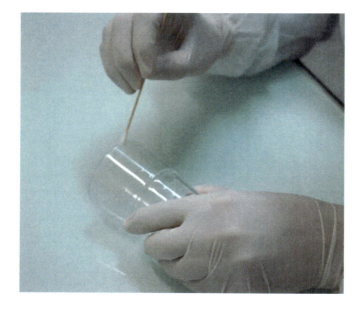

Photo 7. Swab realised on the area in contact with buccal cells.

## 4. ANALYSIS OF TRACES OR STAINS

The DNA analysis is composed of different steps in order to obtain a DNA profile. The first one is the extraction step following by an amplification step and finished by a genotyping or sequencing step.

## a) Extraction

DNA extraction consists in extract DNA from nucleus or mitochondria by different methods. The more used methods are chemical. These methods of reference used in forensic laboratories are numerous (Butler, 2005: chapter 3): Phenol-Chloroform, Chelex 5% or some extraction kits from different suppliers (Qiagen, Promega etc.). Some methods are used specifically for some samples, others are used whatever the samples (blood, hair roots, semen, contact cells, buccal swabs or FTA paper).

For all the methods except Chelex method, this step is preceded by a cell lysis which consists to break membrane cells by using a proteinase K. This protease hydrolyses nucleic acids, in particular the peptide connections located after the hydrophobic amino acids. In order to facilitate the proteinase K action, notably for spermatozoids, the compounds called DiThioThreitol (DTT) is added in order to reduce disulfide bridges of proteins.

*Phenol chloroform method* is used to extracts DNA cells from sexual assault. Samples include often female cells mixed to spermatozoids, a separation between them is mandatory to get a unique DNA profiles. After the lysis, only female cells are lysed, spermatozoids are intact because of the numerous disulfide bridges. Further to centrifugation, male cells can be isolated and lysed with a lysis buffer containing a proteinase k and DTT. The lysis products are processed with Phenol-Chloroform-Isoamylic Alcohol (PCIA). Phenol deproteinized the sample in order to avoid a solubilisation of DNA, chloroform denatures proteins and facilitates the isolation of the aqueous phase from the organic phase and isoamilic alcohol is an anti-foams agent. DNA is concentrated and purified by filtration on a membrane; this membrane isolates DNA from small molecules and recuperates by centrifugation.

*Chelex* is a resin which has a large affinity to groups charged positively into an alkaline pH. Cells are lysed by a thermal shock in presence of chelex resin. By chelating ions from heavy metal, the resin prevents the degradation of DNA at high-temperature in a solution of weak ionic strength. To the sample, a proteinase K and/or DTT can be added to facilitate the lysis.

*Extractions kits* are numerous. These kits used particles which capture DNA in order to purify the samples and eliminate inhibitors. Two kind of particle are used. The first ones are particles of silica which adsorb selectively nucleic acids into ionic controlled conditions. DNA fixes on particles of silica in presence of ethanol and elevated concentration of chaotropics salts. The chaotropic salts induce a modification of spatial structure of water molecules around the particles of silica which allow the specific fixation of DNA. To recuperate the DNA a buffer poor in salt with a alkaline pH is used. The second methods consist in using magnetic particles to capture DNA, and wash buffer to recuperate DNA.

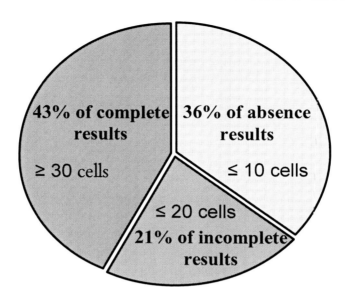

Figure 1. Repartition of the results for contact cells analysis by the method of reference.

### Results of Analysis of Contact Cells by Method of Reference in 2008

In 2008, on 6000 samples of contact cells were analysed (Figure 1): 47% of the samples contained DNA, among these samples, 64% of results were obtained (with a mean level of 0.6ng/ul which corresponds approximately to 100 cells) or with more than ten cells. 36% of absence results contained less than ten cells.

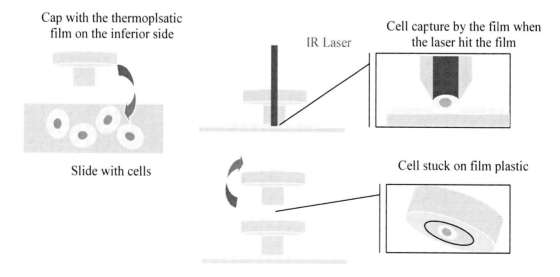

Figure 2. Schematic representation of a laser microdissection sample which allows collecting one to several cells on a same cap.

To obtain a DNA profile, with reference method, twenty cells are mandatory. Usually, after a cells transfer, less than twenty cells are present on the support. With less than twenty cells, it's difficult to obtain an exploitable profile. With less than ten cells, no profile results of the DNA analysis.

Different kinds of object contain systematically less than ten cells like munitions (bullets, cartridges) and, no results were obtained for their analysis.

Therefore a change of strategy is necessary for supports comprising less than twenty cells. Among all the possibility, the laser microdissection method stands out by its simplicity, its reliability and its reproducibility. With this new technique, less than ten cells allow us to get an exploitable and exact DNA profile. This method much more sensitive is used in complement of methods of references. This technique is used to analyse spermatozoa but only in forensic research laboratory and to analyse contact cells for real forensic cases.

Two different laser microdissection methods have been developed based on distinct principles. Laser microdissection techniques are powerful technologies which associate morphological, histochemical and molecular analysis.

The first one called laser cutting microdissection. This method consists in using a pulsed UV-A laser coupled into a microscope and focussed via the objective lenses to a micronsized spot diameter. By activating laser, forces are generated within the narrow laser focal spot that induce ablation of material without degradation of the cells. Using the same laser the separated cell(s) can be lifted up and captured in a collection device. This is a totally non-contact process, as only focussed light is used for the transportation of a selected area into a collection device. This technique is developed in forensic research laboratory essentially to separate male cells and females cells with fluorescence method (Seidl et al. 2005; Miyazaki et al., 2008; Vandewoestyne et al., 2008).

The second one named laser capture microdissection consists in an inverted microscope coupled into an infrared laser. The use of caps composed of a thermoplastic film allows collecting stained cells deposited on a slide by starting up the laser. Further to laser activation, the interest cell(s) adhere(s) to the cap film, not to the slide (see Figure 2). Forensic research laboratory works on it in order to isolate male cells from females cells (Elliott et al., 2003) and also to analyse contact cells for scene crime samples.

With this new technology, complete DNA profile results from the analysis of one to ten cells.

Moreover, advantages are numerous. The visualisation of the cells is direct, no quantification by Quantitative PCR (Polymerase Chain Reaction) is mandatory. The number of collected cells is known. One to several cells can be collected on a same device, or several devices with one cell can be realised in order to obtain a unique DNA profile. Indeed, analysis on one cell involves the getting of a unique DNA profile. And an important point is that no cleaning, no purification of the sample is mandatory because only cells adhere to the film, not the background.

## *Results of Analysis of Contact Cells by Laser Capture Microdissection Laser in 2008*

In 2008, 430 samples containing less than cells were analysed with the microdissection laser method (Figure 3). 61% of samples contained cells. 27% of results were obtained with a mean of three cells collected by microdissection laser.

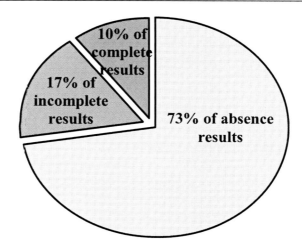

Figure 3. Repartition of the results for contact cells analysis by laser capture microdissection method.

In the case of munitions examples, analysis of contact cells allows obtaining 19% of results with microdissection method.

## b) Amplification – PCR

### i. Polymorph Regions

*The polymorphism of repetition* is characterized by the repetition of short identical sequences present on all the genome which varies from a person to another (minisatellites or microsatellites). The major part of the n-DNA is composed of repetitive units (from 2pb to several hundred). These units are specific to a person and their number allows defining a polymorphism.

- *VNTRs (variable number tandem repeat ou minisatellites).* Sir Alec Jeffreys studying a gene on a non coding DNA region revealed some repeated DNA bases contained in a microsatellite. These repeated units result probably to DNA copy during cellular division. This modification has no effect on function of chromosome, no mechanism of reparation occurs, therefore the modification are transmitted to the next generation. The number of repeated sequences does not follow rules; each minisatellite varies from a person to another that is allowed to identify the persons.
  Usually, repeated units are composed of 15 to 50 bases and these sequences can be repeated sufficiently to obtain a minisatellite (around 20 kilobases).
- *STRs (short tandem repeat or microsatellites).* These repeated units are the most used in forensic analysis (Butler, 2005: chapter 5). These sequences are composed of 3 to 5 bases, the resulted microstallites containing 50 to 300 bases.

Example for one locus with the repeated units (AGAT):

AGGTTT(AGAT)$_8$CGTA : allele 8
AGGTTT(AGAT)$_8$AGATAGATAGATAGATCGTA : allele 12

AGGTTT(AGAT)₈AGATAGATAGATAGATAGCGTA : allele 12.2

Companies sell kit which allows amplifying together several STRs on autosomal chromosomes associated to a marker on sexual chromosome to form a multiplex.
For instance:

- kit AmpFSTR Identifiler - Applied Biosystem:16 loci
- kit AmpFSTR Minifiler - Applied Biosystem: 9 loci
- kit GenePrint$^R$PowerPlex$^{TM}$ 16 System - Promega: 16 loci

Other kits associate STR from Y chromosome like Powerplex$^R$ Y System – Promega: 11 loci on Y chromosome. Some laboratories are developing kits in order to analyse STRs from X chromosome (Edelmann et al., 2008; Becker et al, 2008).

*Restriction polymorphism.* Coding regions represent only ten percent of the genome; so, ninety percent is not implicated in the protein production. In non coding regions, no selection force is present that's why mutation can occur without visible damage. Because of the important rate of mutation, this polymorphism is very widespread and easily transmitted to next generations. As a result (consequently), the non coding regions of genome are more informative to identify a person. Moreover, these non coding regions do not offer information about the physiology or anatomy of the person.

*SNPs (single nucleotide polymorphism).* SNPs correspond to variation of one base pair in the genome for two persons of same specie (Butler, 2005: chapter 8).

These variations are frequent: 1/1000 base pair for human which represents ninety percent of the variation in human genome. SNPs are present in non coding regions, on coding regions and between genes. SNPs are used in order to identify persons or to build genealogical trees.
Example of SNP:

| Person A | AGGTACTCCAT |
|          | TCCATGAGGTA |
| Person B | AGGTATTCCAT |
|          | TCCATAAGGTA |

A modification just for one base can induce significant changes on phenotype like drug tolerance or disease predisposition.

## ii. Polymorphic Regions on m-DNA

*HVI-HVII*

Mt-DNA is transmitted only by the mother: it's specific to maternal lineage and conserved as generations go by. It does not contain repeated units. Analysis consists to study hypervariable areas called HV1 and HV2 (Doutremepuich et al., 2003; Butler, 2005: chapter 10) but these areas can be identical for two individuals without blood relationship that's represents one risk on two thousand. Therefore, in forensic, this analysis is a complementary analysis that allows excluding a person.

But mt-DNA has some advantages because mt-DNA is present in the form of numerous copies in cells: it allows investigating degraded samples and hairs without roots for which no result would be obtained (Martin, 2003).

The two areas analysed HV1 and HV2 contained respectively 393 base pairs and 358 base pairs and are located respectively between the base 15998 and 16391 for HV1 and between the base 49 and 407 for HV2. After sequencing, the analysis consists in comparison to a reference sequence called Anderson sequence. This comparison allows establishing mutations characterising the maternal lieanage of the person. In order to determinate if two persons bellow to the same lineage, their mutation are compared. Two differences implicate exclusion, they don't below two the same lineage, if only one difference is revealed, no conclusion can be done. For the report of result, important precautions must be taken to avoid the mistakes of interpretation.

*Cytochrome b*

Cytochrome b (bases 14841 to 15148) is analysed in order to successfully identify the origin of the sample (human or animal) (De Pancorbo, 2003). This protein is composed of 400 amino acids and involved in the transport of electron and the production of ATP.

When the sequence lines up to Anderson sequence and presents not much or no mutation, the origin is human. In the opposite when the sequence does not line up to Anderson sequence and presents a lot of mutation, the origin is animal. For an animal origin, laboratories use a data base like "BLAST" in order to determine the specie of the revealed sequence.

## c) Applications

### i) Identification of Traces

Collected samples like sperm, contact cells, blood, roots hair, urinary are analysed, the resulted DNA profile can be then compared. The comparison test allows investigator identifying victim samples and assailant samples.

Identification occurs:

- either by comparison to a DNA profile obtained from a buccal swab or from a FTA paper
- or to a data base. Different data base exists as a function of the country, for example the CODIS in USA, the FNAEG in France or Interpol Data base in Europe (Kloosterman and Janssen, 2001; Robert, 2001; Butler, 2005: chapter 18; Doutremepuich, 2006).

### ii) Mass Crash – Cadaver Identification

DNA analysis is realised on a portion of long bones like femur where the cells are protected in cavities and therefore DNA resist more to putrefaction, this sample is better than collect muscles.

n-DNA on autosomal chromosome, on Y chromosome or on m-DNA can be analysed as a function of the case. The results are compared to personal object like brush teeth or brush hair etc or to members of the presumed family in order to establish filiations

Filiation's analysis is very sensitive for many raisons: civil father can not be the biological father or brothers or sisters have different n-DNA or probability has to be superior to 99,999 %. In doubt, it's necessary to complete the investigation with the analysis of chromosome Y or/and m-DNA.

### *iii) Paternity Testing*

The analysis in some countries like France requires a mission of expertise. This paternity testing consists to analyse cells collected on swabs or FTA paper in order to establish filiations.

### *iv) Statistical Analysis*

A comparison between a trace and a DNA profile from a buccal swab (suspect), a comparison for filiations requires statistical analysis. For each analysed locus, laboratories possess population studies in order to determine a comparative probability (Butler, 2005: chapter 20 and 21).

Example: for one person, on the locus TPOX, the DNA analysis revealed two alleles with different sizes: 10-12. This profile is compared to a DNA profile obtained from a blood trace which alleles are 11-12. The conclusion is exclusion: there is no concordance between the two results; the blood trace does not correspond to the compared person. On the other hand, if the results correspond for all the allele analysed, in other words if all the alleles obtained from blood trace are identical to those from person to compared, the conclusion is an inclusion.

The Table 1 presents an example of results obtained after the DNA analysis from a suspect and DNA analysis from a blood trace. For each analysed systems, a comparison is realised between the two DNA profiles.

The comparison between the suspect profile and the blood trace profile reveals four discordances and 11 concordances: the suspect profile is excluded.

**Table 1.**

| Systèmes | Suspect | Blood trace | Concordance | Discordance |
|---|---|---|---|---|
| D8S1179 | 14-15 | 14-15 | x | |
| D21S11 | 28-28 | 28-28 | x | |
| D7S820 | 10-12 | 10-11 | | x |
| CSF1PO | 11-13 | 11-12 | | x |
| D3S1358 | 16-17 | 16-17 | x | |
| TH01 | 8-9 | 8-9 | x | |
| D13S317 | 14-14 | 10-14 | | x |
| D16S539 | 12-13 | 12-13 | x | |
| D2S1338 | 19-24 | 19-24 | x | |
| D19S433 | 14-15 | 14-15 | x | |
| vWA | 15-17 | 15-17 | x | |
| TPOX | 10-12 | 11-12 | | x |
| D18S51 | 17-20 | 17-20 | x | |
| Amelogenine | X-Y | X-Y | x | |
| D5S818 | 10-13 | 10-13 | x | |
| FGA | 19-22 | 19-22 | x | |

The analysis of one allele is not sufficient to conclude for an inclusion. To conclude for an inclusion, an a-posteriori probability has to be calculated as a function of three factors which are the allelic frequency, the number of allele obtained for a DNA profile after analysis of the sample and the a-priori probability which corresponds to the probability for a person to be at the origin of the trace before the analysis, this probability is established by the investigator as the function of the investigation elements.

## 5. VALIDATION AND QUALITY ASSURANCE

Each recognized laboratory has to assure quality in the work and reproducibility in the results. These requirements implicate a specific organization of the staff, the protocols and the equipments/infrastructure (Butler, 2005: chapter 16).

### Organisation of the Laboratory

The laboratory is divided in several departments specialised in a function: the department which receives evidences, the department which investigates biological material, the molecular biology department which realises extraction amplification and genotyping, the quality department which controls and validates the results and the secretary department which writes the report for magistrates and investigators. The direction department composed of an expert is in charge of control these different departments and to sign reports.

Moreover, at the most sensitive step which is the investigation of the trace, the question evidences which the origin is unknown are analysed in a laboratory different from the laboratory where the comparison evidences are analysed. For the question evidences laboratoriess, the victim samples are analysed in a laboratory different from the laboratory where suspect samples are collected.

In all the laboratories which use PCR technique, the risk is contamination by an outsider DNA which is due to the extreme sensitivity of the method. This risk is minimised by separating the different analysis steps (extraction and PCR preparation).

### Training, Protocoles and Procedures

The staff of each department is trained in the laboratory by tutor in order to learn all the protocols and the procedures used by his department. Work instruction which describes the different techniques and protocols are available in each department.

The different protocols are tested and validated to check the performance, the reproducibility and the repeatability of the analysis by the quality department. For instance, for each step of the analysis (trace investigation, extraction and molecular biology), negative controls (no DNA in the sample) are realised in order to determine the absence of cross contamination and the neutrality of the reactive. To this negative control is added a positive control (DNA which profile is known) to check the well sequence of the different analysis.

## Accreditation and Certification

It's important that forensic laboratories work in accordance with a quality reference recognized at a world level like the norm ISO (International Standard Organization). Laboratories can be certificated ISO 9001 which recognizes the organization of the laboratory and accredited ISO 17025 which approves the performance of the laboratory and the competency of its staff and its protocoles. For instance, in some countries like France, the certification is not required. In France, certification and accreditation are controlled each year by independent organism like the AFAQ and the COFRAC respectively.

These accreditation and certification implicate demands notably improve the efficiency of the system of quality management and to respect a quality politic define by the laboratory. The quality politic can include the improvements of protocols, the performance of the results, the respect of delay, the client proximity. The laboratory promises to respect this quality politic.

## 6. Conclusion

In ten years, whatever the country, the genetic analysis in judicial practice allowed to include or to exclude persons accused of murder, rapes or theft etc. The Biologist saw his participation increased within the framework of the penal lawsuit. It ensued from it an obligation of quality as well as of performance in the depiction of the results. The quality of the result fits into a global step of the laboratory within the international frame of reference ISO 17025 and within a specific step by the use of many controls so internal as external. However these analyses will be always dependent on the quality of the samples collect.

## Competing Interests

The authors declare that they have no competing interests. The authors alone are responsible for the content and writing of the paper.

## References

Becker D., Rodig H., Augustin C., Edelmann J., Götz F., Heiring S., Szibor R., Brabetz. W. (2008) Population genetic evaluation of eight X-chromosomal short tandem repeat loci using Mentype Argus X-8 PCR amplification kit. *Forensic Science International: Genetics* 2: 69-74.

Butler J. M. (2005) Forensic DNA typing. *Biology, technology and genetics of STR markers*. Elsevier academic press, second edition.

Doutremepuich F., Heyvang N., Beaufils M., Morales V., Ausset L. et Doutremepuich. C. (2003) L'ADN mitochondrial : étude des régions HVI et HVII en pratique judiciaire, ADN mitochondrial : de l'intérêt scientifique à la pratique judiciaire. Paris, *La documentation Française*, pp. 75-85.

Doutremepuich C. (2006) *Les fichiers des empreintes génétiques en pratique judiciaire.* Paris, La documentation Française.

Edelmann J., Hering S., Augustin C., Szibor R.. (2008) Characterisation of the STR markers DXS10146, DXS10134 and DXS10147 located within a 79.1 Kb region at Xq28. *Forensic Science International*: Genetics 2: 41-46.

Elliott K., Hill D.S., Lambert C., Burroughes T.R. and Gill P. (2003) Use of laser microdissection greatly improves the recovery of DNA from sperm on microscope slides. *Forensic Science International;* 137: 28-36.

Kloosterman A. et Janssen H. (2001). La base de données d'ADN au Pays-Bas, 10 ans d'empreintes génétiques. Paris, *La documentation Française,* pp. 167-173.

Martin P. (2003). L'utilisation de l'analyse de l'ADN mitochondrial dans la science médico-légale, A*DN mitochondrial : de l'intérêt scientifique à la pratique judiciaire.* Paris, La documentation Française, pp. 87-92.

Miyazaki T., Hara M., Ichki A., Yamamoto Y., Takada A., Kido A., Nodera M., Yanagisawa H., Suzuki H. and Saito K. (2008) An efficient novel method for analyzing STR loci from a single sperm captured by laser microdissection. *Forensic Science International;* 1: 437-438.

De Pancorbo M. M. (2003) Utilisation de l'ADN mitochondrial dans l'identification des restes d'origine animale, *ADN mitochondrial De l'intérêt scientifique à la pratique judiciaire.* Paris, La documentation Française, pp. 35-50.

Robert M. (2001) Le fichier national automatisé des empreintes génétiques, 10 ans d'empreintes génétiques. Paris, *La documentation Française*, pp. 189-200.

Seidl S., Burgemeister R., Hausmann R., Betz P. and Lederer T. (2005) Contact-free isolation of sperm and epithelial cells by laser microdissection and pressure catapulting. Forensic Science, *Medecine and Pathology;* 1: 153-158

Vandewoestyne M., Van Hoofstat D., Van Nieuwerburgh F. and Deforce D. (2008) Automatic detection of spermatozoa for laser capture microdissection. *International Journal of Legal Medicine;* 123.

In: Forensic Genetics Research Progress
Editor: F. Gonzalez-Andrade

ISBN: 978-1-60876-198-2
© 2010 Nova Science Publishers, Inc.

**Chapter 5**

# INFLUENCE OF HUMIC ACID ON DNA ANALYSIS

## *Davorka Sutlovic*[*]

*Assistant Professor, University Hospital Split and School of Medicine, Department of Forensic Medicine, Spinciceva 1; 21000 Split; Croatia*

### ABSTRACT

The identification process of dead bodies or human remains is now days conducted in numerous fields of forensic science, archeology and other judicial cases.

A particular problem is the isolation and DNA typing of human remains found in mass graves, due to the degradation process, as well as post mortal DNA contamination with bacteria, fungi, humic acids (HA), metals etc. In this study we investigated the influence of humic acid on the success of DNA extraction, quantification and typing by Real time - PCR and PCR methods.

It was reported that the humic acid if present in the amplification reaction mix inhibited the DNA amplification, but the addition of 50 mg PVPP to the reaction mixture before extraction, appeared to be optimum in overcoming that inhibition.

It was investigated the dose-response effect of humic acid on the Quantification Real Time PCR (QRT-PCR) inhibition and the efficiency of Taq polymerase increment in preventing inhibition by HA in DNA extracted from ancient bones. The addition 10 - 75 ng of synthetic HA (Fluka) can inhibit QRT- PCR while the addition of 100 ng of synthetic HA completely inhibits QRT- PCR. The addition of 1.25 Unit (U) of Taq polymerase per assay appeared to be the optimum amount in overcoming the HA inhibition. The best results were obtained when crude DNA extracts containing humic substances were quantified by QRT-PCR, with adding of 1.25 Unit (U) of extra Taq polymerase per assay.

It was investigated the possible mechanisms of HA interaction with human DNA, and kinetics of QRT-PCR inhibition were investigated. In QRT-PCR with pure human DNA and no HA added, $V_{MAX}$ was 40. With DNA sample containing 4 µg/ml of HA, $V_{MAX}$ was 30.30 while the addition of extra Taq polymerase to the same sample changed

---

[*] E-mail: dsutlov@kbsplit.hr

$V_{MAX}$ into 38.91, amplifying between 80 and 90% of input DNA. The $K_M/V_{MAX}$ ratio in all the samples remained constant, indicating that the mechanism of HA inhibition of QRT-PCR is uncompetitive by nature. Moreover HA shifts the human DNA melting temperature point ($T_m$) from 75°C to 87°C and inhibits DNase I mediated DNA cleavage, most probably affecting the enzyme's activity.

# DNA IN FORENSIC MEDICINE

## 1.1. Problems in Forensic DNA Analysis

The polymerase chain reaction (PCR) is very powerful and sensitive analytical technique with applications in many diverse fields, including molecular biology, clinical diagnosis, population genetics and forensic analysis. Analysis of deoxyribonucleic acid (DNA) by short tandem repeats (STR) polymorphisms has had a major impact on identity testing. Exhumation and war victims identification have a special connotation. Different identification methods are used depending on the case circumstances and the grade of the post mortal body changes [1, 2]. One of the methods is the identification by DNA typing of different biological samples (genotyping).

The problems that forensic scientists are most often faced with, while working with DNA extracted from bones and teeth samples recovered from mass graves or mass disaster sites, are low DNA quantity, high DNA degradation, DNA contamination and presence of inhibitors [1, 3]. Humic substances are ubiquitous in soil and water and can contaminate any exposed material, which in turn renders false negative results [4]. The total DNA extraction from soil always results in co-extraction of some other soil components, mainly humic acid (HA) and other humic substances, which adversely affect the DNA detecting processes [5-7]. Characteristic features of humic substances are their structural heterogeneity (Figure 1.), their property to bind metal ions and to form complexes, and their property to interact with a variety of organic compounds [8]. Humic acid can inhibit PCR, if template DNA is extracted directly from soil [5].

## 1.2. Humic Acid

A humic acid is the fraction of humic substances that is not soluble in water under acidic conditions (pH less than 2) but is soluble at higher pH values. They can be extracted from soil by various reagents and which is insoluble in dilute acid. Humic acids are the major extractable component of soil humic substances. They are dark brown to black in color.

Electron microscope observations revealed the humic acids of different soils to have polymeric structure, appearing in form of rings, chains, and clusters. The sizes of their macromolecules can range from 60 - 500 A, what is mainly decided of by the occuring humification process, which also exerts an influence on their spatial sructure. Compared to other taxonomic units, the polymers of podsol- earth soils showed to most loose structure. It iss apparent that humic substances consist of a heterogeneous mixture of compounds for which no single structural formula will suffice. Humic acids are thought to be complex aromatic macromolecules with amino acids, amino sugars, peptides, aliphatic compounds involved in linkages between the aromatic groups. The hypothetical structure for humic acid, shown in figure, contains free and bound phenolic OH groups, quinone structures, nitrogen and oxygen as bridge units and COOH groups variously placed on aromatic rings.

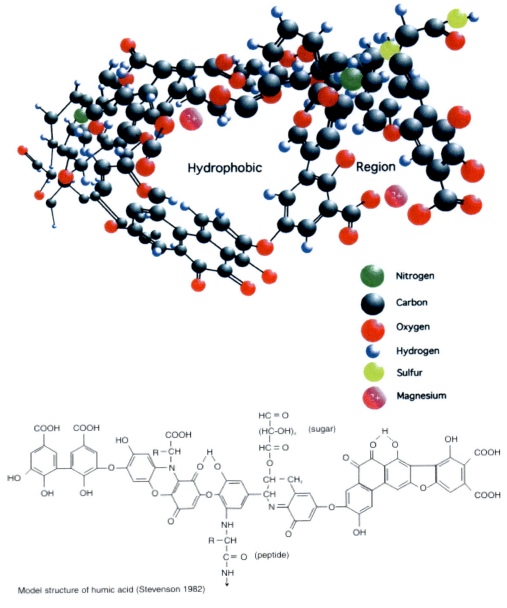

Figure 1. The hypothetical model structure of humic acid (Buffle's model) contains both aromatic and aliphatic structures, both extensively substituted with oxygen - containing functional groups (figure taken from http://www.geochemicaltransactions.com/content/1/1/10/figure).

## 1.3. DNA Extraction Problems

Extraction of DNA from bones may result with co-extraction of HA, which than interferes with DNA detection and measurement [9]. This contamination can inhibit PCR amplification. Many scientists have reported that PCR inhibitors were frequently co-purified with the DNA extracted from a mass grave bone or an ancient bone [10, 11]. Also, scientists have reported about extraction and purification methods of DNA from different samples, but source of samples was not a human. Tebbe and Vahjen, Cullen and Hirsch developed protocol for the extraction and purification of total DNA from soil samples [6]. Tsai and Olson found that the best results were obtained when crude DNA extracts containing HA were purified by using Sephadex G-200 spin columns [7]. Howeler et. al, explained extraction and purification of DNA from compost [12]. Some authors described that the HA could be removed by treatment with polyvinil-polypyrrolidone (PVPP) resin [13].

When the template DNA is extracted directly from soil, HA can inhibit PCR [5]. Also, total DNA extraction from soil always results in co-extraction of other soil components, mainly HA or other humic substances, which negatively interfere with DNA detecting processes [6, 7, 14-16]. Characteristic features of humic substances are their structural heterogeneity, their property to bind metal ions by complex formation and their property to interact with a variety of organic compounds [8]. Humic substances are ubiquitous in soil and water and can contaminate any material exposed to those environments, which cause false negative results [4, 16].

## 1.4. DNA Quantification and Amplification Problems

DNA quantification ensures the optimal use of limited amounts of DNA found in the majority of forensic material evidences, so that DNA is not wasted in expensive repetitive endpoint PCR typing analysis, performed with inappropriate amounts of DNA templates [17]. Furthermore, some DNA quantification designs could also provide additional information about DNA degradation and the presence of possible DNA inhibitors [18, 19].

QRT-PCR can fail because of the presence of inhibitors or the absence of adequate template DNA [20]. It is useful to distinguish two categories of inhibition: (i) inhibitors of Taq DNA polymerase may co-purify with DNA and (ii) the modification of DNA template makes it unrecognizable as substrate for QRT-PCR. Before concluding that amplifiable DNA is not present in a sample, it is necessary to confirm that the inhibitors of Taq polymerase are not present in the preparation.

Quality control PCR can detect inhibitors that could be present in templates. DNA quantification based on the real-time 5' exonuclease detection assay (TaqMan®), using the ABI PRISM® 7000 instrument, has gained a widespread use in many areas for low-copy DNA quantification [19, 21]. Real-time detection is a very fast and accurate technology that does not require post-PCR processing since the detection is done during each PCR cycle. The TaqMan® assay is based on the cleavage of a target-specific probe by the 5'$\to$ 3' exonuclease activity of Taq DNA polymerase, resulting in an increased intensity of reporter emission [22]. The threshold cycle ($C_T$) is inversely proportional to the final target sequence concentration.

Furthermore, a multiplex analysis of multiple targets is possible using dyes with a large difference in emission wavelengths [ FAM, VIC ] [22].

QRT-PCR methods have the ability to quantify trace amounts of human DNA isolated from old bone samples [23, 24]. To enhance the PCR efficiency in samples containing inhibitors, 0.16 mg/mL bovine serum albumin (BSA) and 3.75 U extra AmpliTaq® DNA polymerase were included in the reactions [19]. Altered amplification plots were observed during the analysis of 50 years old saliva stains on stamps and envelopes due to the presence of inhibitors. The addition of BSA and extra Taq amounts has proven efficient in overcoming the effects of inhibitors [17].

This original study examined inhibition mechanisms of HA and its interaction with human DNA. Inhibition is a particularly important problem when extracting DNA from old and ancient material, because severe postmortem DNA changes may prevent amplification, inhibiting both QRT-PCR and PCR due to the absence of adequate template DNA [10]. It is therefore useful to distinguish two mechanisms of inhibition: (i) inhibitors of Taq DNA polymerase co-purify with DNA and (ii) the modification of DNA template makes it unrecognizable as a substrate.

The inhibition mechanism directs the experimental algorithm: if DNA is damaged – the sample is discarded and a new extraction is required; if an inhibitor is present – the sample can be either purified, or, if HA is the inhibitor, additional Taq will overcome the inhibition [9]

QRT-PCR can detect inhibitors possibly present in templates. DNA quantification based on real-time 5' exonuclease detection assay (TaqMan®), using the ABI PRISM® 7000 instrument (Applied Biosystems, Foster City, CA), has gained a widespread use in many areas for lowcopy DNA quantification [17, 19].

Another simple optical method widely employed for determination of DNA stability and interaction with ligands is UV-thermal denaturation [25, 26]. Thermal denaturation of DNA and DNA-ligand complex is usually observed at 260 nm. As a function of the GC/AT ratio, length, and sequence of DNA templates, acquired melting curves assume different shapes. The change of the melting curve shape also indicates intercalation of unspecific DNA ligands [25], the presence of which will subsequently change DNA digestibility by DNase I. [6, 12]. But not all ligands will intercalate. Some will semi-intercalate and some will externally attach to dsDNA.

## 2. EXPERIMENTS

### 2.1. DNA Extraction Test

We developed rapid method for extraction human DNA which contains HA. It could be useful for forensic DNA analysis of biological evidence materials containing very small amounts of DNA which is in used in criminal investigations. We investigated differences between organic extraction using Phenol/Chloroform/Isoamyl Alcohol: 25/24/1 and inorganic extraction using Chelex resin with PVPP resin addition. A model of inhibition samples was used to investigate the effects of HA on extraction of human DNA. The model system employed the HA known impurity that may be present in bone samples. All of our DNA samples for in vitro tests were DNA extracted from 50 mg of ten fresh bones. Bone preparation and DNA extraction were done as described by Burgi SB and Walsh PS [24, 27]. HA was a product of Fluka Inc. (Taufkirchen, Germany). PVPP was a product from MERCK (Darmstadt, Germany).

In this study, we described the effect of PVPP on DNA inorganic extraction by Chelex resin and PCR inhibition. The influence of HA on the PCR efficiency of DNA extracts was monitored with 0.5 and 5 µg of HA / mg dry bones and different amount of PVPP (25 and 50 mg per assay). PCR amplification was performed on the Perkin-Elmer thermal Cycler 9600 using the AmpFlSTR ProfilerPlus™ PCR Amplification from Applied Biosystems, according to the recommended protocols [28]. The amount of DNA was between 1-5 ng. The thermal cycling conditions was: 95°C for 11 min, 28 cycles of [94°C for 1 min, 59°C for 1 min, 72°C for 1 min] and 60°C for 45 min. Typing of PCR products were performed on an ABI Prism 310 Genetic Analyzer (Applied Biosystems) with Data Collection Software. Electropherogram data was analyzed with GeneScan® Software and Genotyper® Software v.2.5.2. for use with Macintosh operating system. Internal standard was Rox-350 [29].

## 2.2. Quantification Test

Human genomic DNA 9947 at 0.1 and 200 ng/µL concentrations (Applied Biosystems, Foster City, CA USA) was used as a DNA standard. HA was a product of Fluka Inc. (Taufkirchen, Germany). Quantifiler™ human DNA quantification kit and AmpliTaq Gold® were from Applied Biosystems. Ten DNA extracts from ancient bone samples (5 DNA samples retrieved from 10-50 years old bones and 5 DNA samples obtained from about 1300 years old bones recovered from church of St Duje, Split, Croatia).

All of our samples were femur bones. After all traces of soft tissue and bone marrow had been removed, using razor blades and sandpaper, the bone was crushed into small fragments and stored in sterile polypropylene tubes at –20°C until analyzed. Further bone preparation and DNA extraction were done as proposed by Alonso A. et al, Burgi SB, Hochmeister MN. et al, Erceg I. et al. and Ausbel FM et al. [1, 24, 30-32].

### 2.2.1. Humic Acid Measurements in DNA Samples from Ancient Bones

HA was evaluated by spectrophotometer measurements [8]. Making serial dilutions of commercial HA mixture created duplicate standard curves. Absorbances at 495 nm were measured in quartz cuvette with HA standards and crude extracts. Measurements were made on spectrophotometer Ultrospec 2000. Pharmacia Biotech (Biochrom) Ltd. Cambridge, England.

### 2.2.2. DNA Quantification

The quantification assay was performed in total volume of 25 µL containing 2 µL of DNA extract, Quantifiler human primer mix and Quantifiler PCR reaction mix according to the manufacture's protocols (16). All reactions without templates served as negative controls.

The influence of HA on the QRT-PCR efficiency of DNA extracts was monitored by duplicate experiments performed both with and without the extra addition of Taq polymerase. First experiment was conducted with increasing amounts of HA (from 1 to 100 ng) and the same amount of DNA (100 pg), while the second experiment was conducted with 100 ng HA and different amounts of DNA (from 12 to 50,000 pg). Two-fold serial dilutions of the genomic DNA were included in each experiment to generate the standard curve for nuclear DNA. All reactions without templates served as negative controls.

The influence of HA on the QRT-PCR efficiency was also monitored by duplicate experiments performed both with and without the extra addition of 1.25; 2.5 and 3.75 U Taq polymerase per assay.

Each probe was labeled with a specific reporter. One TaqMan® MGB probe was labeled with 6-FAM™ dye for detecting the amplified sequence and the other TaqMan® MGB probe was labeled with VIC® dye (a synthetic sequence not found in nature) for detecting the amplified IPC template DNA, both from Applied Biosystems. During the run, charge - - coupled device (CCD) camera detected the fluorescence emission ($R_n$) between 500 nm and 660 nm from each well and collected them by SDS software. The SDS software displayed cycle-by-cycle changes in normalized reporter signal ($R_n$).

The thermal cycling conditions were: 95°C for 10 min, 40 cycles at 95°C for 15 s and 60°C for 1 min. The samples were analyzed according to the manufacture's protocols. Data was collected using the ABI PRISM 7000 Sequence Detection System (Applied Biosystems). Data analysis was performed with ABI PRISM 7000 Sequence Detector Software (SDS) v 1.0 to generate the individual standard curves from each experiment and to calculate the DNA amount from each unknown sample. The $C_T$ value was set to a default threshold of 0.20 for all reactions, and the copy number value for unknown samples was inferred from the regression line of standard curves.

## 2.3. Interaction of Humic Acids with Human DNA - Mechanisms and Kinetics Experiment

Human genomic DNA 9947 at 0.1 and 200 ng/μL concentrations (Applied Biosystems, Foster City, CA) was used as a DNA standard. Quantifiler™ human DNA quantification kit and AmpliTaq Gold® were purchased from Applied Biosystems. HA was a product of Fluka Inc. (Taufkirchen, Germany). DNase I enzyme (114 U/μL) was supplied by Invitrogen (Carlsbad, CA), while Ethidium bromide, $MnCl_2$ and $MgCl_2$ salts were obtained from Sigma-Aldrich (Taufkirchen, Germany).

### 2.3.1. Influence of HA on the QRT-PCR Efficiency

The quantification assay was performed in total volume of 25 μL containing 2 μL of DNA template, Quantifiler human primer mix and Quantifiler PCR reaction mix according to the manufacturer's protocol [22]. Reactions without templates served as negative controls.

Two sets of experiments were conducted as follows: (i) with varied concentrations of DNA (from 12 to 50,000 ng/ml) and fixed concentration of HA (4 μg/ml); (ii) with varied concentrations of both HA (0.04, 0.2 and 2 μg/ml) and DNA (from 31.5 to 500 ng/ml).

In addition, for both sets the influence of HA on the QRT-PCR efficiency was monitored with (concentration of added Taq polymerase was 50 U /ml assay) and without the extra addition of Taq polymerase. The final concentration of Taq polymerase was not known due to the fact that the supplier does not disclose the concentration in the commercial kit. Two-fold serial dilutions of the genomic DNA were included in each experiment to generate the DNA standard curve. For all sets the **K<sub>m</sub>** and V<sub>m</sub> values were determined from Lineweaver-Burk plot.

### 2.3.2. Melting Experiments

Melting experiments were performed on a Varian Cary 3 UV Visible Spectrophotometer (Varian, Palo Alto, CA 94304-1030, USA) equipped with thermostated cuvette holder. The temperature was increased at a rate of 0.5°C/min with a temperature programmer. Thermal denaturation and renaturation of DNA (3.5 µg/ml) without any HA and with HA (in varied concentrations of 7 and 14 µg/ml), were observed at 260 nm.

### 2.3.3. Enzymatic Digestions

DNA was incubated with DNase I (320-400 U/ml) in total volume of 12.5 µl, containing MnCl$_2$ salt, for 10 minutes at 37°C. HA and restriction enzymes were added, respectively. After standard gel electrophoresis (1.5 and 2% agarose gels), inhibition assays were analyzed by UV illumination (312 nm) stained with ethidium bromide.

We monitored the digestion of DNA samples with DNase I in three sets: (i) in respective concentrations of 500, 300 and 100 ng/µl DNA without HA, (ii) in concentration of 500 ng/µl DNA with additions of 4, 8 and 16 µg/ml of HA, respectively, and (iii) in concentration of 500 ng/µl DNA without and with addition of HA, in succeeding concentrations of 0.8, 4 and 8 µg/ml. Fragment lengths were determined by 50 bp marker.

## 3. RESULTS

### 3.1. HA and DNA Extraction

Humic acid had no effect on DNA extraction and PCR amplification by organic extraction. All of ten loci of STR ProfilerPlus kit were successfully amplified. In samples which contain 0.5µg of HA / mg dry bones, and extracted by Chelex (inorganic extraction), several STR loci, longer than 230 base pairs (bp) were not be amplified and typed (Figure 2A).

PVPP had been shown to remove co-extracted humic compounds from soil extracted DNA (8).

PVPP removes HA with phenolic groups from crude DNA extracts via hydrogen bounding and formation of a PVPP-phenolic complexes. By adding, before extraction, of 25 mg PVPP in reaction mixture all of ten loci of STR ProfilerPlus kit were successfully amplified (Figure 2B). Signal of loci longer than 230 bp was not high as signals shorter than 230 bp, but signals in every locus could be determined.

In experiment with higher amount of HA, 5µg of HA / mg dry bones, amplification after extraction was completely inhibited (Figure 3A). A small reduction in PCR inhibition was noted after 25 mg of PVPP was added in reaction mixture before extraction (Figure 3B). The addition of 50 mg PVPP to the reaction mixture appeared to be optimum in overcoming HA inhibition (Figure 3C).

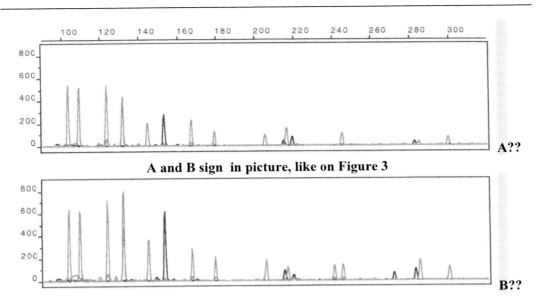

Figure 2. Electropherogram of influence of HA on PCR amplification (DNA from fresh bone extracted by Chelex resin) with the AmpflSTR ProfilerPlus™ Amplification kit. A-with addition of 0.5μg HA/mg dry bone sample, B- with addition of 0.5μg HA/mg dry bone sample and addition of 25 mg PVPP.

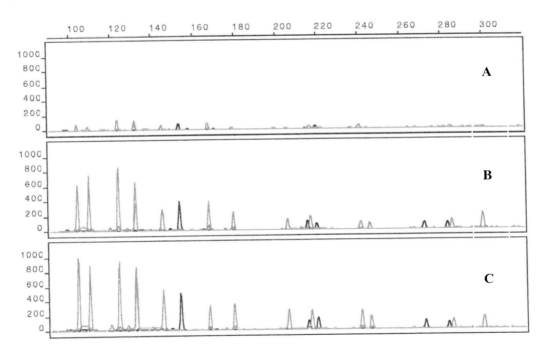

Figure 3. Electropherogram of influence of HA on PCR amplification (DNA from fresh bone extracted by Chelex resin) with the AmpflSTR ProfilerPlus™ Amplification kit. A-with addition of 5μg HA/mg dry bone sample, B- with addition of 5μg HA/mg dry bone sample and addition of 25 mg PVPP, C- with addition of 5μg HA/mg dry bone sample and addition of 50 mg PVPP.

## 3.2. HA and DNA Quantification

### 3.2.1. Results of In vitro Tests on Genomic DNA

The amplification plots of 100 pg human DNA with FAM labeled probe (Figure 4A) and with VIC labeled probe (Figure 4B) show dose-response effect of HA (from 1 to 100 ng) on QRT-PCR inhibition. Amplification plot (Figure 1A) shows lower $\triangle R_n$ values and higher $C_T$ values as the concentration of HA increased. $C_T$ results and corresponding quantification results were relatively stable up to 10 ng HA. Final results were more affected at higher concentrations of HA. As the concentration of HA increased, the PCR efficiency in the Quantifiler kit reactions decreased. The IPC system is more sensitive to PCR inhibition so in samples containing more than 100 ng HA, amplification of IPC detectors failed (Figure 4B).

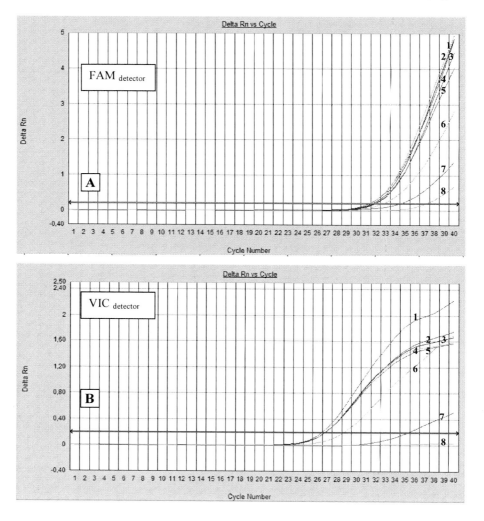

Figure 4. HA inhibition of QRT-PCR. Human DNA (100 pg) was quantified both with and without addition of the HA. Curve 1 - without addition of HA; 2 - addition of 1 ng HA; 3 - addition of 2.5 ng of HA; 4 - addition of 5 ng of HA; 5 - addition of 10 ng of HA; 6 - addition of 50 ng of HA; 7 - addition of 75 ng of HA; 8 - addition of 100 ng of HA; (A) displaying curves and $C_T$ values from experiments by FAM detector. (B) displaying curves and $C_T$ values from experiments by VIC detector.

**Table 1. Quantification of 100 pg human DNA performed in an ABI Prism® 7000 Sequence Detection System (Applied Biosystems) with addition of different amounts of HA**

| Amount (ng) of HA in the sample | Detector* | Threshold cycle value ($C_T$) with extra addition of Taq polymerase ||||
|---|---|---|---|---|---|
| | | none || 1.25 U(units) ||
| | | $C_T$ | Amount (pg) DNA† | $C_T$ | Amount (pg) DNA† |
| 1 | VIC | 26.77 | | 26.54 | |
| | FAM | 31.22 | 96.49 | 31.48 | 80.48 |
| 5 | VIC | 26.89 | | 29.79 | |
| | FAM | 31.81 | 64.40 | 31.54 | 76.97 |
| 10 | VIC | 28.49 | | 27.12 | |
| | FAM | 32.42 | 42.27 | 31.62 | 72.65 |
| 100 | VIC | negative | | 29.79 | |
| | FAM | 37.81 | 0.98 | 31.80 | 64.22 |

\* TaqMan® MGB probe was labeled with 6-FAM™ dye for detecting the amplified sequence and with VIC® dye for detecting the amplified Internal PCR Control DNA.
† Amount (pg) of DNA after adding different amounts of HA in samples containing 100 pg DNA.

The results from this study showed (Table 1) higher $C_T$ values and lower amount of DNA as the concentration of HA increased, while the quantification of samples showed improved amplification efficiency and normal curve shape after adding of extra Taq polymerase. Table 1 (sample 4) shows results of the amplification plot of the human DNA (100 pg), detected with FAM and VIC labeled probes, with the addition of 100 ng of HA and 1.25 U of Taq polymerase. $C_T$ values of the FAM detector decreased from 37.81 to 31.80 and final amount of DNA increased from 0.98 to 64.22 pg after adding extra Taq polymerase. Amplification of Internal PCR Control failed and $C_T$ value of the VIC detector was not detectable with addition of Taq polymerase, the $C_T$ value was 29.79.

In this study we also described the effect of 100 ng of HA on different amounts of DNA on QRT-PCR inhibition (Figure 5 and Table 2). Figure 5A shows amplification plots with normal curve shapes of serial dilutions of human DNA from 50,000 to 12 pg without addition of HA and without addition of extra Taq polymerase. The results of $C_T$ values and DNA amounts are shown in Table 2A. Higher $C_T$ values correspond to lower amounts of DNA. The addition of HA (100 ng) has been used to decrease activity of Taq polymerase and reduce the amount of PCR products. Subsequently the amplification plot had changed (Figure 5B) and the amount of DNA drastically decreased with increased $C_T$ values (Table 2B). In all samples amplification of Internal PCR Control failed and $C_T$ values of the VIC detector were not detectable. Sometimes these can be false negative results.

After the extra addition of 1.25 U of Taq polymerase into the reaction mixture, the curves shape became normal (Figure 5C). $C_T$ values of the VIC detector were detectable and the amount of DNA rapidly increased (Table 2C).

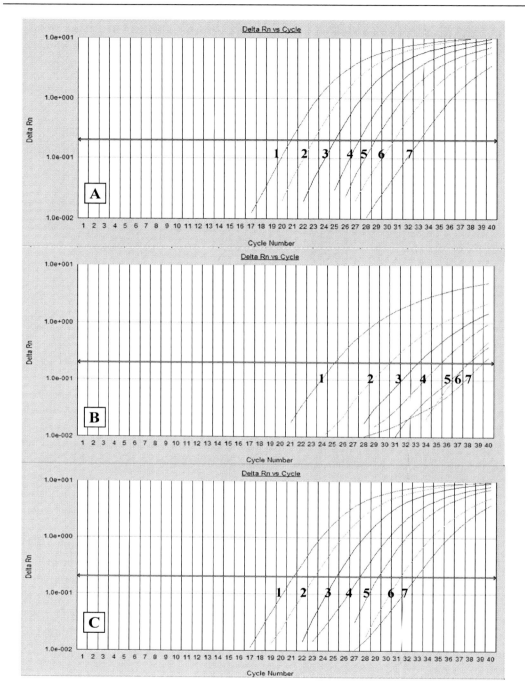

Figure 5. Amplification plot of serial dilutions of human DNA (50,000 to 12 pg shown in table 2) with addition of 100 ng HA and with/without extra addition of Taq polymerase displaying by FAM detector. (A) Amplification plots of human DNA without addition of HA and without extra addition of Taq polymerase. (B) Amplification plots of human DNA with addition of 100 ng HA and without extra addition of Taq polymerase. (C) Amplification plot of human DNA with addition of 100 ng HA and with extra addition of 1.25 U Taq polymerase.

**Table 2. Quantification of serial dilutions of human DNA performed in an ABI Prism® 7000 Sequence Detection System (Applied Biosystems) with addition of 100 ng of HA**

| Sample | Detector* | Threshold cycle value ($C_T$) with addition of HA and extra addition of Taq polymerase ||||||
|---|---|---|---|---|---|---|---|
| | | No HA, no extra Taq || 100 ng HA, no extra Taq || 100 ng HA, 1.25 U Taq ||
| | | $C_T$ | Amount (pg) DNA† | $C_T$ | Amount (pg) DNA‡ | $C_T$ | Amount (pg) DNA‡ |
| 1 | VIC | 38.77 | | negative | | 39.02 | |
|   | FAM | 20.78 | 50,000.00 | 25.14 | 2675.97 | 21.13 | 43,954.30 |
| 2 | VIC | 29.82 | | negative | | 35.72 | |
|   | FAM | 22.97 | 12,500.00 | 30.41 | 67.33 | 23.13 | 10,858.75 |
| 3 | VIC | 26.70 | | negative | | 29.71 | |
|   | FAM | 24.98 | 3,125.00 | 33.16 | 9.90 | 25.18 | 2,597.53 |
| 4 | VIC | 26.31 | | negative | | 27.96 | |
|   | FAM | 27.24 | 781.00 | 38.05 | 0.33 | 27.38 | 558.10 |
| 5 | VIC | 26.41 | | negative | | 27.53 | |
|   | FAM | 28.78 | 195.00 | 35.34 | 2.16 | 29.17 | 160.60 |
| 6 | VIC | 26.53 | | negative | | 28.09 | |
|   | FAM | 30.52 | 49.00 | 37.93 | 0.35 | 31.29 | 36.55 |
| 7 | VIC | 26.47 | | negative | | 27.27 | |
|   | FAM | 33.07 | 12.00 | 39.36 | 0.13 | 32.18 | 12.64 |

\* TaqMan® MGB probe was labeled with 6-FAM™ dye for detecting the amplified sequence and with VIC® dye for detecting the amplified Internal PCR Control DNA.

† Different amounts of input DNA (12 to 50 000 pg).

‡ Measured amounts of DNA after addition of 100 ng of HA in samples with different input DNA concentrations.

### 3.2.2. DNA Quantification from Ancient Bones

The results obtained by using the modified method (addition of extra Taq polymerase) are shown in Table 3 in comparison with different HA content (from 0 to 53.55 ng/µL). At HA concentrations below 5 ng/µL in samples with extra Taq polymerase added, there was some or no effect of HA on DNA quantification. The higher concentrations of HA (samples 4 and 10) produced false negative results, which were reversed ba adding extra Taq polymerase. In 5 DNA extracts (samples 1,5,6,7 and 9) there was no DNA and no influence of HA as inhibitor. In 3 DNA extracts (sample 2, 3 and 8) the quantification was improved after extra Taq polymerase had been added.

**Table 3. Quantification of human DNA extracted from 10 ancient bones performed in an ABI Prism® 7000 Sequence Detection System (Applied Biosystems)**

| Sample | Amount (ng/μL) of HA* | Detector† | Threshold cycle value ($C_T$) with extra addition of Taq polymerase ||||
|---|---|---|---|---|---|---|
| | | | none || 1.25 U ||
| | | | $C_T$ | Amount (pg) DNA | $C_T$ | Amount (pg) DNA |
| 1 | 0.05 | VIC | 29.43 | | 27.80 | |
| | | FAM | negative | - | negative | - |
| 2 | 5.30 | VIC | 30.42 | | 27.89 | |
| | | FAM | 34.14 | 32.11 | 33.66 | 47.29 |
| 3 | 1.33 | VIC | 33.68 | | 28.17 | |
| | | FAM | 34.42 | 25.63 | 33.64 | 47.96 |
| 4 | 18.65 | VIC | negative | | 28.85 | |
| | | FAM | 36.78 | 3.90 | 32.13 | 159.89 |
| 5 | 0.07 | VIC | negative | | 37.26 | |
| | | FAM | negative | - | negative | - |
| 6 | 0 | VIC | negative | | negative | |
| | | FAM | negative | - | negative | - |
| 7 | 0.02 | VIC | 29.83 | | 27.73 | |
| | | FAM | negative | - | negative | - |
| 8 | 0.03 | VIC | negative | | negative | |
| | | FAM | negative | - | 29.45 | 2.90 |
| 9 | 0 | VIC | negative | | negative | |
| | | FAM | negative | - | negative | - |
| 10 | 53.55 | VIC | negative | | 30.55 | |
| | | FAM | negative | - | 27.42 | 6,883.77 |

\* Measured amounts of HA in DNA samples extracted from ancient bones.
† TaqMan® MGB probe was labeled with 6-FAM™ dye for detecting the amplified sequence and with VIC® dye for detecting the amplified Internal PCR Control DNA.
‡ Measured amounts of DNA.

## 3.3. Interaction of Humic Acids with Human DNA - Mechanisms and Kinetics

### 3.3.1. Influence of HA on the QRT-PCR Efficiency

Previously we investigated the effect of 4 μg/ml of HA on QRT-PCR inhibition with varied amounts of DNA. Those results confirmed the inhibitory properties of HA. Amplification plots for serial dilutions of human DNA from 12 to 50,000 ng/ml, without the addition of HA, resulted in a normal curve shape. The addition of HA (4 μg/ml) was supposed to decrease the activity of Taq polymerase and therefore reduce the amount of PCR products.

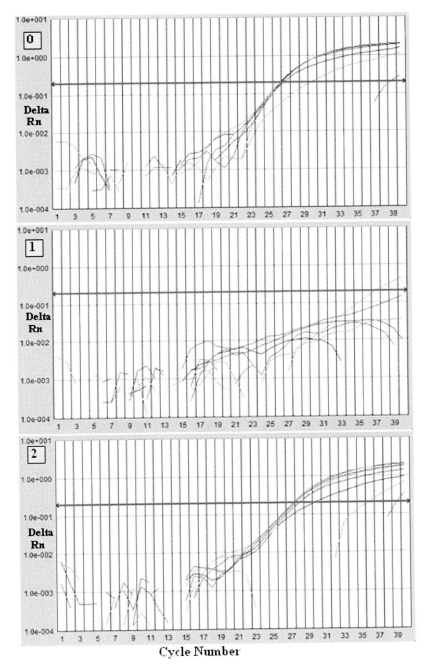

Figure 6.1. HA inhibition of QRT-PCR displaying curves and $C_T$ values from experiments by VIC detector. Serial dilutions of human DNA (12 to 50,000 ng/ml): 0– no HA added; 1- with 4 μg/ml of HA added; 2- with both, 4 μg/ml of HA and extra 50 U/ml of Taq polymerase added.

As projected, the shape of amplification plot did change and the quantity of amplified DNA product drastically decreased, also increasing $C_T$ values. In all samples amplification of Internal PCR Control failed and $C_T$ values of the VIC detector were not detectable. Sometimes, nonetheless, these can be false negative results as described in the assay manual [16]. The extra addition of Taq polymerase (concentration of added Taq polymerase was 50 U /ml assay) to the reaction mixture reversed the curve shapes back to normal. $C_T$ values of the VIC detector were detectable and the amount of DNA rapidly increased. The results are shown using actual Quantifiler data in Figure 6-1 and with Lineweaver-Burk plot in Figure 6-2.

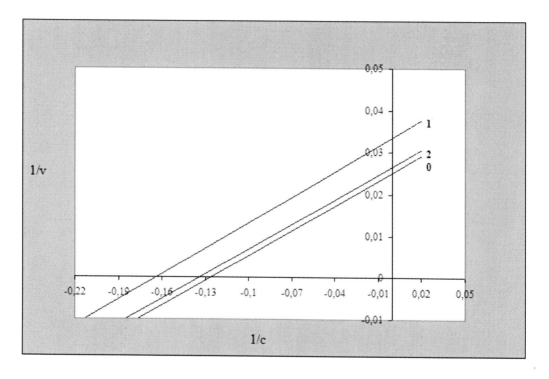

Figure 6.2. Lineweaver-Burk plot of serial dilutions of human DNA (12 to 50,000 ng/ml): 0– no HA added; 1- with 4 µg/ml of HA added; 2- with both, 4 µg/ml of HA and extra 50 U/ml of Taq polymerase added.

In QRT-PCR reaction with pure human DNA and no HA added, $V_{MAX}$ was 40. In DNA sample with 4 µg/ml of HA added, $V_{MAX}$ was 30.30 while the addition of extra Taq polymerase to the same sample changed $V_{MAX}$ to 38.91. The $K_M/V_{MAX}$ ratio was retained at about 0.20 in all the samples.

The interaction of varied concentrations of both HA and human DNA is shown in Figure 7, with the Lineweaver-Burk plot. Using the plot, its slope and x, y-interception points, both inhibition constant, $K_M$, and maximum speed of reaction, $V_{max}$, were determined.

As the HA concentrations increased, $V_{MAX}$ and $K_M$ values equally decreased. DNA sample with 0.04 µg/ml of HA had a $V_{MAX}$ of 30.76; DNA sample with 0.2 µg/ml of HA had a $V_{MAX}$ of 30.49, while the same sample containing 2 µg/ml of HA had a $V_{MAX}$ of 29.85. The $K_M/V_{MAX}$ ratios were approximately 0.23 in all the samples.

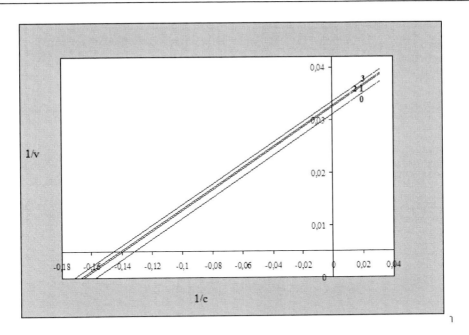

Figure 7. Lineweaver-Burk plot of serial dilutions of human DNA (31.5 to 500 ng/ml): 0- no HA added; 1- 0.04 µg/ml of HA added; 2- 0.2 µg/ml of HA added; 3- 2 µg/ml of HA added.

### 3.3.2. Melting Experiments

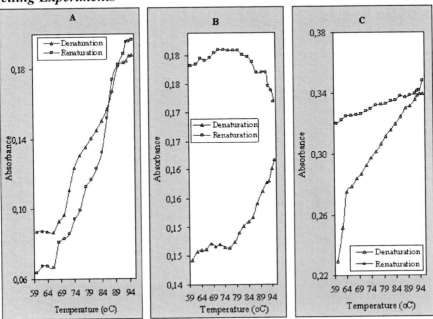

Figure 8. Thermal denaturation (1), and renaturation (2) of human DNA; A- human DNA (3.5 µg/ml) with no HA added; B- human DNA (3.5 µg/ml) with 7 µg/ml of HA added; C- human DNA (3.5 µg/ml) with 14 µg/ml of HA added.

The transition of double stranded DNA into single stranded DNA occurs with the temperature change. Adding the HA into the DNA sample changed the melting point, $T_m$, (Figure 8). Figure 8A shows melting curves of human DNA samples without HA, depicting almost identical curve shapes at heating (denaturation) and cooling (renaturation) steps. When HA was present in the sample, melting curves were neither sigmoid nor reversible (Figure 8B and 8C). After measurements were performed, melting point, $T_m$, was determined by function derivation.

### 3.3.3. Enzymatic Digestions

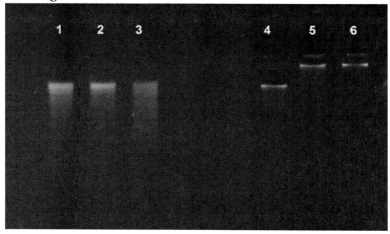

Figure 9. Gel electrophoresis (2 % agarose gel) of human DNA after DNase I digestion and ethidium bromide staining. Lanes 1, 2 and 3- pure DNA digestion in respective concentrations of 500, 300 and 100 ng/ml; lanes 4, 5 and 6- digestion of 500 ng/ml DNA with 4, 8 and 16 μg/ml of HA added respectively.

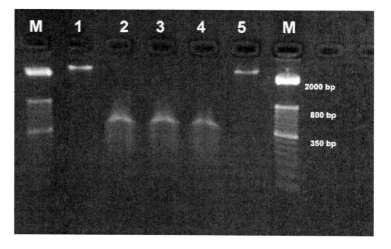

Figure 10. Gel electrophoresis (1.5 % agarose gel) of human DNA (500 ng/ml) after DNase I digestion and ethidium bromide staining. Lane 1- undigested DNA; lane 2- digested DNA without HA; lane 3- digested DNA with 0.8 μg/ml of HA added; lane 4- digested DNA with 4 μg/ml of HA added; lane 5- digested DNA with 8 μg/ml of HA added; M lanes- 50 bp size markers.

Humic acid had an inhibitory effect on DNA digestion by DNase I in samples in which the concentration of HA either equaled or exceeded 8 µg/ml (Figure 9). Observation was similar in samples with varying DNA concentrations. Furthermore, the inhibitory action of HA, in consecutive concentrations of 0.8, 4 and 8 µg/ml, on DNase I activity was determined in samples containing 500 ng/ml human DNA (Figure 10). Fragment lengths of approximately 400 bp were determined by 50 bp size marker.

## 4. Discussion

### 4.1. DNA Extraction

The simple addition of >10 mg PVPP in reaction mixture before inorganic extraction effectively overcomes inhibition of amplification by HA. It is necessary in samples which containing very small amounts of DNA and is becoming widely used in criminal investigations. However, co-extracted HA strongly impair DNA amplification. Using this method the DNA was successfully amplified in all loci. Routine forensic DNA analysis, based on STR markers, could be performed successfully on most evidence materials found at a crime scene[33].

### 4.2. Taq Polymerase Reverses Inhibition of QRT-PCR by Humic Acid

Modified procedure (with addition of extra Taq polymerase) should allow more effective QRT-PCR analysis in HA-containing samples. We demonstrated that the addition of 10 - 75 ng of synthetic HA (Fluka) may inhibit QRT- PCR while the addition of 100 ng of synthetic HA completely inhibits QRT- PCR. The addition of 1.25 Unit (U) of Taq polymerase per assay appeared to be the optimum amount in overcoming the HA inhibition. Weak amplification (high $C_T$ and low $\triangle R_n$ value) of the human DNA and no amplification of the IPC may indicate a partial PCR inhibition in the sample.

In this study, we described the dose-response effect of HA on QRT-PCR inhibition and the effect of adding extra Taq polymerase in overcoming the HA inhibition.

The standard curves display plotted $C_T$ values from experiments versus the log of the initial genomic DNA concentrations (pg). Decreasing amounts of input DNA, consistently revealed higher $C_T$ numbers. In most experiments target was detected down to an amount of DNA in the dilutions series for the standard curve, which indicated that the system is highly sensitive. HA, as a PCR inhibitor, can interfere with the reaction and cause varying levels of reduced PCR efficiency (interfering with polymerase activity), including complete inhibition of QRT-PCR [22]. Signal is detected and decreases in direct proportion to the decrease of PCR product. We have described that HA really inhibits QRT-PCR if present in more than 100 ng per reaction mix. In samples containing less HA, amplification of IPC detectors was inhibited. In our study, the degree of inhibition by adding the HA was in agreement with the successful/unsuccessful amplification of the human DNA. The extra addition of 1.25 U of Taq polymerase to the reaction mixture has proven to be efficient in overcoming the inhibitor.

In all samples the overcoming effect was in a similar range: with extra addition of Taq polymerase about 80 % of input DNA was amplified.

In the second part of this study we tested QRT-PCR method with addition of extra Taq polymerase on DNA samples extracted from ancient bones. The amplification of samples containing inhibitors showed increased amplification efficiency after extra addition of Taq polymerase. Samples containing HA usually were not amplified when analyzed without extra Taq polymerase depending upon the concentration of HA itself. We demonstrated that high amounts of HA could interfere with Taq polymerase, rendering false negative results on the human DNA quantification. A relatively high incidence of PCR inhibitors could be predicted when analyzing bone and ancient DNA samples and other forensic samples. Partial inhibition of Taq polymerase may produce a situation similar to that of low concentration of DNA in a sample. Therefore the use of extra Taq polymerase is considered to be an efficient procedure to overcome false negative results, but our results show that the extra addition of Taq polymerase in DNA extracts from ancient bones effectively overcomes inhibition of QRT-PCR only in some cases. This indicates that the HA is not the only inhibitor in DNA samples from ancient bones. Because of that we evaluated the HA concentration in DNA from ancient bones by spectrophotometer and our results correlated with the finally amplified DNA amount (Table 3). In sample No. 10, which contained the highest concentration of HA, extra addition of Taq polymerase produced the best results when quantified with QRT-PCR.

Alonso et al. included BSA to prevent the action of some inhibitory compounds present in some bone DNA samples [17]. Andreasson, Giambernardi et al. described that the addition BSA has proven efficient in overcoming effects of the inhibitors [19, 21, 34]. In comparison with our study the addition of BSA was not as good as the addition of Taq polymerase (data not shown)[9].

## 4.3. Interaction of Humic Acids with Human DNA - Mechanisms and Kinetics

Forensic analysis of biological evidence containing minute amounts of DNA is widely used in criminal investigations. Therefore, a reliable and highly sensitive DNA quantification system is necessary to ensure the optimum use of limited evidence material. Before concluding that amplifiable DNA is not present in a sample, it is necessary to exclude the presence of any, among many, of Taq polymerase inhibitors. Humic acid, as a PCR inhibitor, can interfere with the reaction (by inhibiting polymerase activity) and cause varying levels of reduced PCR efficiency, including complete inhibition of QRT-PCR [16,17]. After demonstrating that 4 µg/ml of HA completely inhibits QRT-PCR, the addition of 50 U/ml of Taq polymerase per assay appeared to be the optimum amount in overcoming the observed inhibition.

In the light of presented facts we were determined to explain the binding mode and inhibition mechanism of HA, its interactions with human DNA molecules, Taq polymerase and DNase I enzymes. We have also tried to clarify how adding extra Taq polymerase overcomes the HA inhibition.

Glutamine and arginine [35, 36] are side chains in the active site of Taq polymerase. Arginine is a hydrogen ion donor and forms hydrogen bounds through to nitrogen ion, while glutamine can be both a donor and an acceptor of hydrogen ions. Macromolecular structure of HA is based on aromatic, quinonic and heterocyclic rings, which are randomly condensed or linked by ether or aliphatic bridges [8]. Side chains consisting of polysaccharides, peptides and aliphates, as well as chemically active functional groups (carboxylic and carbonyl groups, phenolic and alcoholic hydroxyls), determine the properties of HA. When HA changes from unreactive to reactive form it becomes negatively charged. Broken bonds create places on the HA molecule where positive ions can be absorbed, so it relatively easily interacts with positively charged ions exposed on Taq polymerase active site. Binding to the active sites of Taq polymerase HA probably changes the polarity of the environment and therefore inhibits QRT-PCR.

The described interaction between HA and Taq polymerase is overcomed by providing extra Taq polymerase in the reaction mix. In all our samples the overcoming effect was in a similar range: with extra addition of Taq polymerase, between 80 and 90% of input DNA would amplify.

Substrate binding depends on the extent of the conformational change of the enzyme. Conformation changes depend on the concentration of HA, so if the HA concentration is small, the conformational change of Taq polymerase will probably be small, and HA will not fully inhibit the substrate-binding reaction, leaving some fractions of Taq polymerase in the bound, active state. On the other hand, we speculate, if the concentration of HA increases, conformational changes of Taq polymerase become extensive and reduce the affinity of Taq polymerase for substrate, therefore the inhibition increases as well. Non specific binding of inhibitors might also cause a conformational change of Taq polymerase. This conformational change might decrease not only the enzyme activity, but its substrate-binding affinity as well. In literature this feature is known as mixed inhibition or "nonclassical" competitive inhibition [37].

On the contrary, our study strongly suggests that the inhibition mechanism of HA can be classified as uncompetitive inhibition, where uncompetitive inhibitor binds to enzyme-substrate complex making it un-reactive (Figures 6-1, 6-2 and 7). The result is a decrease in $V_{MAX}$ and an equivalent decrease in $K_M$, without changes in the $K_M/V_{MAX}$ ratio value.

The second inhibition theory could be that HA binds, in two possible ways, to DNA making it unrecognizable as a substrate. We propose the following binding modes: (i) intercalation into DNA strand and (ii) semi-intercalation where HA binds either to the DNA itself or the enzyme (i.e. DNase I).

To test which of these two models is in force, we determined the influence of HA on temperature denaturation and DNase I digestion. The melting curves of double-stranded DNA without HA showed similar denaturation and renaturation shapes (Figure 8A). UV measurements indicate that intercalation or semi-intercalation of HA (7 and 14 µg/ml) into double-stranded DNA significantly influences stability of DNA molecules, which in turn changes shapes of denaturation and renaturation curves (Figure 8B and 8C). Regardless of the input concentration, HA shifts the DNA melting temperature point, $T_m$, from 75°C to 87°C.

In the presence of two different salts, $MgCl_2$ and $MnCl_2$, DNase I cleaves exclusively either single-stranded DNA or double-stranded DNA. Cleavage of single-stranded DNA occurs in $MgCl_2$, and of double-stranded DNA in $MnCl_2$. Since we assumed that HA inhibits DNase I activity, we tested the enzyme's activity in both salts using just double-stranded DNA as substrate, with the addition of HA. Our results showed that only in the presence of

MnCl2, DNase I enzyme cleaved the DNA suggesting that the HA did not intercalate into double stranded DNA, thus confirming the semi-intercalation hypothesis (data not shown).

DNase I enzyme activity was not influenced in the presence of 0.8 or 4 μg/ml HA, while 8 μg/ml of HA completely inhibited the enzyme.

Taq polymerase and DNase I enzymes are inhibited by HA in concentrations of 4 and 8 μg/ml, respectively. There was a good agreement between our results and those of other authors. Using commercial HA, Tebbe and Vahjen [6], found that the minimum inhibitory concentrations (MIC) of 1.08 and 0.54 μg/ml HA inhibited the restriction enzymes. On the other hand, Howeler et al. [12] found that HA concentration of 6.75 μg/ml from compost samples, did not lead to inhibition of restriction enzyme in the reaction vessel. The different results these two studies produced were explained by the different HA sources they used, because it is shown that in a kilo of humic acid there are hardly two identical HA molecules [8, 37]. Neither Tebbe nor Howeler tackled the mechanisms of interaction of HA with human DNA; instead they used DNA from compost, soils or sediments.

## 5. Conclusion

Forensic DNA analysis of biological evidence materials containing very small amounts of DNA is becoming widely used in criminal investigations. Therefore, a reliable and highly sensitive DNA quantification system is necessary to ensure the optimum use of limited material available. Before concluding that amplifiable DNA is not present in a sample, it is necessary to confirm with QRT-PCR that inhibitors of Taq DNA polymerase are not present in the sample. The QRT-PCR quantification system has been proven to be sensitive, reliable, and very useful in routine forensic DNA analysis. Modified procedure (with addition of extra Taq polymerase) should allow more effective QRT-PCR analysis in HA-containing samples. Moreover, the assay will ensure that a minimum amount of DNA is used for a successful amplification and that DNA is retained for repeated analysis.

According to the presented data and previously proposed theories about HA and enzymes that bind to DNA, it was suggested that human DNA is made unrecognizable as a substrate and therefore un-amplifiable. In quantification experiments (QRT-PCR), extra addition of Taq polymerase overcomes HA inhibition, but not completely. Our study suggests that the mechanism of inhibition by HA is probably the result of both substrate change and Taq polymerase inhibition. However, we believe that inhibition mechanisms are even more complex and ample than these two proposed theories, which opens doors to future studies of the subject[38].

## Competing Interests

The authors declare that they have no competing interests. The authors alone are responsible for the content and writing of the paper.

## REFERENCES

[1] Alonso, A, Andelinovic, S, Martin, P, Sutlovic, D, Erceg, I, Huffine, E, et al, DNA typing from skeletal remains: evaluation of multiplex and megaplex STR systems on DNA isolated from bone and teeth samples. *Croat Med J*, 2001. 42(3): p. 260-6.

[2] Evison, M P, Smillie, D M, and Chamberlain, A T, Extraction of single-copy nuclear DNA from forensic specimens with a variety of postmortem histories. *J Forensic Sci*, 1997. 42(6): p. 1032-8.

[3] Primorac, D, Andelinovic, S, Definis-Gojanovic, M, Drmic, I, Rezic, B, Baden, M M, et al, Identification of war victims from mass graves in Croatia, Bosnia, and Herzegovina by use of standard forensic methods and DNA typing. *J Forensic Sci*, 1996. 41(5): p. 891-4.

[4] Kreader, C A, Relief of amplification inhibition in PCR with bovine serum albumin or T4 gene 32 protein. *Appl Environ Microbiol*, 1996. 62(3): p. 1102-6.

[5] Zhou, J, Bruns, M A, and Tiedje, J M, DNA recovery from soils of diverse composition. *Appl Environ Microbiol*, 1996. 62(2): p. 316-22.

[6] Tebbe, C C and Vahjen, W, Interference of humic acids and DNA extracted directly from soil in detection and transformation of recombinant DNA from bacteria and a yeast. *Appl Environ Microbiol*, 1993. 59(8): p. 2657-65.

[7] Tsai, Y L and Olson, B H, Rapid method for separation of bacterial DNA from humic substances in sediments for polymerase chain reaction. *Appl Environ Microbiol*, 1992. 58(7): p. 2292-5.

[8] Zipper, H, Buta, C, Lammle, K, Brunner, H, Bernhagen, J, and Vitzthum, F, Mechanisms underlying the impact of humic acids on DNA quantification by SYBR Green I and consequences for the analysis of soils and aquatic sediments. *Nucleic Acids Res*, 2003. 31(7): p. e39.

[9] Sutlovic, D, Definis Gojanovic, M, Andelinovic, S, Gugic, D, and Primorac, D, Taq polymerase reverses inhibition of quantitative real time polymerase chain reaction by humic acid. *Croat Med J*, 2005. 46(4): p. 556-62.

[10] Goodyear, P D, MacLaughlin-Black, S, and Mason, I J, A reliable method for the removal of co-purifying PCR inhibitors from ancient DNA. *Biotechniques*, 1994. 16(2): p. 232-5.

[11] Akane, A, Matsubara, K, Nakamura, H, Takahashi, S, and Kimura, K, Identification of the heme compound copurified with deoxyribonucleic acid (DNA) from bloodstains, a major inhibitor of polymerase chain reaction (PCR) amplification. *J Forensic Sci*, 1994. 39(2): p. 362-72.

[12] Howeler, M, Ghiorse, W C, and Walker, L P, A quantitative analysis of DNA extraction and purification from compost. J Microbiol Methods, 2003. 54(1): p. 37-45.

[13] Holben, W E, Jansson, J K, Chelm, B K, and Tiedje, J M, DNA Probe Method for the Detection of Specific Microorganisms in the Soil Bacterial Community. *Appl Environ Microbiol*, 1988. 54(3): p. 703-711.

[14] Cullen, D and Hirsch, P, Simple and rapid method for direct extraction of microbial DNA from soil for PCR. *Soil Biol Biochem*, 1998. 30: p. 983-93.

[15] Jacobsen, C S, Microscale detection of specific bacterial DNA in soil with a magnetic capture-hybridization and PCR amplification assay. *Appl Environ Microbiol*, 1995. 61(9): p. 3347-52.

[16] Yeates, C, Gillings, M R, Davison, A D, Altavilla, N, and Veal, D A, PCR amplification of crude microbial DNA extracted from soil. *Lett Appl Microbiol*, 1997. 25(4): p. 303-7.

[17] Alonso, A, Martin, P, Albarran, C, Garcia, P, Primorac, D, Garcia, O, et al, Specific quantification of human genomes from low copy number DNA samples in forensic and ancient DNA studies. *Croat Med J*, 2003. 44(3): p. 273-80.

[18] Alonso, A, Martin, P, Albarran, C, Garcia, P, Garcia, O, de Simon, L F, et al, Real-time PCR designs to estimate nuclear and mitochondrial DNA copy number in forensic and ancient DNA studies. *Forensic Sci Int*, 2004. 139(2-3): p. 141-9.

[19] Andreasson, H, Gyllensten, U, and Allen, M, Real-time DNA quantification of nuclear and mitochondrial DNA in forensic analysis. *Biotechniques*, 2002. 33(2): p. 402-4, 407-11.

[20] Reiss, R A and Rutz, B, Quality control PCR: a method for detecting inhibitors of Taq DNA polymerase. *Biotechniques*, 1999. 27(5): p. 920-2, 924-6.

[21] Andreasson, H and Allen, M, Rapid quantification and sex determination of forensic evidence materials. *J Forensic Sci*, 2003. 48(6): p. 1280-7.

[22] Quantifiler Human DNA Quantification kit, *User's Manual.* 2003.

[23] Hagelberg, E and Clegg, J B, Isolation and characterization of DNA from archaeological bone. *Proc Biol Sci*, 1991. 244(1309): p. 45-50.

[24] Burgi, S, Laboratory manual for Clinical and Forensic Genetics, Clinical Hospital Split. *Laboratory manual* (1997) Sep 23-Oct 3 Split, 1997.

[25] Santella, R M and Li, H J, Studies on interaction between poly(L-lysine58, L-phenylalanine42) and deoxyribonucleic acids. *Biochemistry*, 1975. 14(16): p. 3604-11.

[26] Mukherjee, U and Chatterjee, S N, In-vitro interaction between nitrofurantoin and Vibrio cholerae DNA. *Chem Biol Interact*, 1992. 82(1): p. 111-21.

[27] Walsh, P S, Metzger, D A, and Higuchi, R, Chelex 100 as a medium for simple extraction of DNA for PCR-based typing from forensic material. Biotechniques, 1991. 10(4): p. 506-13.

[28] AmpFlSTR Profiler PCR Amplification Kit: *User's Manual.* 1989.

[29] Butler, J M, McCord, B R, Jung, J M, Wilson, M R, Budowle, B, and Allen, R O, Quantitation of polymerase chain reaction products by capillary electrophoresis using laser fluorescence. *J Chromatogr B Biomed Appl*, 1994. 658(2): p. 271-80.

[30] Hochmeister, M N, Budowle, B, Borer, U V, Eggmann, U, Comey, C T, and Dirnhofer, R, Typing of deoxyribonucleic acid (DNA) extracted from compact bone from human remains. *J Forensic Sci*, 1991. 36(6): p. 1649-61.

[31] Erceg, I, Andjelinovic, S, Sutlovic, D, Rezic, B, Ivkosic, A, and Primorac, D, A one step solution for identification of the skeletal remains. *Second European-American intensive course in clinical and forensic genetics*. Dubrovnik, Croatia, September 3-14. 2001: p. 36.

[32] Ausbel, F, Brent, R, Kingston, R, Moore, D, Seidman, J, and Smith, J, *Current protocols in molecular biology.* 1993.

[33] Sutlovic, D, Gojanovic, M D, and Andelinovic, S, Rapid extraction of human DNA containing humic acid. *Croatica Chemica Acta*, 2007. 80(1): p. 117-120.

[34] Giambernardi, T A, Rodeck, U, and Klebe, R J, Bovine serum albumin reverses inhibition of RT-PCR by melanin. *Biotechniques,* 1998. 25(4): p. 564-6.
[35] Eom, S H, Wang, J, and Steitz, T A, Structure of Taq polymerase with DNA at the polymerase active site. *Nature,* 1996. 382(6588): p. 278-81.
[36] Murali, R, Sharkey, D J, Daiss, J L, and Murthy, H M, Crystal structure of Taq DNA polymerase in complex with an inhibitory Fab: the Fab is directed against an intermediate in the helix-coil dynamics of the enzyme. *Proc Natl Acad Sci U S A,* 1998. 95(21): p. 12562-7.
[37] Stryer, L, *Biochemistry,* 5th Edition. 2002.
[38] Sutlovic, D, Gamulin, S, Definis-Gojanovic, M, Gugic, D, and Andjelinovic, S, Interaction of humic acids with human DNA: proposed mechanisms and kinetics. *Electrophoresis,* 2008. 29(7): p. 1467-72.

In: Forensic Genetics Research Progress
Editor: F. Gonzalez-Andrade

ISBN: 978-1-60876-198-2
© 2010 Nova Science Publishers, Inc.

Chapter 6

# ADVANCES IN DNA TYPING IN SEXUAL ASSAULT CASEWORK

## *María de Fátima Terra Pinheiro*

Laboratório de Biologia e Genética Forense, Instituto de Medicina Legal, Rua Jardim Carrilho Videira, 4050 – Porto, Portugal

## ABSTRACT

Sexual assault is usually a hidden crime where the only witnesses are the victim and the assailant. With this limited initial information, the physical and biological evidence collected from the victim, from the crime scene, and from the suspect will play a prior role in the objective and scientific reconstruction of the events. The obvious first step in finding semen evidence is interviewing the victim. During the investigation of sexual offences, intimate body swabs, clothing and bedding items are routinely submitted for examination. Biological material can accumulate under the fingernail hyponychium of both the victim and/or the suspect and has the potential to provide evidence and intelligence information. In addition to the hairs and debris that may be transferred in other types of violent crime, the rapist often leaves behind a personal biological signature that may include blood, saliva, and most importantly, semen. This semen evidence is frequently a cornerstone in the investigation and prosecution of the case. Bite marks perpetrated in the victim body is another type of sample that can be studied. The presence of a mixture (female/male) can be the unique probative evidence, being a very important statement in a court. The analysis of clothing damage can also be used to corroborate different versions of events. The two commonly used presumptive tests for semen are the Florence and the Brentamine tests. Moreover, prostate specific antigen can be used for forensic identification of semen stains. Confirmatory testing for semen involves the microscopy detection of spermatozoa and its DNA analysis. Identification of one or more intact spermatozoa is conclusive proof of the presence of semen and hence affirms sexual contact. However, the DNA profile identification of the perpetrator must be established. Traditionally, sperm cells are isolated from vaginal cell mixtures by preferential extraction methods. More recently the laser microdissection has proved to be a very powerful tool to isolate specific target cells from a more complex tissue. Autosomal STRs have been used for a long time for human identification and still are a valuable tool in forensic casework. Nevertheless, these markers have some limitations in the analysis of samples concerned to sexual assaults. Since a vast majority of crimes where DNA evidence is helpful, particularly sexual assault, involve males as the perpetrator, DNA tests designed to only examine the male portion can be valuable. A majority of the Y chromosome is transferred directly from father to son without recombination. Therefore, a match between a suspect and evidence only means that the individual in question could have contributed the evidence. A survey was done of alleged victims of sexual assault cases reported to the National Institute of Legal Medicine – North Delegation (Oporto-Portugal) in 2004-2008. Some parameters of interest were analysed, such as the cases that provided: a DNA profile different from the victim (autosomal STR, Y-STR or both); those with more than one perpetrator identified in a mixture; also those where a male profile was identified similar to the suspect one.

## INTRODUCTION

Sexual assault is usually a hidden crime where the only witnesses are the victim and the assailant. With this limited initial information, the physical and biological evidence collected from the victim, from the crime scene, and from the suspect will play a prior role in the objective and scientific reconstruction of the events [Green]. A proper forensic examination may be very detailed and take a long time, and in an emergency situation such as a genital trauma with severe bleeding, the patient's clinical conditions may take precedence over the collection of evidence. However, if there is going to be a prosecution, the case may fail if samples are not processed correctly [Ward et al.].

When examining exhibits from a sexual assault case, one objective of the forensic scientist is to obtain evidence that will support or refute an allegation of non-consensual sexual intercourse. Evidence may be recovered as trace evidence or body fluid stains from the victim, the suspect or the crime scene [French]. The obvious first step in finding semen evidence is interviewing the victim. Initial evidence collection at the crime scene should be guided by the victim's description of the event [Green]. Any material in the victim's hair (pubic, head or body) will be clipped out and retained. The examiner must collect samples from any body cavity or opening where sexual contact was attempted or completed. Semen has also been recovered in cases where the victim believes the assailant wore a condom, so samples should be obtained despite the history of condom use [Green].

There are a number of forensic cases in which the identification of the epithelial cell type, from which DNA originated, would provide important probative evidence. French *et al.* studied three epithelial cell types, and first of all, they state that skin cells differ morphologically from buccal and vaginal cells in that they lack nuclei and are keratinised. Moreover, they have shown that methanol-fixed cell smears stained with the Dane's method reveal consistent differential staining patterns in skin, buccal and vaginal epithelial cells.

Since relatively few genital injuries are discovered at the medical examination, the detection of other marks such as the presence of semen is essential in order to confirm the presumption of sexual assault. For many years, cytological examination and the detection of acid phosphatases were considered as forensic evidence [Khaldi *et al.*]. The discovery of STR markers, the availability of commercial kits for its analysis as well as the development of fluorescence detection instruments, provided forensic laboratories with sophisticated means to achieve its main goals, including the identification of the perpetrator in a sexual assault case.

## TYPE OF SAMPLES

Physical contact can result in the transfer of DNA from one individual to another. In cases of sexual offence this can often be by means of an aggressive or sexual act. Biological material can accumulate under the fingernail hyponychium of both the victim and/or the suspect and has the potential to provide evidence and intelligence information [Malsom *et al.*]. In addition to the hairs and debris that may be transferred in other types of violent crime, the rapist often leaves behind a personal biological signature that may include blood, saliva and, most importantly, semen. This semen evidence is frequently a cornerstone in the investigation and prosecution of the case. Furthermore, intimate body swabs, clothing and bedding items are routinely submitted for forensic examination. The detection of semen on such items and the subsequent use of DNA profiling tests are often of vital importance, together with an evaluation as to the significance of the findings [Allard *et al.*]. Bite marks perpetrated in the victim body is another type of sample that can be studied in sexual assaults. The presence of a mixture (female/male) in the DNA extracted from the moistened swabs, used to collect cells from a bite mark, can be the unique probative evidence. Obviously, this sample doesn't have the same value as, for instance, a vaginal swab in which it was identified a DNA profile similar to the perpetrator one. In this case it could be established a penis penetration occurred in the victim's vagina, a legal condition that must occurred to be considered a rape in some countries. The next step is to demonstrate that the penetration took place without the woman's consent. Generally, this can only be evaluated by the judge since only he has access to the proofs included in the criminal process. The analysis of clothing damage can also be used to corroborate different versions of events and is at its most powerful in elucidating false allegation cases and consent cases, being an integral part of the examinations carried out in sexual assault type cases [Boland *et al.*].

The process of collecting biological samples from the victim usually involves the application of moistened swabs to areas of possible dried stains and the insertion of dry swabs into body cavities to absorb any liquid secretions. Swabs could be initially taken from the vulva, and then from the lower vagina, upper vagina and cervix in ascending order [Green]. Oral and rectal swabs can also be analyzed depending on the sexual aggression. The proper handling and packaging of potential semen evidence cannot be overstressed. In the case of swabs, this requires placement at room temperature during the enough time for the swabs to completely dry. Biological evidence must be packaged in containers that allow air circulation and then, in a proper bag that can be of any type of material, since the samples should be already dry (in our laboratory we have special bags to transport the evidences). Chain of custody must be meticulously documented and the transportation, reception and storage of evidence must also strictly follow known protocols.

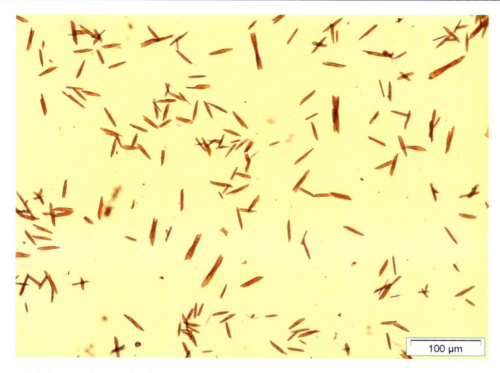

Figure 1. Microscopic examination (10X) of dark brown needle shaped crystals of choline periodide.

## PRESUMPTIVE CHEMICAL TESTS FOR SEMEN

An examination after rape requires the use of a reliable semen detection test that is sensitive and has very good negative predictive power. Presumptive tests should be done before the DNA is extracted from the samples. As screening tests there are, for example, presumptive chemical tests for semen that uses substances within the evidence swabs or stains that allow the identification and/or the individualization of semen. Presumptive testing for semen helps to confirm the sampling location as a potentially positive site.

The two commonly used presumptive tests for semen are both colorimetric. The Florence test identifies the presence of choline and the Brentamine test detects Acid Phosphatase (AP). Both of these assays are qualitative [Green]. Acid phosphatase is not a single enzyme but an array of related isoenzymes from variety of sources. The forensic interest in acid phosphatase in the evaluation of sexual assault evidence is based on the fact that acid phosphatase activity in human semen is 500-1000 times greater than in any other normal bodily fluid. Unfortunately, the use of acid phosphatase as a marker for semen is compromised because the vagina is also a source of the same type of acid phosphatase [Green]. A purple colour indicates the presence of AP. Large areas or clothing can be screened by pressing them against an equal size piece of moistened filter paper and then subjecting the filter paper to the presumptive tests [Butler, JM]. Since seminal and vaginal acid phosphatases cannot be reliably discriminated qualitatively, the only approach to differentiating azoospermic semen from vaginal secretions is the identification of the presence of choline [Green] [Figure 1]. Moreover, prostate specific antigen can be used for forensic identification of semen stains and there are commercial kits that can be used. A previous study has shown that cytology allows the detection of some, but not all types of sperm, up to 72 h whereas a search for acid phosphatase does detect all types of sperm but only in the first 24 h. Regarding PSA detection kit, it allowed all types of semen to be detected up to 48 h [Khaldi *et al.*].

## CONFIRMATORY TESTING FOR SEMEN

A microscopic examination to look for the presence of spermatozoa [Figure 2] is performed in some laboratories on sexual assault evidence and can be very helpful as reference.

However, aspermic or oligospermic males have either no sperm or low sperm count in their seminal fluid ejaculate. In addition, vasectomised males will not release sperm. Therefore, tests that can identify semen-specific enzymes are helpful in verifying the presence of semen in sexual assault cases [Butler]. Confirmatory testing for semen involves the microscopy detection of spermatozoa and its DNA analysis. Identification of one or more intact spermatozoa is conclusive proof of the presence of semen and hence affirms sexual contact. Nevertheless, the DNA profile identification of the perpetrator must be established.

One of the limiting factors for clarifying rape crimes is the lack of spermatozoa collected from vaginal material, which makes the identification of genetic material from the perpetrator difficult. This difficulty is even greater in cases of azoospermic individuals where the loss of viable sperm in the semen is related to the individual's constitution or due to elective surgery (vasectomy). The impossibility of showing the presence of spermatozoa is frequent; however, it does not exclude the presence of male DNA. Besides the technical problems inherent in the kind of material analyzed, the lack of spermatozoa in samples may be explained by several factors such as, among others, the long time period after the intercourse, penetration without ejaculation, or even the azoospermy or oligospermy of the aggressor. In these last two cases, there is much less seminal DNA as the spermatozoa represent the major source of DNA in ejaculates for potential genotyping analysis. Furthermore, there is a great variation in the DNA concentration in semen samples [Soares-Vieira *et al.*]. The reasons for this variation are, for instance, the age, the length of sexual abstinence, the season of the year, the smoking habits and the caffeine intake.

## ISOLATING CELLS

Forensic scientists are sometimes confronted with cellular material originating from an individual, often in trace quantities, that is mixed with cellular material from a different person. DNA profiling of such cellular mixtures will often generate either mixed DNA profiles that require complex statistical calculations or a profile that only represents the major contributor, when the need is to obtain DNA information on the minor contributor [Anoruo *et al.*].

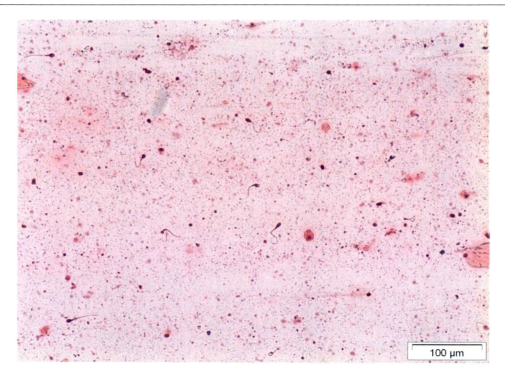

Figure 2. Microscopic examination (10X) of spermatozoa stained with amoniacal erythrosine.

Forensic evidence comprised of biological mixtures is a common occurrence, particularly in sexual assault crimes. Typically the sperm cells are the component of interest, while the victim's cells from vaginal, rectal, oral, or other body swab complicate genotyping of the assailant. The preferential lysis method has been the forensic standard for separating sperm cells from epithelial cells. This method utilizes cell-specific differences in membrane chemical composition by first lysing the nonsperm cells without disrupting the sperm cells, and then washing away any residual exogenous DNA from the intact sperm cells. Although this method can generally provide two cellular fractions, one comprising of sperm cell DNA and the other of non sperm DNA, the separation is not always complete. There may be carryover from one cell fraction to another, making eventual genotype interpretation and a further statistical analysis challenging. Additional limitations to this technique are the premature lysis and loss of sperm cells in the first digestion and the multiple liquid transfers and washing steps that reduce cells recovered. An alternative to a chemical separation, such as the preferential lysis method, can be the separation by direct physical selection of the target cells from a mixture [Sanders *et al.*].

Laser Microdissection systems, combining microscope and laser cutting and isolation beam technology, permit the identification and isolation of tissue sections and single cells, as well as sub-cellular components. In 2003, the British Forensic Science Service investigates Laser Microdissection (LMD) as a tool for forensic DNA analysis for identifying and isolating sperm and epithelial cells in sexual assault samples. As a matter of fact, Elliott *et al.* (2003) using the laser LMD demonstrated its capability to isolate spermatozoa from microscope slides containing sperms and vaginal cells and its significant improvements relative to the preferential lysis method. Microlaser systems are used by the forensic community for the same purpose (Di Martino D *et al.*, Sanders CT *et al.*]. Moreover, it was used: to cut the telogen hair in order to exclusively collect the lower part of the follicle and reduce keratin contamination [Di Martino *et al.*]; to isolate male cells from cellular mixtures using a staining method that detects all cells carrying a Y-chromosome with a digoxigenin labelled chromosome Y cocktail probe [Anslinger *et al.*]; to identify and isolate cells from environmental debris [Lambie-Anoruo *et al.*]; to recognize and isolate trace amounts of cells from somatic cellular mixtures (blood and saliva), and compared its efficiency in generating single-source DNA profiles with current profiling protocols [Anoruo *et al.*]. Despite its advantages, such as: to eliminate traditional DNA extraction methods, to provide the total separation of sperm and epithelial DNA and to decrease analysis times and sexual assault DNA casework, its high cost and the mandatory validation process are its major disadvantages.

## DNA Identification Perspective

Haploid cells, such as spermatozoa, are formed by the biological process of meiosis and contain half genetic material of the donor organism. Spermatozoa are frequently tested in sexual assault cases, and any DNA profiles obtained are likely to form a substantial component of the forensic evidence. A man produces approximately 300 million spermatozoa per ejaculate [Green]. Assuming a DNA content of 3 pg per cell the expectation is that there will be approximately 0.9 mg of DNA per ejaculate. The high cell density of spermatozoa in semen makes it an excellent source of DNA for forensic DNA profiling [Lucy *et al.*]. It is especially important to know how many cells or how much material the laboratory needs to produce a DNA profile in cases of unsolved sexual assault, where the original slides are the only remaining forensic evidence or from cases where only trace amounts of spermatozoa have been isolated from intimate swabs or clothing. It has been widely demonstrated, using commercially available kits, that accurate DNA profiles can be routinely produced from 100 pg or less of purified DNA [Gill *et al.*, Wickenheiser *et al.*].

## Amelogenin System

The ability to designate whether a sample originated from a male or a female source is useful in sexual assault cases, where distinguishing between the victim and the perpetrator's evidence is important. By far the most popular method for sex-typing today is the amelogenin system as it can be performed in conjunction with STR analysis. Amelogenin is a gene that codes for proteins found in tooth enamel. The Forensic Science Service was the first to describe the particular PCR primer sets that are used in forensic DNA laboratories today [Butler]. Since 2000, both Promega and Applied Biosystems have marketed multiplex PCR reactions that permit co-amplification of 15 autosomal STRs in a single reaction along with the amelogenin sex-typing marker, respectively, PowerPlex® 16 and Identifiler™.

## AUTOSOMAL STRs

Autosomal STRs have been used for a long time for human identification and still are a valuable tool in forensic casework, where small amounts of DNA are available [Petricevic *et al.*]. Analysis of mixed samples containing male and female DNA presents certain challenges, even in sexual assault investigations where only one aggressor is involved. At certain times, evidence samples from sexual assault cases contain relatively high quantities of female DNA, compared with male DNA. During analysis for autosomal STR loci, the profile from female DNA often masks the male DNA profile or competes for reagents such that no male profile is obtained [Shewale *et al.*]. In cases where multiple males are involved, the autosomal STR profiles obtained often provide inconclusive results [Shewale *et al.*]. When the mixture contains different male/male proportion of DNA, only the full profile of the major component could, usually, be detected.

## MIXTURES

Physical contact can result in the transfer of DNA from one individual to another. In cases of sexual offence this can often be by means of an aggressive or sexual act. [Malsom *et al.*]. Mixtures can occur in different kinds of samples taken from a sexual victim. The more frequent ones result from swabs collected from any victim body cavity, biological material accumulate under the fingernail and bite marks. The stains found in clothing, bedding and other materials can also be a source of mixtures. Mixtures arise when two or more individuals contribute to the sample being tested [Butler]. If more than two allelic bands per locus are present, a mixture may be inferred. Extra bands may also be present because of somatic/genetic polymorphism and stutters. In addition, allele asymmetry occurs because shared alleles result in 'masking'. The profile appears unbalanced as a result [Gill *et al.*].

Mixed DNA profiles are used in court as evidence to either support the defence or prosecution depending on the background of the case. The presence of alleles matching the suspect supports the hypothesis that contact between the suspect and victim took place; however, the significance of this will depend on the relationship between the suspect and victim prior to the offence. Previous contact can be used as an explanation for the presence of foreign DNA by the defence whereas support for the prosecution is provided when the victim and suspect have had no previous contact [Malsom *et al.*]. Mixtures can be challenging to detect and interpret without extensive experience and careful training. The DNA Commission of the International Society of Forensic Genetics approved guidelines to encourage best practice that can be universally applied to assist with mixture interpretation [Gill *et al.*].

## Y CHROMOSOME STRs

The value of Y chromosome in forensic DNA testing is that it is found only in males. Since a vast majority of crimes where DNA evidence is helpful, particularly sexual assault, involve males as the perpetrator, DNA tests designed to only examine the male portion can be valuable. With Y chromosome tests, interpretable results can be obtained in some cases where autosomal tests are limited by the evidence, such as high levels of female DNA in the presence of minor amounts of male DNA. In addition, the number of individuals involved may be easier to determine with Y chromosome than with autosomal STR mixtures [Butler]. Using Y chromosome specific PCR primers can improve the chances of detecting low levels of perpetrator's DNA in a high background of the female victim's DNA [Hall, Ballantyne]. At present, several commercial available Y-STR multiplex system kits, such as AmpflSTR Y-filer kit (Applied Biosystems) and Power Plex Y System (Promega, Madison, WI, USA), have a wide circulation.

Autosomal STRs only allow reliable identification of minor components in a mixture for ratios up to approximately 1 in 20. However, it has been shown that this ratio can be drastically increased with the use of Y-chromosomal STRs. Parson et al. (2001) described that they were able to detect male contributions and its correct Y-STR haplotype in various male/female DNA mixtures even in the order of up to 1 in 500. They demonstrate that the addition of the PCRx Enhancer to the reaction mix increases the specificity of Y-STR typing of male/female mixture samples. The authors conclude that this method may be a useful tool for the analysis of mixture samples even when the gender-specific Amelogenin marker shows no indication of a male contribution.

Soares-Vieira et al. (2007) using the Y-STRs (DYS19, DYS389I, DYS389II, DYS390, DYS391, DYS392, and DYS393) in DNA analysis of sperm samples from 105 vasectomized men demonstrated a great disparity in DNA concentration. It is referred that this was attributed to variation in the number of epithelial cells and/or leucocytes present in the semen. Such variation in the quantity of epithelial cells and/or leukocytes may be related to several factors, such as the period of sexual abstinence and the presence of infections in the individuals. DNA concentration in these samples ranged from 0.9 to 96.5 mg/mL. Nonsperm cells in semen, including immature germ cells, leukocytes, and epithelial cells, are normally found in a concentration of 15% of the sperm material. The glands of the male genital tract, such as the prostate and seminal vesicle, are the major source of epithelial cells in the semen. The prevalence and clinical significance of leukocytes, immature germ cells, and epithelial cells in semen is currently a subject of controversy. The World Health Organization proposed as normal the limit of $4.7 \times 10^6$ leukocytes/mL of ejaculate [Petricevic et al.]. In addition, the authors concluded that the study of the Y-STR is a very useful method for analyzing small quantities of DNA in mixture samples.

Shewale et al. (2004) in a previous study, have demonstrated that Y-STRs were successfully amplified when mixing male and female DNA at the ratio 1:800 (0.5:400 ng), showing that although there was a much higher concentration of female DNA, this did not inhibit the amplification of the Y-STRs. These authors also showed that the mixture of DNA, from two men who had distinct allele profiles for nine Y-STRs, was successful in the amplification of both haplotypes in mixtures of up to 1:30 (0.2:6.0 ng), although some variation in the degree of amplification had been observed for the minor component. They concluded that their approach is useful in the DNA analysis of multiple rape case samples, wherein one of the aggressors is azoospermic.

Hall and Ballantyne (2003) recognized that depending upon specific situation, some victims of sexual assault provide vaginal samples more than 36–48 h after the incident. In these cases, the ability to obtain an autosomal STR profile of the semen donor from the living victim diminishes rapidly as the post-coital interval (interval between the sexual intercourse and the clinical forensic examination) is extended. Although it may be possible, though unlikely in most instances, to obtain an autosomal STR profile of the semen donor from vaginal samples taken 24–36 h after intercourse, it is normally not possible to do so when the post-coital interval exceeds 48 h. The reasons for the inability to detect the genetic profile of the male donor in extended interval post-coital vaginal samples can be attributed to a combination of sperm loss or lysis and the technological limitations of the DNA typing systems employed [Hall, Ballantyne]. So, no semen will be recovered if none was deposited (sexual dysfunction, condom use), mechanical elimination (drainage, hygiene activities), biological elimination (degradation), physiologic dilution, or any combination of them may yield negative results.

The authors also stated that sperm loss can also occur during the multiple manipulations required of the differential extraction process used to separate the sperm from the non-sperm DNA fractions within the laboratory. In addition to sperm loss, premature lysis of the few remaining fragile sperm during the differential extraction process will result in male DNA becoming admixed with female DNA. These authors analysed post-coital cervicovaginal or lower to mid-vaginal swabs (2x) taken from a female subject at various time intervals after sexual intercourse including 0, 12, 24, 48, 72, 85 h, 4–6 days. The female subject in these experiments abstained from sexual relations for at least 3 days prior to sexual intercourse. The authors realize that using Y chromosome specific PCR primers can improve the chances of detecting low levels of perpetrator's DNA in a high background of the female victim's DNA.

Recently, Mayntz-Press *et at.* (2008) have described that male cells are present in the cervix at least a week after intercourse and yet standard DNA typing systems are unable to discern the male donor profile after 3 days or less. They report the ability to obtain a Y-STR profile from the male donor in extended interval ($\geq$ 3 days) post-coital samples. Therefore, using cervicovaginal swabs collected from volunteers the authors have demonstrated the relative facility of obtaining full Y-STR profiles from cervicovaginal samples recovered 3–4 days after intercourse using both commercial and in-house systems. Partial profiles were also obtainable 5–6 days post-coitus. It was also remarked that more complete profiles were obtained when DNA from the sperm fraction of a differential lysis method was amplified as opposed to the amplification of relatively large quantities of admixed male/female DNA.

However, the conditions for obtaining male DNA samples in rape cases are very much different from the ones developed in experiment conditions, such as the referred in two later studies. In the majority of the rape cases, the aggressor's DNA is obtained from the vaginal fluid where the amount of female DNA is much higher. Another difficulty arises when multiple males are contributors.

The same feature of the Y chromosome that gives it an advantage in forensic testing is also its biggest limitation. A majority of the Y chromosome is transferred directly from father to son without recombination to shuffle its genes and provide greater variety to future generations. Random mutations are the only mechanisms for variation over time between paternally related males. Thus, while exclusions in Y chromosome DNA testing results can aid forensic investigations, a match between a suspect and evidence only means that the individual in question could have contributed the evidence [Butler]. For this reason, inclusions with Y chromosome analysis are not as meaningful as autosomal STR matches from a random match probability point of view [de Knjiff].

## MINI «Y-STRS»

Asamura *et al.* (2007) designed polymerase chain reaction (PCR) primer sets for DYS504, DYS508, DYS522, DYS540, DYS556, DYS570, DYS576 and DYS632 to generate as short amplicon as possible, and attempted to develop two miniYSTR quadruplex systems for degraded DNA. The genetic data for 224 Japanese male individuals has shown the PCR amplification products for the eight loci ranged in length from 95 bp (DYS632) to 147 bp (DYS570). This study demonstrated the usefulness of analyses of degraded DNA samples using the miniY-STR systems evaluated on 27 degraded DNA samples. Despite the demonstrated utility of these markers, specifically in the study of degraded DNA samples, there is no evidence of its value to solve sexual assaults where the DNA of the collected samples is degraded. It should be an interesting study to use these miniY-STR markers to detect the genetic profile of the assailant in the extended interval post-coital vaginal samples, where there is a combination of the sperm loss and its lysis.

## A SURVEY ON SEXUAL ASSAULT CASES

In Portugal the medico-legal expertises are done by the National Institute of Legal Medicine. This Institute has three branches are located in the North, Centre and South of the country. Each branch has four technical forensic services, being the Forensic Genetic and Biology one of them. This laboratory deals with different kinds of issues, such as kinship analysis, individual genetic identification, mainly human remains, and forensic cases. The samples related to sexual assaults are the most analysed in our laboratory connected to the latter.

Complainants of sexual violence can report the incident to the police department or directly to the National Institute of Legal Medicine. When the police are first contacted, the victims are present to this Institute for forensic medical examination in order to be observed and to be collected the necessary evidence. In Portugal, sexual crimes are considered as against the "sexual freedom" when the victims are more than fourteen years old (Penal Code–163° to 170° Articles) and crimes against the "sexual self determination" when the victims are less than fourteen years old (Penal Code–171° to 176° Articles).

The primary methods used for the identification of semen in our laboratory are the Acid Phosphatase with the Brentamine test or the Phosphatesmo KM Paper® kit that is a rapid staining, using qualitative enzymatic staining procedure. Furthermore, the microscopic detection of spermatozoa is done when slides are available. An additional test for the Choline is occasionally also used. If the results of these tests are negative, some of the samples are selected to be submitted to the DNA extraction, according to our perception of their importance in solving the case. The Chelex DNA extraction method is used for the reference samples from the victim and suspect. The use of the differential lysis technique is universal and can work well in most sexual assault cases to separate the female and male fractions from one another. However, this method is frequently ineffective, mainly when there is low number of sperms due to the inevitable contamination of the profile by female DNA. So, we always use the organic extraction method without the differential lysis. This extraction method works well for recovery of high molecular weight DNA. Obviously, in the majority of the cases, we have a mixture which is challenging to interpret, especially when we analyse the autosomal STRs (AmpF/STR® Identifiler™ kit). Our experience shows that the results are better using the organic method since there is less loss of male cells, as previously mentioned. In the case of a mixture we don't assign to the major or minor contributor. So, if the genotype from a suspect is present in the DNA profile from a sample, the suspect cannot be excluded as contributing for the mixture. The next step is to study the Y chromosome STR (AmpFlSTR®Yfiler™). If the profile from the suspect is similar to the sample one, we will not be able to conclude that the two samples could be originated from the same source. Then, we use the distribution of the identified haplotype in a reference database to evaluate how often the two randomly selected haplotypes emerge as the two matched haplotypes found in the case analysed. The European Y-STR Haplotype Database (http://www.ystr.org) is the database used. Nowadays this database includes the minimal haplotype loci (DYS19, DYS389I/II, DYS390, DYS391, DYS392, DYS393, and DYS385 a/b) and the additional loci DYS438, DYS439, DYS437, DYS448, DYS456, DYS458, DYS635, YGATAH4, that are now available in commercial Y-STR kits.

The sexual offences constitute 69% (n= 595) of the cases studied in a total of 860 criminal expertises concluded in a period of five years (2004-2008) [Figure 3].

In 90% of the sexual offences (n= 537) the victims were female with a sex ratio equal to 9.26 (female:male). The assailant was a family member of the victim in 8.9% of the cases (the father in 71.7%). In 50% (n= 297) of the sexual aggressions studied cases, a match was obtained between the DNA profile of the victim and the one provided from samples related to the crime, collected from her body. In 9.6% (n= 57) it wasn't identified any DNA profile. These cases can have some analogy to those in which we have a DNA profile similar to the victim. Finally, in 40.5% of the cases (n= 241) a male DNA profile different from the victim was identified [Figure 4], but only in 47% of the cases (n= 113) it could be possible to compare it to the suspect one. In 81% (n= 92) a match between the two profiles was found [Figure 5].

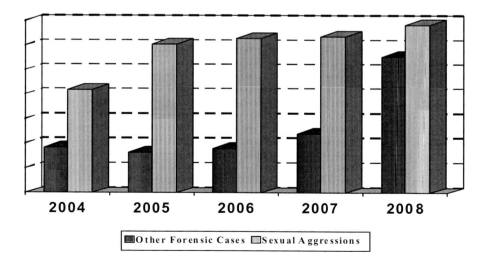

Figure 3. Distribution of sexual offences and other forensic cases (2004-2008).

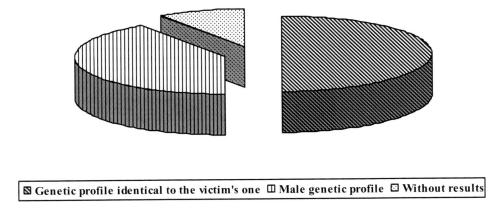

☒ **Genetic profile identical to the victim's one** ☐ **Male genetic profile** ☐ **Without results**

Figure 4. Results obtained by comparing the DNA samples profile with the victim's and suspect's profiles.

Some of these cases are very recent and the criminal investigation was not yet concluded, which can explain the failure in the suspect identification. While in kinship analysis we have, in the beginning of the expertise, all persons involved, in the forensic cases sometimes we never have the suspect. Though, there are cases which are successfully concluded under the laboratory point of view, but they never finished under the criminal investigation perspective.

A DNA database should be a valuable tool in aiding law enforcement to identify the assailants and, consequently, to solve the majority of the cases where a male profile is found in the samples analysed. In Portugal there is a DNA database, since February 2008, and it has two main purposes, civil and criminal identifications. It is supposed that the database will be fully implanted in 2009.

This survey was done on alleged victims of sexual assault cases reported to the National Institute of Legal Medicine – North Branch (Oporto-Portugal) in 2004-2008.

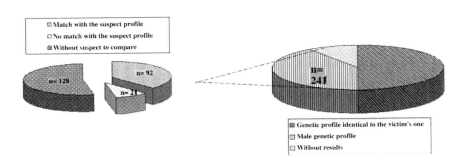

Figure 5. Results obtained by comparing the DNA male samples with the suspect's profile.

## CONCLUSION

A considerable number of sexual assaults are reported to the National Institute of Legal Medicine (North Branch). Despite the use of adequate technology, there are a high number of cases in which the perpetrator's DNA wasn't identified and only a female profile was recognized. An explanation for the similarity between the samples and the victim profiles can be the fact that samples collection was done some days after intercourse. Unfortunately, no information about the post-coital interval is available for the majority of the studied cases. Consequently, the absence of male cells in these cases is unknown. Another reason for this absence can be the fact that the aggression didn't occur. This possibility can be confirmed through additional information provided in the form filled by the doctor. The number of the identified perpetrators is generally low. This number can increase with a use of a DNA database, since the sexual aggression involved recidivist perpetrators. Therefore, when the DNA database is implemented a great part of sexual aggressions and even cold cases might be solved.

## COMPETING INTERESTS

The author declares that they have no competing interests. The author alone is responsible for the content and writing of the paper.

## REFERENCES

Allard, JE; Baird, A; Davidson, G; Jones, S; Lewis, J; McKenna, L; Weston, C; Scrimger, D; Teppett, G. A comparison of methods used in the UK and Ireland for the extraction and detection of semen on swabs and cloth samples. *Science and Justice* (2007) 47: 160–167.

Anoruo, B; van Oorschot, R; Mitchell, J; Howells, D. Isolating cells from non-sperm cellular mixtures using the PALM® microlaser micro dissection system. *Forensic Science International* (2007) 173: 93–96.

Anslinger, K; Mack, B; Bayer, B; Rolf, B; Eisenmenger, W. Digoxigenin labelling and laser capture microdissection of male cells. *Int J Legal Med* (2005) 119: 374–377.

Asamura, H; Sakai, H; Ota, M; Fukushima, H. MiniY-STR quadruplex systems with short amplicon lengths for analysis of degraded DNA samples. *Forensic Science International: Genetics* (2007) 1: 56–61.

Anoruo, B; van Oorschot, R; Mitchell, J; Howells, D. Isolating cells from non-sperm cellular mixtures using the PALM® microlaser micro dissection system. *Forensic Science International* (2007) 173: 93–96.

Boland, CA. Clothing damage analysis in alleged sexual assaults—The need for a systematic approach. *Forensic Science International* (2007) 167: 110–115.

Butler, JM. Forensic DNA Typing. Second Edition. *Elsevier Academic – MA.* (2005).

French, CEV; Jensen,CG; Vintiner, SK; Elliot, DA; McGlashan, SR. A novel histological technique for distinguishing between epithelial cells in forensic casework. *Forensic Science International* (2008) 178: 1–6.

de Knijff, P. *Profiles in DNA*, 7, 3–5. (2003). Available online at: http://www.promega.com/profiles.

Di Martino, D; Giuffre, G; Staiti, N; Simone, A; Todaro, P; Saravo, L. Laser microdissection and DNA typing of cells from single hair follicles. *Forensic Science Internatinal* (2004) 146S S155–S157.

Di Martino, D; Giuffre, G; Staiti, N; Simone, A; Le Donne, M; Saravo, L. Single sperm cell isolation by laser microdissection. *Forensic Science Internatinal* (2004) 146S S151–S153.

Elliott, K; Hill, DS; Lambert, C; Burroughes, TR; Gill, P. Use of laser microdissection greatly improves the recovery of DNA from sperm on microscope slides. *Forensic Science International* (2003) 137: 28–36.

Gill, P; Whitaker, J; Flaxman, C; Brown, N; Buckleton, J. An investigation of the rigor of interpretation rules for STRs derived from less than 100 pg of DNA. *Forensic Science International* (2000) 112 (1): 17–40.

Gill, P; Brenner, CH; Buckleton, JS; Carracedo, A; Krawczak, M; Mayr, WR; Morling, N; Prinz, M; Schneider, PM; Weir, BS. DNA commission of the International Society of Forensic Genetics: Recommendations on the interpretation of mixtures. *Forensic Science International* (2006) 160: 90–101.

Green, W. Sexual Assault and semen persistence. Encyclopedia of Forensic Sciences, Three-Volume Set. (2000). http://books.elsevier.com/bookscat/links/details.asp?isbn=0122272153. 397-403

Kathleen, A; Mayntz-Press, Sims, LM; Hall, A; Ballantyne, J. Y-STR Profiling in Extended Interval (‡3 days) Postcoital Cervicovaginal Samples. *J Forensic Sci* (2008). March 2008 Vol. 53, No. 2

Khaldi, N; Miras, A; Botti, K; Benali, L; Gromb, S. Evaluation of Three Rapid Detection Methods for the Forensic Identification of seminal Fluid in Rape Cases. *J Forensic Sci* (2004) Vol. 49, N° 4

Hall, A; Ballantyne, J. Novel Y-STR typing strategies reveal the genetic profile of the semen donor in extended interval post-coital cervicovaginal samples. *Forensic Science International* (2003) 136: 58–72.

Lambie-Anoruo, BL; Prince, DV; Koukoulas, I; Howells, DW; Mitchell, RJ; Van Oorschot, RAH. Laser microdissection and pressure catapulting with PALM1 to assist typing of target DNA in dirt samples, *Int. Congr. Ser.* (2006) 1288 559–561.

Lucy, D; Curran, JM; Pirie, AA; Gill P. The probability of achieving full allelic representation for LCN-STR profiling of haploid cells. *Science and Justice* (2007) 47:168–171.

Malsom, S; Flanagan, N; McAlister, C; Dixon, L. The prevalence of mixed DNA profiles in fingernail samples taken from couples who co-habit using autosomal and Y-STRs. (2008). Forensic Science International: Genetics. *Journal homepage:* www.elsevier.com/locate/fsig

Parson, W; Niederstätter, H; Köchl, S; Steinlechner, M; Berger, B. When autosomal short tandem repeats fail: optimized primer and reaction design for Y-chromosome short tandem repeat analysis in forensic casework. *Croation Med J* (2001) 42: 285-287.

Petricevic, SF; Brigth, JA; Cockerton, SL. DNA profiling of trace DNA recovered from bedding. *Forensic Science Internatinal* (2006) 159:21–6.

Sanders, CT; Sanchez, N; Ballantyne, J; Peterson, DA. Laser Microdissection Separation of Pure Spermatozoa from Epithelial Cells for Short Tandem Repeat Analysis. *J Forensic Sci* (2006) Vol. 51, N° 4.

Shewale, JG; Sikka, SC; Schneida, E; Sinha, SK. DNA profiling of azoospermic semen samples from vasectomized males by using Y-Plex TM 6 amplification Kit. *J Forensic Sci* (2003) 48(1):127–9.

Shewale, JG; Nasir, H; Schneida, E; Gross, AM; Budowle, B; Sinha SK. Y Chromosome STR system, Y-PlexTM 12, for forensic casework: development and validation. *J Forensic Sci* (2004) 49(6):1278–90.

Soares-Vieira, JA; Billerbeck, A; Elisa, C; Iwamura, ESM; Zampieri, RA; Gattás, GJF; Munoz, DR; Hallak, J; Mendonca, BB; Lucon, AM. Y-STRs in Forensic Medicine: DNA Analysis in Semen Samples of Azoospermic Individuals. *J Forensic Sci* (2007) Vol. 52 No. 3.

Ward, S. Sexual assault and rape. Obstetrics, *Gynaecology and Reproductive Medicine* (2007) 17:11

Wickenheiser, RA. Trace DNA: a review, discussion of theory, and application of the transfer of trace quantities of DNA through skin contact. *J Forensic Sci* (2002) 47 (3): 442–450.

In: Forensic Genetics Research Progress
Editor: F. Gonzalez-Andrade

ISBN: 978-1-60876-198-2
© 2010 Nova Science Publishers, Inc.

*Chapter 7*

# ANALYSIS OF REDUCED SIZE STR AMPLICONS AS TOOLS FOR THE STUDY OF DEGRADED DNA

*Miriam Baeta[1], Carolina Nuñez[1], Fabricio González-Andrade[1-2],\**
*Santiago Gascón[1], and Begoña Martínez-Jarreta[1]*

[1]Forensic Genetics Laboratory, Forensic Medicine Department, University of Zaragoza,
Calle Domingo Miral s/n, Zaragoza 50.009, Spain
[2]Department of Medicine, Metropolitan Hospital,
Av. Mariana de Jesús Oe8, Quito, Ecuador

## ABSTRACT

Polymorphic Short Tandem Repeats (STRs) markers have become a very useful tool in forensic analysis of human DNA. Multiplex PCR amplification of STR loci enables to obtain genetic information from almost any source of biological material. However, some forensic evidences, can be so extremely degraded (e.g. certain mass disasters, old and bad preserved remains, etc) that STR typing is unsuccessful. In these situations DNA typing can be challenging and it could be difficult to obtain quality profiles (ej: loss of signal of larger sized loci is frequently observed as a result of DNA fragmentation, etc.). Recent efforts have focused on the use of nuclear Single Nucleotide Polymorphism (SNP) markers as an alternative and more recently, on reducing the size of STR markers (miniSTRs). The development of miniSTRs is accomplished by simply moving the primer binding sites closer to the STR repeat region, and creating DNA fragments that are shorter than traditional STR markers. MiniSTRs markers have shown to be very successful at recovering DNA profiles from highly degraded samples The possibility of obtaining nuclear MiniSTRs profiles corresponding to conventional STR markers is also considered a great advantage as most of the National intelligence DNA banks are based on them. In this chapter we will review the development and use of miniSTRs loci in forensic genetics from its first application in the analysis of Branch Davidian fire in Waco to its incorporation in commercial kits. We will not only focus on autosomal

---

\* E-mail: fabriciogonzaleza@yahoo.es

miniSTRs but also on the recent development of miniY-STRs and miniX-STRs. Advantages and disadvantages of these markers in Forensics will be considered and compared to those of traditional STR markers. Finally, we will review potential applications and future perspectives of their use in Forensic Genetics.

## INTRODUCTION

Polymorphic Short Tandem Repeats (STRs) markers have become a very useful tool in forensic analysis of human DNA. Multiplex PCR amplification of STR loci enables to obtain genetic information from almost any source of biological material. However, it is common in criminalistics to find forensic evidences that are so extremely degraded (e.g. certain mass disasters, old and bad preserved remains) that STR typing is unsuccessful. During the decomposition of a sample, DNA molecules are gradually degraded in small fragments by the action of endogenous nucleases. The degradation process depends on environmental conditions, such as temperature, humidity, pH, soil chemistry or UV radiation, which can cause molecular damage on the DNA over time, through hydrolysis and oxidation processes. Degradation will limit the amount of amplifiable DNA available, as DNA will be fragmented in small size fragments, and just few of them will have the complete target sequence to be typed. In addition, there can be PCR inhibitors such as humic acid or derived degradation products, coextracted with the DNA, which can impede the PCR reaction (Fondevila et al. 2008).

In these situations it is frequent to observe a loss of signal of larger sized loci, due to DNA fragmentation or, in other cases, to the presence of inhibitors (see Figure 1A). The progressive loss of signal, as size locus increases, can be seen in the electropherogram as a decay curve. The peak height is inversely proportional to the amplicon length, so larger loci will have lower signal, even falling below the detection threshold (see Figure 1B). As a result, degraded samples often result in partial genetic profiles with allele and/or complete locus dropout (Cotton et al. 2000, Wallin et al. 1998).

## DEGRADED DNA TYPING

Forensic laboratories have faced the problem of typing degraded DNA samples in different ways. When samples are so degraded that STR typing methods are ineffectual, one possible approach to obtain results is to analyze the mitochondrial DNA (mtDNA) hypervariable regions (Stone et al. 2001, Bender et al. 2000). As the mitochondrial DNA is present in a high number within cells, with hundreds or thousands of copies per cell, there is a high likelihood of success in typing degraded samples. Furthermore, the haploid and maternal transmission between generations facilitates the comparison among maternal relatives, since they should have an identical mtDNA. However, mtDNA analysis has the disadvantage of being a time-consuming and labor-intensive process. But the principal limitation in forensic mtDNA testing is the difficulty to differenciate among individuals who share common HVI/HVII haplotypes, resulting in a low power of discrimination (Just et al. 2004, Parsons et al. 2001).

Recent efforts have focused on studying shorter regions of DNA, such as Single Nucleotide Polymorphism (SNP) or smaller STR markers (miniSTRs), as alternative approaches to analyse degraded DNA (Dixon et al. 2006). The utility of autosomal (Whitaker et al. 1995), mitochondrial (Quintans et al. 2004) and Y chromosomal SNPs (Bouakaze et al. 2007) have been proved in challenging samples typing.

SNPs markers offer a good alternative to STR analysis because of their small size (<150bp), abundance and possibility to automation (Odriozola et al, 2009). But unfortunately, SNP analysis has the setback of requiring the study of a high number of loci (45-50) to reach match probabilities comparable with STR multiplexes (Butler et al 2007).

Reducing the size of STR (miniSTR) to amplicon sizes less than 200 bp has become a successful method of typing small fragments of DNA. It is especially appropriate for degraded DNA evidence, for example from mass disasters or anthropological remains.

The development of miniSTRs is accomplished by simply moving the primer binding sites closer to the STR repeat region, and creating DNA fragments that are shorter than traditional STR markers (Figure2). It is important to have in mind that repeat information is independent of amplicon size, which will be defined by primers position.

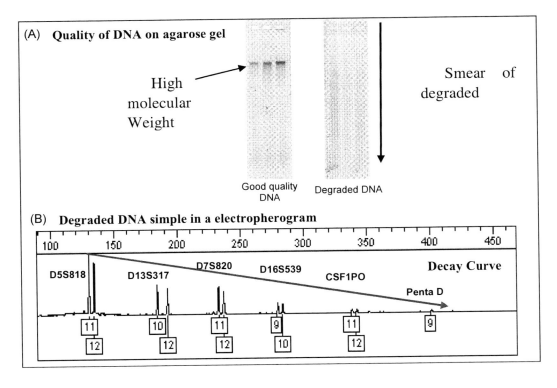

Figure 1. (A) Quality of DNA sample on agarose gel. Degraded DNA is fragmented into small pieces that will be seen on the gel as a smear. (B) Decay curve: progressive loss of signal as size locus increase, the larger loci often fall below the detection threshold. Modified from Butler J, 2005.

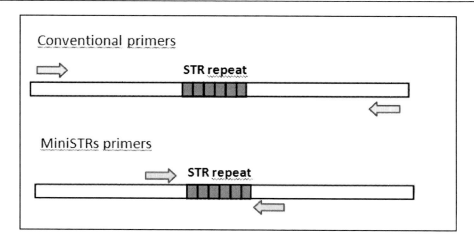

Figure 2. Methodology used to reduce amplicons.

Recently there has been some debate about which new markers should be implemented to increase the success of typing degraded DNA: conventional STRs, miniSTRs, or SNPs. The EDNAP and ENFSI groups concluded that miniSTR analysis, in general, is the most effective approach for degraded DNA (Dixon et al. 2006).

## MINISTRS TIMELINE

The first evidence that smaller STRs worked better than larger loci was the successful analysis of severely degraded samples taken from the scene of the Branch Davidian fire in Waco (Texas) (Whitaker et al. 1995).

Afterwards some authors started to generate new primer pairs of STRs in monoplex reactions which showed an improvement in the efficiency of amplification, especially in degraded samples (Yoshida et al. 1997; Ricci et al. 1999).

Wiegand and Kleiber (2001) demonstrated that highly degraded DNA, as well as very low amounts of DNA, could be more successfully typed using some new redesigned PCR primers. These new primers were closer to the STR repeat compared to the established sequences that generated longer amplicons for the same loci. Later, these results were confirmed by a study where a multiplex reaction for the TH01, TPOX, CFS1PO, and vWA loci was performed with newly designed pair of primers (Tsukada et al. 2002).

Butler et al. (1998) started to work in mass spectrometry typing and multiplexing using small STR amplicons. New primer sets for Y chromosome and CODIS STR loci were designed and tested using conventional capillary electrophoresis instrumentation, showing reliable STR typing (Ruitberg et al. 2000).

Following the World Trade Center attacks, it quickly became evident that traditional methods for DNA typing were not likely to be fully successful in identifying all of the recovered remains. Thus, a big effort was made to improve and develop new technologies of DNA analysis to identify the huge number of victims (Holland et al. 2003). Indeed, the short STRs methodology was accelerated to be used in aid of victim's identifications.

## Table 1. Miniplex systems described.

| Author/s | Name | Included markers |
|---|---|---|
| Schumm et al. 2004<br>Bode Plexes were used in the WTC victim's analysis (2002) by the Forensic Institute of NYC. | BodePlex 1: | D13S317, D21S11, D7S820, D16S539, CSF1PO |
| | BodePlex 2: | TPOX, FGA, D7S820, D18S51 |
| Butler et al. 2003<br>In D3S317, D5S818 y VWA there is no concordance with commercial systems due to the presence of delections and dimers formation (Drabek et al. 2004) | Miniplex 1 | CSF1PO, TH01, TPOX |
| | Miniplex 2 | D5S818, D8S1179, D16S539 |
| | Miniplex 3 | FGA, D7S820, D21S11 |
| | Miniplex 4 | VWA, D13S317, D18 |
| | Miniplex 5 | Penta D, Penta E, D2S1338 |
| | Big Mini | CSF1PO, FGA, TH01, TPOX, D7S820, D21S11 |
| Chung et al. 2004 | Miniplex 2 | D5S818, D8S1179, D16S539 |
| | Miniplex 4 | VWA, D18S51, D13S317 |
| | Miniplex 5 | Penta D, Penta E, D2S1338 |
| | Big Mini | Multiplex 1: TH01, TPOX, CSF1PO<br>Multiplex 2: FGA, D21S11, D7S820 |
| Coble et al. 2005<br>Development of potential miniSTRs, candidates with more heterozigosity which produced < 125 bp amplicons. | Miniplex 1 | D10S1248, D14S1434, D22S1045 |
| | Miniplex 2 | D1S1677, D2S441, D4S2364 |
| Gill P et al. 2006<br>EDNAP/ENFSI recommendations for the development of new miniSTRs. | Miniplex 1 | D10S1248, D14S1434, D22S1045 |
| | Miniplex 2 | D12S391, D1S1656, TPOX |
| Wiegand et al. 2005 | Pentaplex | Amelogenin, TH01, D3S1358, VWA, FGA |
| | Multiplex 2 | TH01, D3S1358, VWA, FGA |
| | Blue kit | D3S1358, VWA, FGA |
| Butler et al. 2005a | Mini SGM | TH01, Amelogenin, FGA, D18S51, D16S539, D21S1138 |
| | Mini NC01 | D10S1248, D14S1434, D22S1045 |
| Hill et al. 2006.<br>Development of 27 new MiniSTR loci for improved analysis of degraded DNA samples. Poster B105 at AAFS Congress, Seattle, 2006. | NC01 | D10S1248, D14S1434, D22S1045 |
| | NC02 | D4S2364, D2S441, D1S1677 |
| | NC03 | D3S3053, D6S474, D20S482 |
| | NC04 | D1GATA113, D2S1776, D4S2408 |
| | NC05 | D1S1627, D5S2500, D8S1115, |
| | NC06 | D3S4529, D6S1017, D9S2157 |
| | NC07 | D9S1122, D10S1435, D12ATA63 |
| | NC08 | D17S1301, D18S853, D20S1082 |
| | NC09 | D6S1027, D17S974, D11S4463 |
| Hill C et al. 2006<br>Loci rejected and reasons for not considering them. | | D9S324: allelic displacement, presence of complex repetitions.<br>D10S1430: presence of complex repetitions.<br>D10S2327: profiles with three and four alleles.<br>D14S297: poor heterozigosity.<br>D15S817: profiles with three and four alleles. |

Butler and McCord developed five multiplex assays that covered all of the CODIS STR loci as well as D2S1338, Penta D, and Penta E, and they termed such systems as "miniSTRs" or "miniplexes" (Butler et al. 2003) (Table 1). They combined two sets of primers to develop the "Big Mini", which was used by the Office of Chief Medical Examiner of New York (NY OCME). However, the miniSTR concept still needed to be further studied to increase the sensitivity and be capable of working robustly on an industrial scale in order to process thousands of samples from the WTC site. Based on this strategy two "BodePlexes" were developed and used on samples from the WTC investigation (Schumm et al. 2004).

Since then, several miniplexes have been developed and evaluated to improve the strategy (Chung et al. 2004; Drabek et al. 2004; Coble et al. 2005; Opel et al. 2006; Hill et al. 2008).

Recently, the EDNAP and ENFSI groups recommended the implementation of miniSTRs as the way forward to increase both the robustness and sensitivity of forensic DNA analysis (Gill et al. 2006b).

An important progress for miniSTR technology was the development of the "MiniFiler" kit by Applied Biosystems, a 9-plex kit that proved its concordance with conventional STR typing kits (Hill et al. 2007).

## Pros and Cons of MiniSTRs

As it was previously commented, miniSTRs markers provide a very useful tool for analysing degraded DNA samples. Their small size increases success rate of degraded DNA analysis, allowing the recovery of valuable information from casework samples, which would gave negative or very partial results if analysed with STR markers (Wiegand et al. 2001, Tsukada et al. 2002, Coble et al. 2005, Grubwieser et al. 2006)

The usefulness of miniSTR assays has been confirmed in intra- and inter-laboratory studies involving degraded bones and aged blood and saliva stains (Opel et al. 2006, Butler et al. 2003). In all cases, miniSTR markers gave higher success rates in recovering information than conventional STR kits. Their efficacy has also been validated in telogen hairs, samples frequently found in crime scenes (Hellmann et al. 2001). Until the development of miniSTRs markers, it was complicated to obtain DNA profiles from these samples, because nuclear DNA from keratinized cells was highly degraded (about 100 bp in size), and as result, the use of conventional STRs would show a low success rate or even fail.

MiniSTRs loci also provide a very sensible approach that permits to obtain genetic profiles from low amounts of DNA. Whereas traditional STR testing works best with about 1-2 nanograms of DNA, miniplexes can get valuable results from 0.25-0.5 nanograms of DNA, or even from less than this quantity of DNA. Furthermore, the new miniSTR systems will also significantly increase the success of amplification of samples containing PCR inhibitors, such as humic acids or heme groups, which adversely affect the STR multiplex systems (Eisenberg et al. 2007).

The compatibility of several miniplexes with commercial STR kits has been tested to check possible discrepancies due to allele dropouts. A high concordance of results between the two methods was established (Drabek et al. 2004, Hill et al. 2007). This compatibility with STRs will allow the comparison between miniSTRs, and CODIS and international databasing standards, reducing the possibility of discrepancies.

Actually these new markers are not meant to replace the current CODIS loci, but complement them, especially in cases where additional genetic information is needed. For example, in situations where there are closely related individuals involved, such as complex paternity cases (e.g., incest) or mass disasters, the use of miniSTRs will increase the discriminating power of the multiplexes. In fact, the implementation of miniSTRs will augment both the robustness and sensitivity of analysis, providing additional statistical support for an association. Indeed, the kit Minifiler (Applied Biosystems) offers highly discrimination results with probability of Identity values of less than $1 \times 10^{-10}$ for US populations.

Moreover, miniSTRs constitutes a good alternative to mtDNA typing in degraded samples, as the results obtained by mtDNA analysis cannot always be compared with DNA profiles from routine casework or from databases.

Furthermore, new laboratory equipment or additional staff training is not necessary to work with miniSTRs, because the same methodology as STRs is used. Consequently, the implementation of these markers in laboratories will not cause further technical or economical difficulties. Besides, alternative technologies such as high-speed microfluidic and time-of-flight mass spectrometric can be applied to these miniplexes (Butler et al. 1998, 2001, Schmalzing et al. 1997).

Unfortunately, the miniSTRs have some disadvantages. A major inconvenient is the small number of miniSTRs that can be coamplified in the same multiplex reaction. As a result of the size reduction, the different miniSTR loci have a similar size range (~100bp), causing their overlapping within the same fluorescent dye lane. For this reason, there will be typically one miniSTR locus per dye color (instead of the 4 or more loci included in STRs multiplex). This will decrease the power of discrimination of multiplexes; for example, a 6-miniplex with 100% amplification success will give less genetic information than a 16-plex where the six largest amplicons loci have dropped out (Parsons et al. 2007). One way to overcome this limitation is to combine the typical 5-dye fluorescent system with the addition of non-nucleotide linkers. This will allow the simultaneous amplification and efficient separation of the different miniSTR loci, without the risk of overlapping.

Another important limitation is that not all STRs can be reduced in size. For example, some of the CODIS core loci have large allele ranges that make not viable the design of smaller amplicons (e.g. FGA, with a range size of 156 pb). In other cases, it is not possible to bring primers as close as possible to the STR repeat region, because the flanking sequences contain polymorphic nucleotides, partial repeats, mononucleotide repeat stretches, or insertions/deletions that could prevent stable primer annealing. This is the case of D7S820 locus that contains a poly-T stretch, located 13 nucleotides downstream of the core repeat, and that can have eight, nine, or ten T's. Consequently, the reverse primer for this marker has to be outside the poly-T stretch to retain this variation and permit full concordance with commercial STR kit results. The design of primers for other loci also shows similar problems. FGA has a partial repeat and the mononucleotide repeat stretch "TTTC TTCC TTTC TTTTTT" downstream of the core repeat. In order to avoid this problematic region, the reverse primer for FGA binds 23 nucleotides away from the end of the repeat, limiting the size reduction (Butler et al. 2003).

Another point to be considered is the fact that different primers are used in STR and miniSTR typing, so possible genotyping inconsistencies can be observed due to allele dropout. Indeed if some point mutations, insertions or deletions happened in the STR flanking regions, but outside of the miniSTR primer binding sites, STR primer annealing could be prevented. Consequently an allelic dropout could appear, causing potential discrepancies with miniSTR results, since the individual would be erroneously considered homozygous for this locus. For example, loci D8S1179 and vWA have some polymorphic nucleotides in the flanking region that will affect STR amplification causing allele dropout, but it will not have effect on miniSTR typing (Alves et al. 2001, Han et al. 2001, Budowle et al. 2001).

Another problem of concordance can be seen in D13S317 locus typing. This locus has a four-base deletion of TGTC that is 24 bases downstream from the core. The miniSTR reverse primer is located between the repeat region and the potential deletion sequence, thus its amplification will not be affected by the mutation. On the contrary, STR primers are located outside of the deletion region, so in presence of the deletion, the amplification product will be 4bp shorter than in miniSTR typing (Boutrand et al. 2001).

A different problem to solve is the potential contamination derived from the high number of cycles used in the amplification (28-35 cycles). Since such a small sample is being amplified, this can be easily contaminated by exogenous DNA. Moreover, it is important to consider that despite the high sensitivity of the method, PCR inhibition problems can occur. Although shorter fragments are supposed to amplify more efficiently and be more resistant to Taq polymerase inhibition, the presence of inhibitors can also affect the PCR (Parsons et al. 2007).

## NULL ALLELES IN MINISTRS

As we mentioned above, occasionally, sequence variation (point mutations or indels) could occur in the flanking region of commonly used STR loci. As result, the primer annealing to the STR locus during amplification can be prevented, resulting in a null allele. This phenomenon can result highly problematic in the interpretation of results, since a heterozygote for a detected allele and a null allele can be erroneously considered as homozygote for the detected allele. Other possible causes of microsatellite null alleles are the preferential amplification of short alleles (large allele dropout) or PCR failure due to low quality or quantity of DNA (Wattier et al. 1998, Wanderler et al. 2003).

There are various approaches to estimate the frequencies of null alleles. Chakraborty (1992) and Brookfield (1996) estimated null allele frequencies through statistical analysis of STR typing data, assuming that the heterozygote deficiency is caused by null alleles and not by other genotyping errors. They predicted potential null alleles comparing the observed and expected heterozygosities based on Hardy–Weinberg (HW) equilibrium. The statistical methods are indirect approaches to the detection of microsatellite null alleles. In fact, the best approach is a molecular study by directly sequencing the null allele.

Understandably the presence of null alleles will have a strong impact in population genetic databases, as they can bias allele frequencies and produce an apparent deficiency of heterozygosity (or excess of homozygosity), compared with Hardy-Weinberg expectations. This can be solved by doing less rigorous searches in databases.

On the other hand, null alleles will also create difficulties in forensic studies since they can lead to incorrect exclusions of samples that are from the same source but appeared to be different. Indeed, they can cause false parentage exclusion if the parent and child in question show an apparent homozygosis for different alleles (Dakin et al. 2004).

After detecting a null allele in a STR locus, there are several possible solutions to correct it, such as discarding the problematic locus, redesigning the primers, using degenerate primers (that include the problematic primer binding site variant), or adjusting allele and genotype frequencies based on the estimated null allele frequency (Butler 2005b).

It is important to consider all known information about flanking sequence variation in the design of primers to avoid possible null alleles. Furthermore, primer concordance studies are indispensable to look for possible discrepancies between commercial kits and miniplexes.

## Standardization of STR Loci

EDNAP and ENFSI have collaborated to standardize DNA profiles in Europe, so comparisons between laboratories become straightforward (Gill et al. 2006a). Most of this standarization effort has focused on STR loci (Chakraborty et al, 1999; Gill, 2002; Butler, 2006) and as a result they have become nearly the gold standard in Forensic Genetics. Intelligent banks for Criminal purposes have been built on a consensus set of 13 core STR markers (CODIS system) established by the FBI Laboratory (Budowle et al, 1998). This core includes the 13 STR loci, CSF1PO, FGA, TH01, TPOX, VWA, D3S1358, D5S818, D7S820, D8S1179, D13S317, D16S539, D18S51, and D21S11.

Nowadays a number of different STR multiplexes are in use for Forensic casework. In fact, even though there are seven Interpol STR loci established (Schneider et al. 2001; Martin et al. 2001), for instance, most European laboratories show a much higher degree of compatibility because they use the same multiplex systems as AmpFlSTR® SGM Plus, AmpFlSTR® Identifiler, or PowerPlex 16® System. However, it is still necessary to modify existing multiplexes to increase success rates in degraded DNA typing (Schneider et al 2004).

The rapid implementation of new loci in National databases would be possible as a result of the high level of scientific and technical standardisation reached in forensic laboratories. Nevertheless, due to the differences between countries in the choice of loci included in National DNA databases it is important to adapt new multiplexes to national requirements. The most practical strategy would be to design multiplexes that incorporate new loci, in addition to those currently used, rather than discarding the existing loci. Furthermore, if miniSTRs were included in the multiplexes already established higher success rates could be achieved with degraded samples.

Other issues to solve are legislative and political considerations. In fact, in some countries this would mean to alter the existing legislation to be able to include new markers.

Recently, it has been proposed to connect database laboratories using virtual networks, instead of using a centralised database. With this system, each country would maintain control over their databases and access to other databases information according to local legislative requirements. Additionally, searches would not be limited to the Interpol core loci.

Databases should be dynamic and keep up with the scientific development of Forensic Genetics. Thus, new genetic markers could be changed or included if one of these reasons exists:

1. To improve the system's discrimination power.

2. To improve the analytical sensitivity of low copy number.
3. To improve the robustness or quality of the results.

Since national DNA databases have been built using different multiplexes, it is not realistic to suggest the retirement of existent loci in favour of new ones. For this reason, the investigation of new core loci has been proposed, making possible to laboratories to expand their multiplexes while maintaining their existing set of STRs. These new core loci will be decided by the EDNAP group in collaboration with the ENFSI group. Afterwards some less value loci could be retired, even though the information after their analysis stayed as a remnant in databases.

## ENFSI/EDNAP Recommendations about the Incorporation of New MiniSTRs

1. MiniSTRs will be adopted as the approach to increase the robustness and sensitivity of DNA analysis.
2. Core loci in national databases will be retained and transformed into miniSTRs by re-engineering, moving the primers closer to the repetitive region (Drabek et al. 2004; Hellman et al. 2001).
3. It is recommended the adoption of a new multiplex called Miniplex 1 (Table 2), with D12S1248, D22S1045, D2S441 markers between 70 and 125 bp. Also, DS441 instead of D14S1434, because the second one has a low discrimination power in comparison with the other loci (D2S441, PD = 1/2500; D14S1434, PD = 1/7).
4. A secondary loci list which could be converted into miniSTRs has been compiled. This multiplex 2 includes D12S391, D1S1656, and TPOX markers. The first ones are miniSTRs between 120 and 180 bp. These loci are not in consensus, but they are recommended as additional loci to increase the multiplex size (Hellman et al. 2001; Gill et al. 1998; Shigeta et al. 2002).
5. The new multiplexes should be similar in sensitivity to that already existent, which means they should be able to detect DNA in quantities less than 250 pg, using standard PCR amplification methods. The main purpose is to facilitate partially degraded DNA detection, taking into account the correct balance of multiplex size versus its efficiency.
6. It is suggested that ENFSI/EDNAP evaluate new multiplexes following the proposed recommendations.

Table 2. Miniplex I (recommended by ENFSI/EDNAP) is derived from miniplex NC01 developed by NIST (Coble et al. 2005; Butler et al. 2003).

| STR | Repetition | Motif | Chromosomic position | Observed size pb | Observed heterozigosity |
|---|---|---|---|---|---|
| D22S1045 | Tri | TAA | Crom 22, 35.78 Mb | 76 109 | 0,784 |
| D2S441 | Tetra | TCTA | Crom 6, 68.21 Mb | 78 – 110 | 0,774 |
| D10S1248 | Tetra | GGAA | Crom 10, 130.57 Mb | 83 - 123 | 0,792 |

## NEW AUTOSOMAL MINISTRS STRATEGIES

Different strategies for the development of a new generation of STRs have been proposed (Gill et al. 2006a). Two different but parallel strategies have been adopted according to the different requirements within Europe.

The first strategy employs a 13 STR loci-multiplex that includes three mini-STRs: D12S1248, D22S1045, and D2S441. Laboratories that prefer this strategy will typically wish to work with a single multiplex for all evidential types and will routinely analyse a significant proportion of highly degraded samples. The intention here is that the new multiplex will quickly replace the current multiplex.

On the other hand, the second strategy is to modify a multiplex of six high molecular weight STRs (commonly used), to create smaller amplicons. This will be combined with an additional two loci of high discriminating power, D12S391 and D1S1656. Additionally, it has been proposed to reduce TPOX size. In this case, this new multiplex will be used in conjunction with existing multiplex systems rather than acting as a replacement

These different approaches arise mainly from differences in the emphasis of the type of evidential material that is routinely analysed and in laboratory practices. However, there is full agreement that the overriding requirement is that both strategies must converge to achieve the aim of increasing the number of universal loci to be used throughout Europe, through the use of a new multiplex of 15 STR loci of international level (Gill et al. 2006a).

These new miniSTRs should not replace the actual STRs collection, but complement it, in particular in disaster cases where highly degraded DNA exists (Gill et al. 2004).

Butler (2002) suggested the development by re-engineering of a miniplex that included the 13 CODIS STRs. This system -named "autoplex"-, should have lower allelic ranges, a reduction of "stutters", should cover all 22 autosomal chromosomes and sexual chromosomes, and should exhibit more robust characteristics.

## OTHER MINISTRS MULTIPLEXES

Until recently, most studies focused on developing autosomal miniSTRs multiplexes to improve recovery rates from difficult samples. Nevertheless, new efforts have been made to develop alternative procedures for the analysis of degraded DNA, with the successful characterization of Y-chromosome and X-chromosome miniSTRs.

Forensic interest in gonosomal polymorphisms (Y and X chromosomes) has increased notably in the last years, especially Y chromosome studies (Roewer et al, 2001). The singular features of this chromosome, which include haploidy, paternal inheritance and lack of recombination through most of its length, make the Y chromosome a powerful tool for forensic, genealogical and evolutionary studies (Jobling et al. 1997, de Knijff et al. 1997; González-Andrade et al, 2009a). A high amount of Y-STRs and population data have been published (Redd et al. 2002, Hanson et al. 2006, Roewer et al. 2001; González-Andrade et al, 2009b; Martínez-Jarreta et al, 2005). Although there are some commercial kits such as AmpflSTR Y-filer kit (Applied Biosystems) and Power Plex Y sytem (Promega) for routine casework, they are not optimized for working with degraded DNA samples. This is especially accentuated in STR loci exceeding 200 bp, where the possibility of allelic dropout is high, due to DNA fragmentation. For this reason and with the aim of increasing the success rate of Y-STR typing for degraded DNA, several miniY-chromosomal STR multiplex have been developed.

One of the first studies on Y-chromosome miniSTRs was carried out by Park et al. (2007), creating two Y-miniplexes of 21 reduced Y-STR loci. They included the 17 Y-STR loci of the commercial kit AmpFlSTR® Yfiler™ (DYS19, DYS385, DYS389-I, DYS389-II, DYS390, DYS391, DYS392, DYS393, DYS437, DYS438, DYS439, DYS448, DYS456, DYS458, DYS635, and GATA H4.1) and other four loci (DYS388, DYS446, DYS447, and DYS449) to augment the discrimination capacity. At the end, they were able to reduce the size of 9 Y-STRs (DYS385, DYS390, DYS391, DYS392, DYS438, DYS439, DYS448, and DYS635); the other primers could not be redesigned because of the prior small size of the amplicon size or other motifs. According to the study, the Y-miniplexes will increase the number of analyzed loci, increasing the discrimination power of the Y-STR profiles. However, they need to be fully forensically validated, requiring a primer concordance study and an evaluation of non-human samples.

Other research group headed by Asamura (2007) has also developed their own Y-miniplexes, concretely two quadruplex systems, which include DYS504, DYS508, DYS522, DYS540, DYS556, DYS570, DYS576 and DYS632. As a result, they obtained PCR amplification products for the eight loci ranged in length from 95 bp (DYS632) to 147 bp (DYS570). Their miniplexes proved to be helpful tools for forensic analysis of degraded DNA samples. Afterwards, the same working group designed new multiplexes for 16 polymorphic Y-STR loci: DYS441, DYS446, DYS462, DYS481, DYS485, DYS495, DYS505, DYS510, DYS511, DYS549, DYS575, DYS578, DYS593, DYS618, DYS638, and DYS643 (products from 91 bp to 151 bp). These new miniplexes were more efficient than the kit AmpflSTR Yfiler when typing degraded DNA (Asamura et al. 2008).

Regarding to the X-chromosome, so far, it has played a minor role in forensic science. Nevertheless, it can be efficiently used to complement the analysis of other genetic markers (autosomal, Y-chromosomal and mtDNA) in forensic casework. It is a very potent tool in complex kinship and deficiency paternity, when the disputed child is female; and in forensic casework to identify the female DNA profile in mixture analysis (Szibor et al. 2003). Although many X-STRs have been validated for forensic testing, additional population studies are needed (Bini 2005, Pereira 2007). As well as in autosomal and Y chromosome STRs, shorter amplicons are necessary to efficiently analyze degraded DNA. Asamura et al. (2006) have designed an effective system for analyzing X-chromosomal short tandem repeats in highly degraded DNA. They generated two miniX-multiplex PCR systems for DXS7423, DXS6789, DXS101, GATA31E08, DXS8378, DXS7133, DXS7424, and GATA165B12. This new miniplexes showed a high effectiveness in analyzing degraded DNA.

Another common problem with degraded DNA samples is to reliably determine their gender. The amelogin test is routinely used to define the sex of DNA samples in forensic cases as it is integrated in most commercial kits. The amelogin gene has two homologous alleles, one on the X chromosome and the other on the Y chromosome, AMELX and AMELY, respectively. Since females have two X-chromosomes, in the typing there will be just one peak corresponding to the AMELX, whereas males (XY) will also have an AMELY peak. However, it has been reported that there can be misleading results, because of primer binding mutations or large-scale deletions in Y chromosome. As a result, males with deletions in the amelogenin gene on the Y chromosome can be erroneously typed as females. To solve this problem, a new PCR multiplex has been designed by Esteve et al. (2008). It includes 4 mini-X-STR loci and fragments of SRY and amelogenine genes, with product sizes less than 140bp. This short size will be positive to detect the gender when working with degraded DNA.

## FUTURE

It is likely that miniSTRs will play a role in the future of degraded DNA analysis probably helping to recover information that would be lost with larger loci from conventional megaplex amplification. Nevertheless, new miniSTRs should not replace the actual STRs collection, but complement it. Furthermore it would be interesting to cover the same loci with STR and miniSTRs primers, so they could be used in routine or difficult cases, respectively. Reasonably, concordance studies would be needed to make possible the comparison of results from both typing methods.

At present, new markers with smaller allele ranges, low stutter and improved characteristics are being studied as possible miniSTRs candidates, which could increase the chance of success in highly degraded samples and the resulting power of discrimination of existing multiplexes.

## COMPETING INTERESTS

The authors declare that they have no competing interests. The authors alone are responsible for the content and writing of the paper.

## REFERENCES

Alves C, Amorim A, Gusmao L, Pereira L. VWA STR genotyping: further inconsistencies between Perkin-Elmer and Promega kits. *Int J Legal Med*, 2001; 115(2):97–9.

Asamura H, Sakai H, Kobayashi K, Ota M, Fukushima H. MiniX-STR multiplex system population study in Japan and application to degraded DNA analysis. *Int J Legal Med* 2006 120:174–181.

Asamura H, Sakai H, Ota M, Fukushima H. MiniY-STR quadruplex systems with short amplicon lengths for analysis of degraded DNA samples. *Forensic Sci Int Genet*, 2007; 1:56–61.

Asamura H, Fujimori S, Ota M, Oki T, Fukushima H. Evaluation of miniY-STR multiplex PCR systems for extended 16 Y-STR loci. *Int J Legal Med*, 2008; 122(1):43-9.

Bender K, Schneider PM, Rittner C. Application of mtDNA sequence analysis in forensic casework for the identification of human remains. *Forensic Sci Int*, 2000;113(1–3):103–7.

Bini C, Ceccardi S, Ferri G, Pelotti S, Alù M, Roncaglia E, Beduschi G, Caenazzo L, Ponzano E, Tasinato P, Turchi C, Buscemi L, Mazzanti M, Tagliabracci A, Toni C, Spinetti I, Domenici R, Presciuttini S. (2005) Development of a heptaplex PCR system to analyse X-chromosome STR loci from five Italian population samples. *A collaborative study Forensic Sci Int*, 2005;153(2-3):231-6.

Bouakaze C, Keyser C, Amory S, Crubézy E, Ludes B.First successful assay of Y-SNP typing by SNaPshot minisequencing on ancient DNA. *Int J Legal Med.* 2007 Nov; 121(6):493-9.

Boutrand L, Egyed B, Furedi S, Mommers N, Mertens G, Vandenberghe A. Variations in primer sequences are the origin of allele dropout at lociD13S317 and CD4. *Int J Legal Med*, 2001; 114(4–5):295–7.

Brookfield JFY. (1996) A simple new method for estimating null allele frequency from heterozygote deficiency. *Molecular Ecology*, 1996; 5: 453–455.

Budowle B, Moretti TR, Niezgoda SJ, Brown BL. CODIS and PCR-based short tandem repeat loci: law enforcement tools. *Second European Symposium on Human Identification 1998*, Madison, Wisconsin: Promega Corporation, 1998. pp. 73-88.

Budowle B, Masibay A, Anderson SJ, Barna C, Biega L, Brenneke S, Brown BL, Cramer J, DeGroot GA, Douglas D, Duceman B, Eastman A, Giles R, Hamill J, Haase DJ, Janssen DW, Kupferschmid TD, Lawton T, Lemire C, Llewellyn B, Moretti T, Neves J, Palaski C, Schueler S, Sgueglia J, Sprecher C, Tomsey C, Yet D. *STR primer concordance study. Forensic Sci Int.* 2001 Dec 15;124(1):47-54.

Butler JM, Li J, Shaler TA, Monforte JA, Becker CH. Reliable genotyping of short tandem repeat loci without an allelic ladder using time-of-flight mass spectrometry. *Int J Legal Med*, 1998;112(1):45–49.

Butler JM, Becker CH. Improved analysis of DNA short tandem repeats with time-of-flight mass spectrometry. Washington, DC: Science and Technology Research Report, *National Institute of Justice.* 2001 Oct.

Butler JM. MiniSTR Development to Aid Testing of Degraded Samples. *Poster in NIJ's 3rd WTC Kinship and DNA Analysis Panel.* 2002. Albany, New York.

Butler JM, Shen Y, McCord BR. The development of reduced size STR amplicons as tools for the analysis of degraded DNA. *J Forensic Sci* 2003; 48(5):1054–64.

Butler JM. NIST On-Going Projects to Aid the Human Identity Testing Community. *Talk at NIJ DNA Grantees meeting* (Washington, D.C.) 2005a.

Butler J. Forensic DNA Typing – Biology, *Technology, and Genetics of STR Markers Second Edition*, Academic Press, 2005b.

Butler J. Genetics and genomics of core short tandem repeat loci used in human identity testing. *J Forensic Sci* 2006; 51 (2): 253-65.

Butler JM, Coble MD, Vallone PM. STRs vs. SNPs: thoughts on the future of forensic DNA testing. *Forensic Sci Med Pathol* (2007) 3:200–205.

Chakraborty R, De Andrade M, Daiger SP, Budowle B. Apparent heterozygote deficiencies observed in DNA typing data and their implications in forensic applications. *Annals of Human Genetics*,1992; 56:45–57.

Chakraborty R, Stivers DN, Su B, Zhong Y, Budowle B. The utility of short tandem repeat loci beyond human identification: implications for development of new DNA typing systems. *Electrophoresis* 1999; 20 (8): 1682-96.

Chung D, Drábek J, Opel K, Butler J, McCord B. A study on the effects of degradation and template concentration on the amplification efficiency of the STR Miniplex primer sets. *J Forensic Sci* 2004; 49 (4): 733-40.

Coble MD, Butler JM. Characterization of new miniSTR loci to aid analysis of degraded DNA, *J. Forensic Sci,* 2005; 50: 43–53.

Cotton E.A., Allsop R.F., Guest J.L., Frazier R.R.E., Koumi P., Callow I.P., Seager A., Sparkes R.L. Validation of the AMPFlSTR(R) SGM Plus™ system for use in forensic casework. *Forensic Science International,* 2000;112: 151–161.

Dakin EE, Avise JC. Microsatellite null alleles in parentage analysis. *Heredity* 2004; 93: 504–509.

de Knijff P, Kayser M, Caglià A, Corach D, Fretwell N, Gehrig C, Graziosi G, Heidorn F, Herrmann S, Herzog B, Hidding M, Honda K, Jobling M, Krawczak M, Leim K, Meuser S, Meyer E, Oesterreich W, Pandya A, Parson W, Penacino G, Perez-Lezaun A, Piccinini A, Prinz M, Roewer L, et al.. Chromosome Y microsatellites: population genetic and evolutionary aspects. *Int J Legal Med,* 1997; 110(3):134-49.

Dixon LA, Dobbins AE, Pulker HK, Butler JM, Vallone PM, Coble MD, Parson W, Berger B, Grubwieser P, Mogensen HS, Morling N, Nielsen K, Sanchez JJ, Petkovski E, Carracedo A, Sanchez-Diz P, Ramos-Luis E, Brion M, Irwin JA, Just RS, Loreille O, Parsons TJ, Syndercombe-Court D, Schmitter H, Stradmann-Bellinghausen B, Bender K, Gill P. Analysis of artificially degraded DNA using STRs and SNPs – results of a collaborative European (EDNAP) exercise. *Forensic Sci Int,* 2006; 164(1):33-44.

Drabek J, Chung DT, Butler JM, McCord BR. Concordance study between miniplex STR assays and a commercial STR typing kit. *J Forensic Sci,* 2004;49(4):859–60.

Eisenberg AJ., Planz J V. Field Test of Current Technology Used in the Identification of Unidentified Remains. *2007 National Criminal Justice Reference Service* 2004-DN-BX-K214.

Esteve Codina A, Niederstätter H, Parson W. "GenderPlex" a PCR multiplex for reliable gender determination of degraded human DNA samples and complex gender constellations. *Int J Legal Med,* 2008 Dec.

Fondevila M, Phillips C, Naverán N, Cerezo M, Rodríguez A, CalvoR, Fernández LM, Carracedo A, Lareu M.V. Challenging DNA: Assessment of a range of genotyping approaches for highly degraded forensic samples. *Forensic Science International* 2008; 1 (Suppl.): S26-28.

Gill P. Role of short tandem repeat DNA in forensic casework in the UK-past, present, and future perspectives. Biotechniques 2002; 32 (2): 366-72.

Gill P Fereday L, Morling N, Schneider P. New multiplexes for Europe-amendments and clarification of strategic development. *Forensic Sci Int,* 2006a; 163: 155-7.

Gill P, Fereday L, Morling N, Schneider P. The evolution of DNA databases-Recommendations for new European STR loci. *Forensic Sci Int,* 2006b; 156: 242-4.

González-Andrade F, Sánchez D, Penacino B, Martínez-Jarreta B. Two fathers for the same child: a deficient paternity case of false inclusion with autosomic STRs. *Forensic Sci Int Genet,* 2009a; 3 (2): 138-40.

González-Andrade F, Roewer L, Willuweit S, Sánchez D, Martínez-Jarreta B. Y-STR variation among ethnic groups from Ecuador: Mestizos, Kichwas, Afro-Ecuadorans and Waoranis. *Forensic Sci Int Genet,* 2009b; 3 (3): e83-91.

Grubwieser P, Muhlmann R, Berger B, Niederstatter H, Pavlic M, Parson W. A new ''miniSTR-multiplex'' displaying reduced amplicon lengths for the analysis of degraded DNA, *Int. J. Legal Med,* 2006; 120: 115–120.

Han GR, Song ES, Hwang JJ. Non-amplification of an allele of the D8S1179 locus due to a point mutation. *Int J Legal Med* 2001; 115(1):45–7.

Hanson EK, Berdos PN, Ballantyne J.Testing and evaluation of 43 "noncore" Y chromosome markers for forensic casework applications. *J Forensic Sci,* 2006; 51(6):1298-314.

Hellmann A, Rohleder U, Schmitter H, Wittig M.STR typing of human telogen hairs – a new approach. *Int J Legal Med,* 2001;114(4-5):269-73.

Hill C, Coble D, Butler JM. *Development of 27 new miniSTR loci for improved analysis of degraded DNA samples.* Poster B105 at AAFS Congress, Seatle, 2006.

Hill C, Kline M., Mulero J., Lagace R.E., Chang C., Hennessy L., Butler J. Concordance study between the AmpFlSTR MiniFiler PCR Amplification Kit and conventional STR typing kits. *J. Forensic Sci,* 2007; 52(4): 870-873.

Hill C, Kline M, Coble M, Butler J. Characterization of 26 miniSTR loci for improved analysis of degraded DNA samples. *J Forensic Sci,* 2008; 53 (1): 73-80.

Holland M, Cave C, Holland C, Bille T. Development of a quality, high throughput DNA analysis procedure for skeletal samples to assist with the identification of victims from the World Trade Center attacks. *Croat Med J,* 2003; 44 (3): 264-72.

Jobling MA, Pandya A, Tyler-Smith C. The Y chromosome in forensic analysis and paternity testing. *Int J Legal Med,* 1997; 110:118–124.

Just R.S., Irwin J.A., O'Callaghan J.E., Saunier J.L., Coble M.D., Vallone P.M., Butler J.M., Barritt S.M., Parsons T.J. Toward increased utility of mtDNA in forensic identifications, *Forensic Sci. Int,* 2004; 146 (Suppl.): S147–S149.

Martin P, Schmitter H, Schneider P. A brief history of the formation of DNA databases in forensic science within Europe. *Forensic Sci Int,* 2001; 119: 225–231.

Martínez-Jarreta B, Vásquez P, Abecia E, Budowle B, Luna A, Peiró F. Characterization of 17 Y-STR loci in a population from El Salvador (San Salvador, Central America) and their potential for DNA profiling. J Forensic Sci, 2005; 50 (5): 1243-6.

Odriozola A, Aznar JM, Valverde L, Cardoso S, Bravo ML, Builes JJ, Martínez B, Sanchez D, González-Andrade F, Sarasola E, González-Fernánez MC, Jarreta BM, De Pancorbo MM. SNPSTR rs59186128_D7S820 polymorphism distribution in European Caucasoid, Hispanic, and Afro-American populations. *Int J Leg Med*, 2009; [Epub ahead of print].

Opel KL, Chung DT, Drábek J, Tatarek NE, Jantz LM, McCord BR. The application of miniplex primer sets in the analysis of degraded DNA from human skeletal remains. *J Forensic Sci,* 2006; 51(2):351-6.

Park MJ, Lee HY, Chung U, Kang SC, Shin KJ. Y-STR analysis of degraded DNA using reduced-size amplicons. *Int J Legal Med,*2007; 121:152–157.

Parsons TJ, Coble MD. Increasing the forensic discrimination of mitochondrial DNA testing through analysis of the entire mitochondrial DNA genome. *Croat Med J,* 2001; 42:304–309.

Parsons TJ, Huel R, Davoren J, Katzmarzyk C, Milos A, Selmanović A, Smajlović L, Coble MD, Rizvić A.Application of novel "mini-amplicon" STR multiplexes to high volume casework on degraded skeletal remains. *Forensic Sci Int Genet.* 2007 Jun;1(2):175-9.

Pereira R, Gomes I, Amorim A, Gusmao L. (2007) Genetic diversity of 10 X chromosome STRs in northern Portugal. *Int J Legal Med;* 121:192–197.

Quintáns B, Alvarez-Iglesias V, Salas A, Phillips C, Lareu MV, Carracedo A. Typing of mitochondrial DNA coding region SNPs of forensic and anthropological interest using SNaPshot minisequencing. *Forensic Sci Int,* 2004; 140(2-3):251-7.

Redd AJ, Agellon AB, Kearney VA, Contreras VA, Karafet T, Park H, de Knijff P, Butler JM, Hammer MF. Forensic value of 14 novel STRs on the human Y chromosome. *Forensic Sci Int,* 2002; 130(2-3):97-111.

Ricci U, Giovannucci M, Klintschar M. Modified primers for D12S391 and a modified silver stainning technique. *Int J Legal Med,* 1999; 112: 342-4.

Roewer L, Krawczak M, Willuweit S, Nagy M, Alves C, Amorim A, Anslinger K, Augustin C, Betz A, Bosch E, Cagliá A, Carracedo A, Corach D, Dekairelle AF, Dobosz T, Dupuy BM, Füredi S, Gehrig C, Gusmaõ L, Henke J, Henke L, Hidding M, Hohoff C, Hoste B, Jobling MA, Kärgel HJ, de Knijff P, Lessig R, Liebeherr E, Lorente M, Martínez-Jarreta B, Nievas P, Nowak M, Parson W, Pascali VL, Penacino G, Ploski R, Rolf B, Sala A, Schmidt U, Schmitt C, Schneider PM, Szibor R, Teifel-Greding J, Kayser M. Online reference database of European Y-chromosomal short tandem repeat (STR) haplotypes. *Forensic Sci Int,* 2001; 118(2-3):106-13.

Ruitberg C, Butler J. New Primer Sets for Y Chromosome and CODIS STR Loci. In: *11th International Symposium on Human Identification,* 2000.

Schmalzing D, Koutny L, Adourian A, Belgrader P, Matsudaira P, Ehrlich D. DNA typing in thirty seconds with a microfabricated device. *Proc Natl Acad Sci USA* 1997;94:10273–8.

Schneider P, Martin P. Criminal DNA databases: the European situation. *Forensic Sci Int,* 2001; 119: 232–238.

Schneider P, Bender K, Mayr W, Parson W, Hoste B, Decorte R, et al.. STR analysis of artificially degraded DNA results of a collaborative European exercise. *Forensic Sci Int,* 2004; 139: 123-34.

Schumm J, Wingrove R, Douglas E. Robust STR multiplexes for challenging casework samples. *Progress in Forensic Genetics ICS,* 2004; 1261: 547-9.

Shigeta Y, Yamamoto Y, Doi Y, Miyaishi S, Ishizu H. Evaluation of a method for typing the microsatellite D12S391 locus using a new primer pair and capillary electrophoresis, *Acta Med. Okayama* 56 (2002) 229–36.

Stone AC, Starrs JE and Stoneking M. Mitochondrial DNA analysis of the presumptive remains of Jesse James. *Journal of Forensic Sciences,* 2001; 46:173-176.

Szibor R, Krawczak M, Hering S, Edelmann J, Kuhlisch E, Krause D. Use of X-linked markers for forensic purposes. *Int J Legal Med,* 2003 117:67–74.

Tsukada K., Takayanagi K., Asamura H., Ota M., Fukushima H. Multiplex short tandem repeat typing in degraded samples using newly designed primers for the TH01, TPOX, CSF1PO, and vWA loci, *Legal Med,* 2002; 4: 239–245.

Wallin J M; Buoncristiani M R; Lazaruk K D; Fildes N; Holt C L; Walsh P S. TWGDAM validation of the AmpFISTR blue PCR amplification kit for forensic casework analysis. *Journal of forensic sciences* 1998; 43(4):854-70.

Wandeler P, Smith S, Morin PA, Pettifor RA, Funk SM. Patterns of nuclear DNA degeneration over time – a case study in historic teeth samples. *Molecular Ecology* 2003;12(4):1087-93.

Wattier R, Engel CR, Saumitou-Laprade P, Valero M. Short allele dominance as a source of heterozygote deficiency at microsatellite loci: experimental evidence at the inucleotidelocus Gv1CT in Gracilaria gracilis (Rhodophyta). *Mol Ecol,* 1998; 7:1569–1573.

Whitaker J, Clayton T, Urquhart A, Millican E, Downes T, Kimpton C, et al.. Short tandem repeat typing of bodies from a mass disaster: high success rate and characteristic amplification patterns in highly degraded samples. *BioTechniques,* 1995; 18(4): 670-7.

Wiegand P, Kleiber M. Less is more—length reduction of STR amplicons using redesigned primers, *Int. J. Legal Med*, 2001; 114: 285–287.

Yoshida K, Sekiguchi K, Kasai K, Sato H, Seta S, Sensabaugh G. Evaluation of new primers for CSF1PO. *Int J Legal Med,* 1997; 110: 36-8.

In: Forensic Genetics Research Progress
Editor: F. Gonzalez-Andrade

ISBN: 978-1-60876-198-2
© 2010 Nova Science Publishers, Inc.

*Chapter 8*

# THE STUDY OF ANCIENT DNA IN FORENSIC GENETICS

## *Cecilia Sosa\* and Begoña Martínez-Jarreta*

Forensic Genetics Laboratory, Forensic Medicine Department, University of Zaragoza, Calle Domingo Miral s/n, Zaragoza 50.009, Spain

## ABSTRACT

The vertiginous progress in molecular biological techniques has enabled the retrieval and analysis of DNA from very diverse ancient specimens. This has broadened the spectrum of possibilities for Paleobiology and Genetic Anthropology and many exciting reports have come through. However, along with the technical progresses, the field has revealed certain peculiarities and drawbacks that on occasions could raise reasonable doubts on the authenticity of reported results. In this paper a review of the history of this challenging field is summarized. Since this is a vast and ever growing speciality, we will focus on the study of ancient DNA from human skeletal remains and on its Forensic applications. Particularities of bone diagenesis related to DNA preservation, features of ancient DNA molecules, unique characteristics, preservation conditions of skeletal remains, etc., are factors that make genetic typing of ancient bones and teeth a challenging task. The main technical issues on DNA analysis, such as molecular damage, exogenous contamination and presence of amplification inhibitors, are addressed in this chapter, emphasising in those practices that prevent from false-positive results and enable to demonstrate the authenticity of findings.

---

\* E-mail: cecis@unizar.es

## 1. INTRODUCTION

*Remains of ancient biomolecules that have long been trapped in human skeletons have finally started to become accessible to science. Working at the cutting edge of genetic technologies, scientists are making a fiction dream come true. There is still a long way to walk and no one technique or protocol can be considered as a panacea.*

The first attempts to analyse *ancient DNA (aDNA)* date back to the early 80s decade. Thanks to the vertiginous progress in molecular biological techniques, it has been possible to retrieve and study DNA from very diverse ancient specimens. The advent of new methods and techniques has allowed shedding light on an increasing number of investigations. In the specific field of Genetic Anthropology, it has meant the resolution of human identification and genealogic issues, and has allowed gaining insights on phylogenetic and evolutionary pathways. Probably the most remarkable result in this area has been the recovery of mitochondrial DNA (mtDNA) from Neanderthal individuals, which allowed the resolution of a long-discussed issue. From the works of Krings et al., (1997) it is now clear that Neanderthals were extinct without contributing mtDNA to modern humans.

The study of ancient DNA could be defined as the genetic analysis of ancient remains. Strictly, the adjective "ancient" relates to the historical period beginning with the earliest known civilizations and extending to the fall of the Western Roman Empire (in 476 A.D.). Yet, the studies on aDNA have far exceeded those limits. The temporal definition of the term is still vague and up to now, no concise range has come through. On the furthermost end, there have been some spectacular reports on DNA extracted from specimens dated up to 135 millions of years BP (Golenberg et al., 1990, DeSalle et al., 1992, Cano et al., 1993, Woodward et al., 1994b). However, these reports were very soon on debate, since it has been argued that the molecular preservation of geologically ancient DNA (i.e., more than 1 million years old) is not possible (Hebsgaard et al., 2005) and that a more reasonable limit would be 100,000 years (Lindahl, 1993a) or even 50,000 years (Marota & Rollo, 2002). On the nearest end, the limit to the term "aDNA" is even vaguer, since it is sometimes applied even to modern samples with a high extent of degradation due to the similitude of the study strategies.

The possibility to assess aDNA has widened the spectrum for the recent disciplines of Palaeobiology and Genetic Anthropology and is being applied to several other fields: in forensic sciences, enabling human identification (either in crime scene investigations or identification of historic persons); conservation genetics; phylogenetic studies, kinship affiliations, Phylogeography; Palaeoepidemiology; Anthropology (diet and behaviour of human and animals); studies of domestication of animals and plants; etc. This has been possible in part thanks to the generation of protocols suitable for the extraction of DNA from almost any kind of ancient biological material, ranging from human and animal remains (mummified tissues, soft tissue, hairs, bone, teeth, etc) to plants or seeds, coprolites, amber-embedded specimens, microorganisms, organisms persisting in permafrost and even sediments.

Nevertheless, along with the technical progresses the field has revealed some peculiarities and encountered certain drawbacks that on occasions have raised reasonable doubts on the authenticity of the results reported by researchers. Some of them were pointed out at the very beginning of these studies, as early as in 1988 by Pääbo and colleagues (1988). In a research paper in which they report the retrieval of a mtDNA sequence from a 7000-year old human brain, they rose the three major problems of aDNA: molecular damage, and therefore, the negative correlation between efficiency of amplification and amplicon size; contamination (even more risky when working with human remains); and inhibition of amplification, along with some practical solutions. They also discussed about authentication of the sequences obtained. Two decades have passed, and research in ancient DNA is still struggling with these problems.

After a brief revision of notable events and investigations that provided the basis of research on molecular anthropology, we will focus on human aDNA derived from skeletal remains (i.e., bones and teeth). Nevertheless, many issues and general methodological approaches that we will discuss here are common to other types of ancient samples.

## 2. HISTORY OF A RECENT DISCIPLINE

The history of Molecular Archaeology is intimately linked to the development of Molecular Biology since the studies in aDNA benefited from the advances in that area. In the late 1970s research on fossil macromolecules was already being carried out with the aim of understanding molecular evolution (Weiner et al., 1976, Prager et al., 1980). It was very early in the 1980s decade that DNA was extracted successfully from muscle of a museum 140yr-old quagga - an extinct zebra-like equid - and two sequences of 229 bp mtDNA were obtained from the cloned DNA (Higuchi et al., 1984). Although there are records of a Chinese report on DNA recovery a few years earlier (cited in, Pääbo et al., 1989, Hummel, 2003), that of Higuchi and colleagues, which was published on Nature and in English and therefore reached the non Chinese-speaking scientific community, became a referent of the beginning of the "ancient DNA era". Less than one year later, DNA retrieved from a 2,400-yr-old mummy of a child was cloned (Pääbo, 1985), being the first ancient DNA analysis on human remains. The same year, Johnson et al. (1985) isolated DNA from several mammoth specimens of up to 53,000 yrs old. The recovery of ancient DNA from a 8,000-yr-old human brain was reported soon after (Doran et al., 1986). In spite of the fact that these works were innovative and pioneer in demonstrating that the recovery of DNA molecules from ancient specimens was possible, they were limited by the number of genome copies retrieved and the impossibility to reproduce the results.

A major breakthrough that revolutionized and propelled the recently born discipline of Molecular Palaeontology was the advent of the polymerase chain reaction (PCR, Saiki et al., 1985, Mullis & Faloona, 1987) and its prompt application to aDNA investigations. In 1988, Pääbo et al. (1988) amplified short sequences (not bigger than 200 bp) of mitochondrial DNA (mtDNA) from a 7,000-yr-old human brain. The additional value of that work is that it pointed out the major problems that are encountered when working with aDNA, which the use of PCR augments. A contribution with far-reaching implications for anthropological and forensic investigations was the recovery of DNA from the hard tissues (i.e., bones and teeth) of ancient human remains, since these are the most common remnants of human life, and are deemed to confer relative protection to biomolecules because of their rigid structure. In the same year, two groups reported the successful recovery and posterior amplification by PCR of mtDNA from human bones ranging from 300 to 6000 years of age (Hagelberg et al., 1989,

Horai et al., 1989). Similarly, teeth also revealed as a good reservoir of ancient DNA (Hanni et al., 1990, Woodward et al., 1994a).

It was not until the advent of molecular fingerprinting that the identification of an individual from skeletal remains was possible. In 1985, Jeffreys et al. (1985b) realized that the study of highly polymorphic repetitive motifs in the DNA or minisatellites were suitable for individual identification and linkage analysis, and coined the term "DNA fingerprint". That technique, which was soon adopted in forensic genetics (Gill et al., 1985, Jeffreys et al., 1985a) was first applied on genetic studies of skeletal remains in 1991 when Hagelberg et al. (1991b) identified a murder victim by bone DNA analysis. Its application to historic human remains came one year later with the identification of the remains of Josef Mengele (Jeffreys et al., 1992). In the following years, these techniques were also applied to the identification of persons from the Vietnam War (Holland et al., 1993) and of the remains of the Romanov family (Gill et al., 1994). Afterwards, Genetic Anthropology continued nourishing from the advances in molecular biology that were applied to forensic science. Thus, the field incorporated the use of real time PCR for DNA quantification, multiplex PCR for the study of short tandem repeats (STR) of autosomic and sexual chromosomes, single nucleotide polymorphisms (SNP) of nuclear and mitochondrial DNA, and the most modern sequencing techniques (cyclic-array, hybridization, real-time sequencing, etc).

The history of aDNA studies has been rapid in its technical progress and development and very stimulating in its findings, although there have been some highly controversial issues that are worth highlighting. The first report on the recovery of geologically ancient DNA (i.e., more than 1 million years old) was that of Golenberg et al., (1990) who claimed to have amplified a 800-bp chloroplast DNA fragment from fossil leaf samples from a 17-20 Myr old Magnolia. This finding soon aroused doubts about the authenticity of the results on the grounds of molecular preservation (Pääbo, 1991, Lindahl, 1993b). Indeed, the results could not be replicated and most likely represented bacterial contamination (Sidow et al., 1991). In 1994, Woodward et al., (1994b) surprised the scientific community publishing a short sequence (less than 200 bp) of the mitochondrial gene encoding cytocrome b, from DNA extracted from bones of a purported 80-million-year-old dinosaur. The paper was greeted with skepticism and the replies were immediate, criticizing the data analysis, claiming that the putative dinosaur mtDNA sequences were probably the result of contamination or that it might represent ancient integrations of mtDNA into the human nuclear genome (Allard et al., 1995, Hedges & Schweitzer, 1995, Henikoff, 1995, Zischler et al., 1995). In other papers an attempt was made to sequence cytocrome b gene from a dinosaur egg, but it was openly concluded that the results obtained represented contamination (Yin et al., 1996, Wang et al., 1997). Another group of works that have given rise to debate are those reporting the recovery of aDNA from amber-preserved specimens. Thus, the recovery of antediluvian DNA and its correspondent sequences was reported in several investigations on amber fossil insects and leaves dating up to 120-135 million of years (DeSalle et al., 1992, Cano et al., 1993, Poinar et al., 1993). Although amber is deemed to confer extraordinary preservation conditions (Cano, 1996), unsuccessful attempts of replication of those early works ruined the promising possibility of obtaining DNA fragments of substantial length amenable to amplification (Austin et al., 1997a, Walden & Robertson, 1997). This has led Lindahl (1993a, 1993b) to refer to the works on antediluvian DNA as "anecdotal" and even "fiasco". It is surprising that even in recent years a purported mtDNA sequence of an 800,000-year-old mammoth has been published (Poulakakis et al., 2006). This paper, like others before, raised controversy and many methodological mistakes were pointed out (Binladen et al., 2007, Orlando et al., 2007). Although not exempt from the common issues of authentication, the exception to the accepted timescale of DNA preservation seems to be the successful retrieval of ancient DNA from permafrost (i.e., soil or rock that is permanently frozen). In this special environment (the coldest one on earth) microbial nucleic acids are claimed to be able to survive up to 3 million years (for a review see, Willerslev et al., 2004).

Following the initial enthusiasm and the belief that the investigations on aDNA had no temporal limit, the field reached a more realistic scenario after the evidence that the DNA molecule suffered natural decay and that preservation was subject to certain environmental conditions. In the case of bones and teeth, it is important to know the processes by which the whole sample degrades in order to understand the peculiarities of DNA preservation in these tissues.

## 3. BONE DIAGENESIS AND DNA PRESERVATION

Bones and teeth are the human remains most commonly available after a certain period of time for genetic analyses. Mature bone, dentin and cementum are composed of an inorganic component, mainly hydroxyapatite, which provides strength, deposited over an organic network that provides flexibility. The most abundant protein is type I collagen, which represents around 90% of the weight of the organic phase of a compact bone (Hedges et al., 1995). The non-collagenous protein fraction is composed by several other proteins (albumin, osteonectin, etc.) although it is mainly represented by osteocalcin (Hauschka, 1980). Bones and teeth, intrinsically rigid because of their high mineral level, would provide a unique shield to protect cellular DNA from environmental distress. The natural locus for DNA in bones and teeth is inside its cellular components: osteocytes, osteoblasts and osteoclast in bones, and odontocytes in teeth, although it could also be found in blood and lymphatic cells or even epithelial cells remaining adhered to the surfaces. Nevertheless, immediately after death, and along the transition from living animal to fossil, taphonomic and diagenetic processes take place. These changes will alter the microscopic structure of bones and teeth and alter the environment that surrounds DNA.

In a simplistic definition it can be said that taphonomy considers modifications on bone assemblages, whereas diagenesis relates to physical, chemical and biological changes that occur in the bone during its degradation. Nevertheless, from a holistic approach, diagenesis is difficult to define, and it can be better assessed if diagenetic parameters –understood as single measurable aspects of a bone sample that reflect the extent of diagenesis– are considered (Hedges et al., 1995, Hedges, 2002). The time of burial or environmental deposition, temperature, geochemistry (pH, concentration of solutes), hydrology, early taphonomy, are some of the environmental factors that influence the type and extent of digenetic processes (Hedges, 2002, Smith et al., 2007). Thus, it has been stated that bones begin with similar values of diagenetic parameters, but may differ widely when recovered (Hedges, 2002). Some of the proposed diagenetic parameters have been histological preservation, protein content, crystallinity and porosity (Bell, 1990, Hedges et al., 1995). Hedges et al., (1995) evaluated different diagenetic parameters and concluded that porosity is the simplest and most direct measure indicating the degree of diagenetic change in the bone; a finding that has been corroborated recently (Smith et al., 2007). Moreover, most of the proposed diagenetic parameters seem to vary in a correlated manner, although site-dependent mechanisms exist (Hedges, 2002).

Given that bones and teeth are comprised of a mineral and an organic fraction, diagenesis will affect both, adding nuances to its definition. The effects of diagenesis on the bone have been summarized by Collins et al (2002) in three pathways: chemical degradation of either the organic fraction or the mineral phase, and microbial attack (biodegradation). Either by dissolution of the mineral phase or by biodegradation, the initial phase in bone deterioration generally is demineralization (the area of damage being more localized in the latter). This mineral transformation will expose the collagen (and other proteins) to accelerated chemical and biological degradation (Collins et al., 2002).

In an attempt to address the question as to what extent DNA will be preserved, and to find screening methods to assess DNA survival, many researchers have studied the relationships between diagenetic parameters, DNA recovery and typing efficiency. It is clear that the time of deposition in the environment is not the determining factor in ancient DNA preservation, and environmental conditions have special relevance (Hagelberg et al., 1989, 1991a, Hedges, 2002, Gilbert et al., 2003a). The presence of DNA has been demonstrated by histochemical analyses within the osteocytic lacunae of ancient bones buried by the 79 A.D. Vesuvius eruption (Guarino et al., 2000). And recently, the presence of mineralized osteocytes –the most abundant cell in mature compact bone- have been demonstrated in fossil human and mammal bones of more than 200,000yrs (Bell et al., 2008). The authors suggested that these cellular structures, which presented partially preserved cytoskeleton, could represent the location of ancient proteins and DNA. However, when these structures disappear because of diagenetic changes, DNA is released into the bone interstice and interacts with other components. If other biomolecules in the bone are well preserved, the same condition could be expected for DNA. In solution, organic biopolymers are fragile molecules, whereas in fossils, they can sometimes escape complete degradation (Geigl et al., 2004). The knowledge of the conditions under which biomolecules are preserved reveals essential for the recovery of genetic information (Hagelberg et al., 1991a, Collins et al., 2002). One of the first relationships found was that of the state of preservation of proteins and the state of DNA integrity (Poinar et al., 1996, Poinar & Stankiewicz, 1999). For example, the degree of racemization of aminoacids, by which L-aminoacids produce D-enantiomers, was inversely correlated with the recovery of DNA, with low D/L ratios indicating the presence of well preserved proteins (Poinar et al., 1996). The application of the degree of racemization as an index of DNA preservation in bone assumes similar rates of DNA depurination and amino acid racemization (in aqueous solution at neutral pH) (Bada et al., 1994). Nevertheless, this methodological approach to assess DNA survival has been debated and was deemed a not reliable proxy for the extent of DNA depurination in bones (Collins et al., 1999). Another approach to characterize organic molecular preservation was through pyrolysis of the sample followed by gas chromatography and mass spectrometry (Py-GC/MS), which was proposed as a way to identify samples from which DNA may be retrieved (Poinar & Stankiewicz, 1999). However, the correlation found in that paper between the amount of pyrolysis products and DNA yield was not always conclusive, and led the authors to state that the observation of Py-GC/MS products compatible with collagen does not guarantee DNA survival. Nevertheless, the relation between the preservation of DNA and proteins is consistent and it has been corroborated recently. The percentage of collagen in ancient bones was found to be positively correlated to their DNA content, and proposed as an initial screening tool (Götherström et al., 2002). Indeed, it has been demonstrated that in aqueous solution the triple helices of collagen form complexes with the double helices of DNA, and that one DNA molecule could interact with up to 15 collagen molecules, in very packed structures (Mrevlishvili & Svintradze, 2005, Svintradze et al., 2008). So it is feasible that factors affecting collagen or DNA, affect the other component collaterally. Research has also been conducted on osteocalcin, the major non-collagenous protein in bone. Osteocalcin has been demonstrated to survive particularly well in fossil bone, probably because its packaging inside the bone (Collins et al., 2000, Nielsen-Marsh et al., 2002, 2005). Nevertheless, a recent work found that intact osteocalcin molecule survives less in archaeological samples than collagen and mtDNA (Buckley et al., 2008). This finding would rule out the study of osteocalcin survival as a screening method of DNA preservation, and the authors suggested that further research should be conducted on collagen survival instead.

On the other hand, it is known that DNA has a strong affinity for the inorganic mineral phase, which makes bound DNA more resistant to degradation than free DNA (Paget et al., 1992). Götherström et al. (2002) found a negative correlation between the presence of DNA and the crystallinity of hydroxyapatite of the ancient bone, and suggested that DNA may be stabilized by adsorption to hydroxyapatite. Consistent with this concept, is the finding of well preserved ancient DNA packed in crystal aggregates in fossil bones (Salamon et al., 2005). It has been reported that fossil DNA remains insoluble after the common extraction procedures, as demonstrated by Southern hybridization (Geigl, 1997, 2002). According to the results of Götherström et al., (2002) hydroxyapatite and collagen play an important role in the preservation of DNA in bone, since recovery of DNA was related directly with collagen index and inversely related to the crystallinity of hydroxyapatite. It is clear that DNA molecules interact with all the components of bone, and that the specific inter-molecular relationships are complex. Histological approaches provide useful information on the general preservation of the structures in bone and histochemistry even allow the detection of particular biomolecules, such as collagen and DNA. Indeed, histochemical and histological analyses have correlated well with the success of DNA extraction and amplification (Colson et al., 1997, Cipollaro et al., 1998, Cipollaro et al., 1999, Guarino et al., 2000, Haynes et al., 2002).

Another proposed indicator for the likelihood of survival of biomolecules in the fossil record is the determination of the thermal age of the sample which is calculated from the thermal history of the burial site and its geographical location (Smith et al., 2003). When the authors analysed published data of aDNA amplifications considering the chronological age and the thermal age of the samples, a consistent correlation was only observed with the thermal age, with only thermally young material yielding amplifiable aDNA. Therefore, they suggested that in the absence of convincing screening methods, a thermal age limit of 19,000 yr at 10°C should be considered. Better amplification efficiencies have been obtained from bones buried at low than at moderate temperatures (Burger et al., 1999). Moreover, the temperature of storage after bone removal from the burial site similarly influences DNA degradation (Burger et al., 1999).

When the recovery of DNA from ancient specimens is successful, there is still the possibility of it being damaged or highly degraded, and therefore, not amenable to amplification.

## 4. CHARACTERISTICS OF aDNA AND ITS STUDY

The study of aDNA faces some difficulties and drawbacks that are typical, and that were already highlighted in 1988 in the seminal article of Pääbo and colleagues (1988). These problems can be grouped into DNA damage, contamination by exogenous DNA and inhibition of amplification. To varying extents depending on the nature of the sample, they must be considered in every attempt to study archaeological remains.

### 4.1. DNA Damage

Nucleic acids in solution, like all biological macromolecules, undergo spontaneous decomposition. DNA molecules suffer the effects of hydrolysis and oxidation, which have been thoroughly reviewed by Lindahl (1993a). Hydrolytic deamination of cytosine to uracil, and oxidation of guanine to 8-hydroxyguanine, are the major types of spontaneous damage in cells (Lindahl, 1993a). These mutations lead to baseless sites or miscoding lesions that result in single-strand breaks. Under physiological conditions these mutations are effectively dealt with by enzymatic pathways. Nevertheless, the post-mortem loss of enzymatic regulation enhances the activity of endo and exonucleases which hydrolyze DNA, resulting in fragmentation of the strands (Bar et al., 1988). Fragmentation of DNA by non specific hydrolysis affects primarily the longer fragments (Bar et al., 1988). In the absence of mechanisms of repair, the effects of damage accumulate giving place to strand breaks and sequence errors in such a degree that it is believed that less than 1% of the DNA molecules extracted from archaeological specimens are undamaged (Pääbo et al., 1989). Based on controlled conditions of pH and temperature, it has been calculated that DNA would be completely destroyed by hydrolytic damage in about 100,000 yrs (Pääbo & Wilson, 1991, Lindahl, 1993a), and therefore, that is the theoretical limit established for aDNA studies. Nevertheless, as mentioned in the previous section, there are many factors influencing DNA survival from bones. It has been suggested that thermal age of the sample should be considered and that the limit of DNA survival should be defined by the thermally oldest material from a specific area (Smith et al., 2003). However, in the opinion of Hansen et al. (2006) it is impossible to generalize since the different types of damage (which in turn depend on environmental factors) would influence the long-term survival of DNA.

The high incidence of spontaneous DNA damage adds difficulty to the study of aDNA and determines the adoption of different strategies to overcome those problems (Table 1). Single-strand breaks are the predominant damage associated to spontaneous degradation, and they can produce regions of single-stranded DNA linking double-stranded DNA segments (Mitchell et al., 2005). This kind of damage has been restored with the use of polymerases and ligases (Pusch et al., 1998, Di Bernardo et al., 2002, Pusch et al., 2002) although they are not very widespread methods.

The high molecular damage determines the approaches of DNA study. When nuclear DNA is present, the analysis of mini STRs of autosomic and sexual chromosomes is the option of preference. However, most studies are based in mtDNA sequences (specifically, the analysis of short overlapping fragments), since its preservation is more feasible. A frequent feature of PCR products from fossil remains is their heterogeneity, which are generally due to regular DNA polymerase errors as well as miscoding lesions in the original DNA sequences (Pääbo et al., 1989, Handt et al., 1994, 1996, Hansen et al., 2001). In addition to the intrinsic degradation, environmental factors cause extra damage, which can be similar to spontaneous damage (free-radical-mediated pathways) or of other kind (alkylations, cross-linking, etc.). Moreover, damage can be provoked by DNA handling during extraction and purification (Mitchell et al., 2005). Finally, amplification artefacts can also lead to sequence misinterpretations (Hebsgaard et al., 2005). Extensive molecular degradation could facilitate recombination during amplification ("jumping PCR") leading to the production of false sequences (Pääbo et al., 1990). The use of novel techniques such as 454 pyrosequencing and single primer extension-based approach, has allowed the identification of cytosine deamination (C > U) as the major cause of nucleotide misincorporations in aDNA (Briggs et al., 2007, Brotherton et al., 2007). Transitions are the predominant miscoding lesion observed in PCR products from aDNA and they have been classified in Type 1 (AT → GC) and Type 2 (CG → TA) transitions, under the assumption that they are indistinguishable (Hansen et al., 2001). Both types have been reported in aDNA extracts (Pääbo, 1989, Gilbert et al., 2003a, 2003b, Binladen et al., 2006) and it has been determined that Type 2 transitions are the dominant miscoding lesion (Stiller et al., 2006, Gilbert et al., 2007). On the other hand, it has been argued that Type 1 transitions do not represent true aDNA damage but could represent damage inflicted during the extraction process or PCR-generated errors, mainly due to DNA polymerase incorporation of incorrect bases (Hansen et al., 2001, Hofreiter et al., 2001, Gilbert et al., 2007). The use of sequencing-by-synthesis technology on permafrost-preserved bones has allowed identifying the strand of origin of the sequences, thus minimizing the need of pooling transitions into complementary pairs (Gilbert et al., 2007). In mtDNA, miscoding lesions are not distributed at random but concentrate in "hotspots", i.e., specific nucleotide positions that undergo a higher rate of damage than the rest (Gilbert et al., 2003b). However (and despite previous contradictory results (Gilbert et al., 2003a)) it has been demonstrated using next generation sequencing techniques that the distribution of damage is similar in both strands of mtDNA (Gilbert et al., 2007). On the other hand, it has been determined by GC/MS that the dominant oxidative damage to aDNA is the occurrence of hydantoin derivatives of pyrimidines, which block strand elongation by DNA polymerases (Höss et al., 1996).

Another frequent damage found in aDNA is the formation of cross-links. Cross-links in DNA can be on the same strand of DNA (intrastrand), between the two complementary strands (interstrand), or between a base on DNA and a reactive group on a protein (DNA-protein) (McHugh et al., 2001). The presence of cross-links has been reported in several works on aDNA (Pääbo, 1989, Poinar et al., 1998, Hansen et al., 2006). The products of the Maillard reaction (formed by condensation reactions between sugars and amino-groups) are recognized to produce cross-linking of macromolecules such as proteins and nucleic acids (Bucala et al., 1984, Poinar et al., 1998). Proteins can crosslink to DNA directly through oxidative free radical mechanisms or indirectly through a chemical linker and these events can occur after the exposure of a variety of agents, including ionizing radiation (Barker et al., 2005). The presence of interstrand cross links have been reported in permafrost samples, with a higher prevalence than single-strand breaks (Hansen et al., 2006). Cross-links may be protective for DNA as they prevent strand separation and degradation. Nevertheless, they block DNA amplification and their in vitro repair is problematic (Mitchell et al., 2005).

**Table 1. Common DNA damage found in ancient remains and possible methodological strategies to overcome them**

| Problem | Possible strategies |
|---|---|
| DNA fragmentation | ▪ MiniSTRs<br>▪ SNPs<br>▪ Low Copy Number approach<br>▪ mtDNA: small, overlapping fragments |
| Miscoding lesions and PCR errors | ▪ High fidelity polymerases<br>▪ Analysis of overlapping fragments<br>▪ Cloning of PCR products<br>▪ Treatment with uracil-$N$-glycosylase |
| Cross-links | ▪ Use of PTB |

It is worth noting that, despite posing technical problems, the typical degradation and miscoding lesions of aDNA are useful tools of validation of the results (see *Authentication of aDNA analysis*).

## 4.2. Contamination

The risk of obtaining false positive results in aDNA study is high because of the (expected) low copy number of DNA present in the sample, and the enormous amplification power of PCR. Indeed, modern undamaged DNA will outcompete damaged aDNA and be preferentially amplified (Austin et al., 1997b). In the studies of human aDNA, the problem of contamination is critical since the most probable source of contamination of samples and in the laboratories is from humans. Of course, microbiological contamination is ubiquitous but somehow negligible, since the systems used for human typing are species-specific. Indeed, it has been suggested that fungal and bacterial DNA should not be considered contaminant DNA in human aDNA studies (Yang & Watt, 2005). For clarity's sake, contamination of an ancient sample with exogenous DNA can be divided in pre-laboratory and post-laboratory.

Pre-laboratory contamination includes that acquired during excavations, handling, transport and storage of the sample, which are instances in which usually many people participate and manipulate the samples and where the sterile conditions necessary for aDNA studies are of difficult imposition and therefore, not always observed. It has been suggested that contaminating DNA enters the bones and teeth due to their intrinsic porosity, and porosity is a sign of diagenetic damage; thus, ancient remains would be very prone to exogenous contamination (Gilbert et al., 2005b). Then, it is important that field archaeologists are aware of the relevance of the introduction of contamination at these first stages on the overall success of the aDNA study, and general guidelines for sample collection have been proposed (Yang & Watt, 2005). This type of contamination is problematic as it will not be detected through the systematic use of negative controls and reagent blanks (Richards et al., 1995, Kolman & Tuross, 2000, Malmström et al., 2005). Repeated extractions from different samples (bones, teeth) of the same individual could help to solve this problem. Another way of detecting the presence of modern contaminating DNA is through the verification of an inverse correlation between amplification efficiencies and size of the amplification products, which has been called "appropriate" or "asymmetric" molecular behaviour (Pääbo, 1989, Cooper & Poinar, 2000, Noonan et al., 2005, Malmström et al., 2007). It is important to bear in mind the possibility of "ancient contamination", that is, contamination with human DNA that would also behave as ancient because of the environmental conditions of which could have been subjected. In studies on human remains this kind of contamination is almost impossible to detect by the analysis of a single individual. However, it can be detected when genealogic information is available.

Once in the laboratory, human contamination is also possible. Therefore, when working with human aDNA some recommendations need to be attended very thoroughly. One of the first logical approaches is that all the laboratory personnel, and all the persons involved in the previous handling of the sample (as far as possible) should be typed, and the results obtained should always be compared with them in the first place. Although in most cases the amount of DNA present in ancient bones or teeth is minimal, cross-contamination between samples should not be underestimated since significant amounts can be retrieved from certain especially well preserved samples. The problem of contaminating human DNA coming from reagents and disposable lab material purchased as sterile from different laboratory suppliers has been addressed in detail by Hummel (2003). The inclusion of negative controls and reagent blanks from extraction to the last step of the analysis process is imperative to detect this type of contamination. Nevertheless, the absence of amplifiable DNA in negative controls does not necessarily means absence of contamination. As mentioned above, one possibility is that the bone samples are contaminated with modern DNA. Another possibility is the existence of exogenous DNA in the extraction or PCR reagents but in such low amounts that it adheres to tube walls in the reagent blanks, whereas it is "dragged" by amplifiable authentic DNA, a phenomenon that has been called "carrier effect" (Cooper, 1992, Handt et al., 1994).

The most significant source of contamination in the laboratory is the carry-over of PCR products, which occurs when amplification products are introduced to a pre-PCR analysis step (Hummel, 2003). All possible efforts should be undertaken to avoid this type of contamination following certain strategies such as physical separation of pre- and post-PCR areas and daily one-way movement up the contamination gradient. Contamination is a very problematic issue in the studies on aDNA and many individual methods performed in order to detect it may fail (Kolman & Tuross, 2000). Thus, the interpretation of results should be carried out taking into consideration all the information available from that sample, including its genealogic and phylogenetic sense. Some of the possible sources of contaminating human DNA in studies on ancient human remains are outlined in Table 2 along with general recommendations to avoid them.

## 4.3. Inhibition

PCR amplification of aDNA extracts can be inhibited by substances that can be co-purified along with DNA and affect DNA polymerases function or by physical prevention of denaturation of DNA during PCR cycles. Inhibition of PCR amplification could lead to the report of false-negative results, or to results being interpreted as non preservation of DNA. A variety of compounds have been identified as PCR inhibitors, many of which are or could be present in bones and teeth, such as calcium ions, humic and fulvic acids and collagen (Tuross,

1994, Wilson, 1997, Scholz et al., 1998, Radström et al., 2004, Sutlovic et al., 2005). Crosslinks can prevent separation of the DNA strands thus preventing amplification (Poinar et al., 1998, Hansen et al., 2006). Many measures have been proposed to overcome the different types of PCR inhibition, such as extract purification and dilution, addition of extra *Taq* DNA polymerase, use of BSA as a facilitator of amplification, use of polyvinylpyrrolidone (PVP), cetyltrimethylammonium bromide (CTAB) (Hänni et al., 1995, Wilson, 1997, Ye et al., 2004, Rohland & Hofreiter, 2007). Treatment with N-phenacylthiazolium bromide (PTB), which breaks Maillard products, has been shown to allow DNA amplification in ancient remains (Poinar et al., 1998). Certain types of damage in the DNA molecules such as accumulation of hydantoins resulting from the oxidation of pyrimidines could also block *Taq* DNA polymerase (Pääbo et al., 2004). It has been demonstrated that even the high fragmentation of the aDNA molecules could inhibit amplification (Pusch et al., 1998, Ricaut et al., 2005).

Table 2. Possible sources of human DNA contamination and general guidelines to avoid it

|  | Sources of human DNA contamination | General guidelines to avoid contamination |
|---|---|---|
| Pre-laboratory | Excavation<br>Anthropological examination<br>Storage | On site:<br>• Use disposable gloves and face masks<br>• Use sterile bags or envelopes for storage<br>In the lab:<br>• Clean and remove outer surface (scraping, sanding) |
| In the lab | Personnel | • Use disposable gloves, coats, face masks<br>• Every person working in the lab should be typed |
|  | Reagents<br>Disposable material | • Use sterile, certified DNA-free reagents and materials<br>• Autoclave/sterilize<br>• Aliquot reagents<br>• Include negative controls and reagent blanks |
|  | Cross-contamination between samples | • Dedicated lab for aDNA studies<br>• Handle one sample at a time<br>• Clean equipment and work surfaces between samples<br>• Change gloves between samples<br>• Store samples separately |
|  | PCR product carry-over | • Physically separated pre- and post-PCR areas<br>• Dedicated equipment and labware for each area<br>• Pre- to post-PCR traffic |

# 5. AUTHENTICATION OF aDNA ANALYSES

Proving that the results obtained are authentic is crucial in aDNA studies, because the field faces many problems inherent to molecular degradation and methodological issues such as contamination, as discussed previously. Furthermore, when the studies are on human remains, strict adherence to established authentication criteria is essential, since the most probable contamination source is from humans. Pääbo et al., (1988) were pioneers in detecting these problems and suggesting measures to overcome them. The concern of the scientific community on the authenticity of the results reported is reflected by the increasing number of papers published on this topic. Current criteria of authenticity are summarized in Table 3 (Cooper & Poinar, 2000, Montiel et al., 2001, Pääbo et al., 2004, Hebsgaard et al., 2005, Willerslev & Cooper, 2005).

Some of these proposed criteria are not always easy to accomplish when working with very valuable or unique remains since the availability of material is often a restriction. Thus, replication of results inside the laboratory and independent replication in a second one could be not possible, as well as collateral studies such as biochemical or microscopic studies. The requirements demanded to validate results have been considered "inherently problematic" (Gilbert et al., 2005a) or even "counter-productive", since authentic results on human aDNA that are impossible to authenticate because of the minute amounts available would be dismissed (Chilvers et al., 2008). The criteria should assist in determining the authenticity of the studies and not be used as a simple checklist (Gilbert et al., 2005a). The authors also called for a cognitive approach of the own data, giving consideration on a case-by-case basis; opinion that we share.

**Table 3. Summary of currently accepted criteria of authenticity**

| Criteria of authenticity |
|---|
| - Physically isolated pre- and post-PCR facilities |
| - Clean laboratories and practices, decontamination of specimens, reagents and lab ware, use of disposable lab coats, face masks, gloves |
| - Daily movement up the contamination gradient |
| - Extraction negative controls and PCR reagent blanks |
| - Quantification of starting templates |
| - Asymmetric molecular behaviour<br>    Verification of inverse relationship between amplicon length and PCR efficiency. |
| - Extraction from different samples of the same individual |
| - Intra-laboratory reproducibility |
| - Inter-laboratory reproducibility of results |
| - Cloning and sequencing of PCR products |
| - Assessment of biochemical preservation<br>    Measure diagenetic parameters, aminoacid racemization, etc. to provide an idea of global preservation status of the specimen. |
| - Study of associated remains<br>    Survival of similar DNA targets in associated faunal samples could support authenticity. |
| - Uracil-N-glycosylase (UNG) treatment<br>    Removal of deamination products of cytosine. |
| - Phylogenetic (and genealogic) sense<br>    Of special importance in studies on human aDNA. |
| - Dating of specimen |

# CONCLUSION

The possibility of performing genetic analysis on archaeological and fossil specimens has enabled shedding light to many issues that were previously difficult to elucidate. The field is not devoid of problems, most of them arising from the inherent molecular damage, and many false results or artefacts may be obtained that could mask the true sequences. Nevertheless, the development of new methodologies and the adoption of suitable laboratory practices and approaches enable obtaining results that can be demonstrated as authentic. Thus, the analysis of human aDNA is promising although maximum methodological cautions and considerations should be taken into account and a rigorous assessment of the authenticity of the results should be made for each individual case. In this chapter a picture of the state of art on ancient DNA typing has been offered. A summary of methodologies with comments on their advantages and drawbacks was also presented. Ancient molecules keep secrets of our past and keep challenging our present.

## COMPETING INTERESTS

The authors declare that they have no competing interests. The authors alone are responsible for the content and writing of the paper.

## REFERENCES

Allard, M. W., Young, D. & Huyen, Y., (1995). Detecting dinosaur DNA. *Science 268 (5214)*, 1192; author reply 1194.

Austin, J. J., Ross, A. J., Smith, A. B., Fortey, R. A. & Thomas, R. H., (1997a). Problems of reproducibility--does geologically ancient DNA survive in amber-preserved insects? *Proceedings. Biological Sciences 264 (1381)*, 467-474.

Austin, J. J., Smith, A. B. & Thomas, R. H., (1997b). Palaeontology in a molecular world: the search for authentic ancient DNA. *Trends in Ecology & Evolution 12 (8)*, 303-306.

Bada, J. L., Wang, X. S., Poinar, H. N., Pääbo, S. & Poinar, G. O., (1994). Amino acid racemization in amber-entombed insects: implications for DNA preservation. *Geochimica et Cosmochimica Acta 58 (14)*, 3131-3135.

Bar, W., Kratzer, A., Machler, M. & Schmid, W., (1988). Postmortem stability of DNA. *Forensic Science International 39 (1)*, 59-70.

Barker, S., Weinfeld, M. & Murray, D., (2005). DNA-protein crosslinks: their induction, repair, and biological consequences. *Mutation Research 589 (2)*, 111-135.

Bell, L. S., (1990). Palaeopathology and diagenesis: an SEM evaluation of structural changes using backscattered electron imaging. *Journal of Archaeological Science 17*, 85-102.

Bell, L. S., Kayser, M. & Jones, C., (2008). The mineralized osteocyte: a living fossil. *American Journal of Physical Anthropology 137 (4)*, 449-456.

Binladen, J., Wiuf, C., Gilbert, M. T., Bunce, M., Barnett, R., Larson, G., Greenwood, A. D., Haile, J., Ho, S. Y., Hansen, A. J. & Willerslev, E., (2006). Assessing the fidelity of ancient DNA sequences amplified from nuclear genes. *Genetics 172 (2)*, 733-741.

Binladen, J., Gilbert, M. T. & Willerslev, E., (2007). 800,000 year old mammoth DNA, modern elephant DNA or PCR artefact? *Biology Letters 3 (1)*, 55-56; discussion 60-53.

Briggs, A. W., Stenzel, U., Johnson, P. L., Green, R. E., Kelso, J., Prufer, K., Meyer, M., Krause, J., Ronan, M. T., Lachmann, M. & Pääbo, S., (2007). Patterns of damage in genomic DNA sequences from a Neandertal. *Proceedings of the National Academy of Sciences of the United States of America 104 (37)*, 14616-14621.

Brotherton, P., Endicott, P., Sanchez, J. J., Beaumont, M., Barnett, R., Austin, J. & Cooper, A., (2007). Novel high-resolution characterization of ancient DNA reveals C > U-type base modification events as the sole cause of post mortem miscoding lesions. *Nucleic Acids Research 35 (17)*, 5717-5728.

Bucala, R., Model, P. & Cerami, A., (1984). Modification of DNA by reducing sugars: a possible mechanism for nucleic acid aging and age-related dysfunction in gene expression. *Proceedings of the National Academy of Sciences of the United States of America 81 (1)*, 105-109.

Buckley, M., Anderung, C., Penkman, K., Raney, B. J., Götherström, A., Thomas-Oates, J. & Collins, M. J., (2008). Comparing the survival of osteocalcin and mtDNA in archaeological bone from four European sites. *Journal of Archaeological Science 35 (6)*, 1756-1764.

Burger, J., Hummel, S., Hermann, B. & Henke, W., (1999). DNA preservation: a microsatellite-DNA study on ancient skeletal remains. *Electrophoresis 20 (8)*, 1722-1728.

Cano, R. J., Poinar, H. N., Pieniazek, N. J., Acra, A. & Poinar, G. O., Jr., (1993). Amplification and sequencing of DNA from a 120-135-million-year-old weevil. *Nature 363 (6429)*, 536-538.

Cano, R. J., (1996). Analysing ancient DNA. *Endeavour 20 (4)*, 162-167.

Cipollaro, M., Di Bernardo, G., Galano, G., Galderisi, U., Guarino, F., Angelini, F. & Cascino, A., (1998). Ancient DNA in human bone remains from Pompeii archaeological site. *Biochemical and Biophysical Research Communications 247 (3)*, 901-904.

Cipollaro, M., Di Bernado, G., Forte, A., Galano, G., De Masi, L., Galderisi, U., Guarino, F. M., Angelini, F. & Cascino, A., (1999). Histological analysis and ancient DNA amplification of human bone remains found in Caius Iulius Polybius house in Pompeii. *Croatian Medical Journal 40 (3)*, 392-397.

Colson, I. B., Bailey, J. F., Vercauteren, M. & Sykes, B. C., (1997). The preservation of ancient DNA and bone diagenesis. *Ancient Biomolecules 1*, 109-117.

Collins, M. J., Waite, E. R. & van Duin, A. C., (1999). Predicting protein decomposition: the case of aspartic-acid racemization kinetics. *Philosophical transactions of the Royal Society of London. Series B, Biological sciences 354 (1379)*, 51-64.

Collins, M. J., Gernaey, A. M., Nielsen-Marsh, C. M., Vermeer, C. & Westbroek, P., (2000). Slow rates of degradation of osteocalcin: Green light for fossil bone protein? *Geology 28 (12)*, 1139-1142.

Collins, M. J., Marsh, C. M. N., Hiller, J., Smith, C. I., Roberts, J. P., Prigodich, R. V., Wess, T. J., Csapò, J., Millard, A. R. & Walker, G. T., (2002). The survival of organic matter in bone: a review. *Archaeometry 44 (3)*, 383-394.

Cooper, A., (1992). Removal of colourings, inhibitors of PCR, and the carrier effect of PCR contamination from ancient DNA samples. *Ancient DNA Newsletter 1*, 31-32.

Cooper, A. & Poinar, H. N., (2000). Ancient DNA: do it right or not at all. *Science 289 (5482)*, 1139.

Chilvers, E. R., Bouwman, A. S., Brown, K. A., Arnott, R. G., Prag, A. J. N. W. & Brown, T. A., (2008). Ancient DNA in human bones from Neolithic and Bronze Age sites in Greece and Crete. *Journal of Archaeological Science 35 (10)*, 2707-2714.

DeSalle, R., Gatesy, J., Wheeler, W. & Grimaldi, D., (1992). DNA sequences from a fossil termite in Oligo-Miocene amber and their phylogenetic implications. *Science 257 (5078)*, 1933-1936.

Di Bernardo, G., Del Gaudio, S., Cammarota, M., Galderisi, U., Cascino, A. & Cipollaro, M., (2002). Enzymatic repair of selected cross-linked homoduplex molecules enhances nuclear gene rescue from Pompeii and Herculaneum remains. *Nucleic Acids Research 30 (4)*, e16.

Doran, G. H., Dickel, D. N., Ballinger, W. E., Jr., Agee, O. F., Laipis, P. J. & Hauswirth, W. W., (1986). Anatomical, cellular and molecular analysis of 8,000-yr-old human brain tissue from the Windover archaeological site. *Nature 323 (6091)*, 803-806.

Geigl, E., (1997). DNA diagenesis in lower palaeolithic bone. *Ancient Biomolecules 1 (3)*, 240-241.

Geigl, E., Baumer, U. & Koller, J., (2004). New approaches to study the preservation of biopolymers in fossil bones. *Environmental Chemistry Letters 2*, 45-48.

Geigl, E. M., (2002). On the circumstances surrounding the preservation and analysis of very old DNA. *Archaeometry 44 (3)*, 337-342.

Gilbert, M. T., Hansen, A. J., Willerslev, E., Rudbeck, L., Barnes, I., Lynnerup, N. & Cooper, A., (2003a). Characterization of genetic miscoding lesions caused by postmortem damage. *American Journal of Human Genetics 72 (1)*, 48-61.

Gilbert, M. T., Willerslev, E., Hansen, A. J., Barnes, I., Rudbeck, L., Lynnerup, N. & Cooper, A., (2003b). Distribution patterns of postmortem damage in human mitochondrial DNA. *American Journal of Human Genetics 72 (1)*, 32-47.

Gilbert, M. T., Bandelt, H. J., Hofreiter, M. & Barnes, I., (2005a). Assessing ancient DNA studies. *Trends in Ecology & Evolution 20 (10)*, 541-544.

Gilbert, M. T., Rudbeck, L., Willerslev, E., Hansen, A. J., Smith, C., Penkman, K. E. H., Prangenberg, K., Nielsen-Marsh, C. M., Jans, M. E., Arthur, P., Lynnerup, N., Turner-Walker, G., Biddle, M., Kjølbye-Biddle, B. & Collins, M. J., (2005b). Biochemical and physical correlates of DNA contamination in archaeological human bones and teeth excavated at Matera, Italy. *Journal of Archaeological Science 32 (5)*, 785-793.

Gilbert, M. T., Binladen, J., Miller, W., Wiuf, C., Willerslev, E., Poinar, H., Carlson, J. E., Leebens-Mack, J. H. & Schuster, S. C., (2007). Recharacterization of ancient DNA miscoding lesions: insights in the era of sequencing-by-synthesis. *Nucleic Acids Research 35 (1)*, 1-10.

Gill, P., Jeffreys, A. J. & Werrett, D. J., (1985). Forensic application of DNA 'fingerprints'. *Nature 318 (6046)*, 577-579.

Gill, P., Ivanov, P. L., Kimpton, C., Piercy, R., Benson, N., Tully, G., Evett, I., Hagelberg, E. & Sullivan, K., (1994). Identification of the remains of the Romanov family by DNA analysis. *Nature Genetics 6 (2)*, 130-135.

Golenberg, E. M., Giannasi, D. E., Clegg, M. T., Smiley, C. J., Durbin, M., Henderson, D. & Zurawski, G., (1990). Chloroplast DNA sequence from a miocene Magnolia species. *Nature 344 (6267)*, 656-658.

Götherström, A., Collins, M. J., Angerbjörn, A. & Lidén, K., (2002). Bone preservation and DNA amplification. *Archaeometry 44 (3)*, 395-404.

Guarino, F. M., Angelini, F., Odierna, G., Bianco, M. R., Di Bernardo, G., Forte, A., Cascino, A. & Cipollaro, M., (2000). Detection of DNA in ancient bones using histochemical methods. *Biotechnic & Histochemistry 75 (3)*, 110-117.

Hagelberg, E., Sykes, B. & Hedges, R., (1989). Ancient bone DNA amplified. *Nature 342 (6249)*, 485.

Hagelberg, E., Bell, L. S., Allen, T., Boyde, A., Jones, S. J. & Clegg, J. B., (1991a). Analysis of ancient bone DNA: techniques and applications. *Philosophical transactions of the Royal Society of London. Series B, Biological sciences 333 (1268)*, 399-407.

Hagelberg, E., Gray, I. C. & Jeffreys, A. J., (1991b). Identification of the skeletal remains of a murder victim by DNA analysis. *Nature 352 (6334)*, 427-429.

Handt, O., Höss, M., Krings, M. & Pääbo, S., (1994). Ancient DNA: methodological challenges. *Experientia 50 (6)*, 524-529.

Handt, O., Krings, M., Ward, R. H. & Pääbo, S., (1996). The retrieval of ancient human DNA sequences. *American Journal of Human Genetics 59 (2)*, 368-376.

Hanni, C., Laudet, V., Sakka, M., Begue, A. & Stehelin, D., (1990). Amplification de fragments d'ADN mitochondrial a partir de dents et d'os humains anciens. *Comptes Rendus d'Academie de Science de Paris 310*, 365-370.

Hänni, C., Begue, A., Laudet, V., Stéhelin, D., Brousseau, T., Amouyel, P. & Duday, H., (1995). Molecular typing of neolithic human bones. *Journal of Archaeological Science 22 (5)*, 649-658.

Hansen, A., Willerslev, E., Wiuf, C., Mourier, T. & Arctander, P., (2001). Statistical evidence for miscoding lesions in ancient DNA templates. *Molecular Biology and Evolution 18 (2)*, 262-265.

Hansen, A. J., Mitchell, D. L., Wiuf, C., Paniker, L., Brand, T. B., Binladen, J., Gilichinsky, D. A., Ronn, R. & Willerslev, E., (2006). Crosslinks rather than strand breaks determine access to ancient DNA sequences from frozen sediments. *Genetics 173 (2)*, 1175-1179.

Hauschka, P. V., (1980). Osteocalcin: a specific protein of bone with potential for fossil dating. In: Hare, P. E., Hoering, T. C.&King Jr, T. (Eds.), *Biogeochemistry of amino acids*. John Wiley, New York, pp. 75-82.

Haynes, S., Searle, J. B., Bretman, A. & Dobney, K. M., (2002). Bone Preservation and Ancient DNA: The Application of Screening Methods for Predicting DNA Survival. *Journal of Archaeological Science 29 (6)*, 585-592.

Hebsgaard, M. B., Phillips, M. J. & Willerslev, E., (2005). Geologically ancient DNA: fact or artefact? *Trends in Microbiology 13 (5)*, 212-220.

Hedges, R. E. M., Millard, A. R. & Pike, A. W. G., (1995). Measurements and Relationships of Diagenetic Alteration of Bone from Three Archaeological Sites. *Journal of Archaeological Science 22 (2)*, 201-209.

Hedges, R. E. M., (2002). Bone diagenesis: an overview of processes. *Archaeometry 44 (3)*, 319-328.

Hedges, S. B. & Schweitzer, M. H., (1995). Detecting dinosaur DNA. *Science 268 (5214)*, 1191-1192; author reply 1194.

Henikoff, S., (1995). Detecting dinosaur DNA. *Science 268 (5214)*, 1192; author reply 1194.

Higuchi, R., Bowman, B., Freiberger, M., Ryder, O. A. & Wilson, A. C., (1984). DNA sequences from the quagga, an extinct member of the horse family. *Nature 312 (5991)*, 282-284.

Hofreiter, M., Jaenicke, V., Serre, D., Haeseler Av, A. & Pääbo, S., (2001). DNA sequences from multiple amplifications reveal artifacts induced by cytosine deamination in ancient DNA. *Nucleic Acids Research 29 (23)*, 4793-4799.

Holland, M. M., Fisher, D. L., Mitchell, L. G., Rodriquez, W. C., Canik, J. J., Merril, C. R. & Weedn, V. W., (1993). Mitochondrial DNA sequence analysis of human skeletal remains: identification of remains from the Vietnam War. *Journal of Forensic Sciences 38 (3)*, 542-553.

Horai, S., Hayasaka, K., Murayama, K., Wate, N., Koike, H. & Nakai, N., (1989). DNA amplification from ancient human skeletal remains and their sequence analysis. *Proceedings of the Japan Academy Series B 65*, 229-233.

Höss, M., Jaruga, P., Zastawny, T. H., Dizdaroglu, M. & Pääbo, S., (1996). DNA damage and DNA sequence retrieval from ancient tissues. *Nucleic Acids Research 24 (7)*, 1304-1307.

Hummel, S., (2003). *Ancient DNA typing: methods, strategies and applications*. Springer-Verlag, Berlin.

Jeffreys, A. J., Brookfield, J. F. & Semeonoff, R., (1985a). Positive identification of an immigration test-case using human DNA fingerprints. *Nature 317 (6040)*, 818-819.

Jeffreys, A. J., Wilson, V. & Thein, S. L., (1985b). Hypervariable 'minisatellite' regions in human DNA. *Nature 314 (6006)*, 67-73.

Jeffreys, A. J., Allen, M. J., Hagelberg, E. & Sonnberg, A., (1992). Identification of the skeletal remains of Josef Mengele by DNA analysis. *Forensic Science International 56 (1)*, 65-76.

Johnson, P. H., Olson, C. B. & Goodman, M., (1985). Isolation and characterization of deoxyribonucleic acid from tissue of the woolly mammoth, Mammuthus primigenius. *Comparative Biochemistry and Physiology. B 81 (4)*, 1045-1051.

Kolman, C. J. & Tuross, N., (2000). Ancient DNA analysis of human populations. *American Journal of Physical Anthropology 111 (1)*, 5-23.

Krings, M., Stone, A., Schmitz, R. W., Krainitzki, H., Stoneking, M. & Pääbo, S., (1997). Neandertal DNA sequences and the origin of modern humans. *Cell 90 (1)*, 19-30.

Lindahl, T., (1993a). Instability and decay of the primary structure of DNA. *Nature 362 (6422)*, 709-715.

Lindahl, T., (1993b). Recovery of antediluvian DNA. *Nature 365 (6448)*, 700.

Malmstrom, H., Stora, J., Dalen, L., Holmlund, G. & Gotherstrom, A., (2005). Extensive human DNA contamination in extracts from ancient dog bones and teeth. *Molecular Biology and Evolution 22 (10)*, 2040-2047.

Malmstrom, H., Svensson, E. M., Gilbert, M. T., Willerslev, E., Gotherstrom, A. & Holmlund, G., (2007). More on contamination: the use of asymmetric molecular behavior to identify authentic ancient human DNA. *Molecular Biology and Evolution 24 (4)*, 998-1004.

Marota, I. & Rollo, F., (2002). Molecular paleontology. *Cellular and Molecular Life Sciences 59 (1)*, 97-111.

McHugh, P. J., Spanswick, V. J. & Hartley, J. A., (2001). Repair of DNA interstrand crosslinks: molecular mechanisms and clinical relevance. *The Lancet Oncology 2 (8)*, 483-490.

Mitchell, D., Willerslev, E. & Hansen, A., (2005). Damage and repair of ancient DNA. *Mutation Research 571 (1-2)*, 265-276.

Montiel, R., Malgosa, A. & Francalacci, P. (2001). Authenticating Ancient Human Mitochondrial DNA. *Human Biology 73(5)*, 689-713.

Mrevlishvili, G. M. & Svintradze, D. V., (2005). DNA as a matrix of collagen fibrils. *International Journal of Biological Macromolecules 36 (5)*, 324-326.

Mullis, K. B. & Faloona, F. A., (1987). Specific synthesis of DNA in vitro via a polymerase-catalyzed chain reaction. *Methods in Enzymology 155*, 335-350.

Nielsen-Marsh, C. M., Ostrom, P. H., Gandhi, H., Shapiro, B., Cooper, A., Hauschka, P. V. & Collins, M. J., (2002). Sequence preservation of osteocalcin protein and mitochondrial DNA in bison bones older than 55 ka. *Geology 30 (12)*, 1099-1102.

Nielsen-Marsh, C. M., Richards, M. P., Hauschka, P. V., Thomas-Oates, J. E., Trinkaus, E., Pettitt, P. B., Karavanic, I., Poinar, H. & Collins, M. J., (2005). Osteocalcin protein sequences of Neanderthals and modern primates. *Proceedings of the National Academy of Sciences of the United States of America 102 (12)*, 4409-4413.

Noonan, J. P., Hofreiter, M., Smith, D., Priest, J. R., Rohland, N., Rabeder, G., Krause, J., Detter, J. C., Pääbo, S. & Rubin, E. M., (2005). Genomic sequencing of Pleistocene cave bears. *Science 309 (5734)*, 597-599.

Orlando, L., Pages, M., Calvignac, S., Hughes, S. & Hanni, C., (2007). Does the 43 bp sequence from an 800,000 year old cretan dwarf elephantid really rewrite the textbook on mammoths? *Biology Letters 3 (1)*, 57-59; discussion 60-53.

Pääbo, S., (1985). Molecular cloning of Ancient Egyptian mummy DNA. *Nature 314 (6012)*, 644-645.

Pääbo, S., Gifford, J. A. & Wilson, A. C., (1988). Mitochondrial DNA sequences from a 7000-year old brain. *Nucleic Acids Research 16 (20)*, 9775-9787.

Pääbo, S., (1989). Ancient DNA: extraction, characterization, molecular cloning, and enzymatic amplification. *Proceedings of the National Academy of Sciences of the United States of America 86 (6)*, 1939-1943.

Pääbo, S., Higuchi, R. G. & Wilson, A. C., (1989). Ancient DNA and the polymerase chain reaction. The emerging field of molecular archaeology. *The Journal of Biological Chemistry 264 (17)*, 9709-9712.

Pääbo, S., Irwin, D. M. & Wilson, A. C., (1990). DNA damage promotes jumping between templates during enzymatic amplification. *The Journal of Biological Chemistry 265 (8)*, 4718-4721.

Pääbo, S., (1991). Amplifying DNA from archeological remains: a meeting report. *PCR Methods and Applications 1 (2)*, 107-110.

Pääbo, S. & Wilson, A. C., (1991). Miocene DNA sequences - a dream come true? *Current Biology 1 (1)*, 45-46.

Pääbo, S., Poinar, H., Serre, D., Jaenicke-Despres, V., Hebler, J., Rohland, N., Kuch, M., Krause, J., Vigilant, L. & Hofreiter, M., (2004). Genetic analyses from ancient DNA. *Annual Reviews of Genetics 38*, 645-679.

Paget, E., Jocteur Monrozier, L. & Simonet, P., (1992). Adsorption of DNA on clay minerals: protection against DNaseI and influence on gene transfer. *FEMS Microbiology Letters 97 (1-2)*, 31-39.

Poinar, H. N., Cano, R. J. & Poinar, G. O., (1993). DNA from an extinct plant. *Nature 363 (6431)*, 677-677.

Poinar, H. N., Höss, M., Bada, J. L. & Pääbo, S., (1996). Amino acid racemization and the preservation of ancient DNA. *Science 272 (5263)*, 864-866.

Poinar, H. N., Hofreiter, M., Spaulding, W. G., Martin, P. S., Stankiewicz, B. A., Bland, H., Evershed, R. P., Possnert, G. & Pääbo, S., (1998). Molecular coproscopy: dung and diet of the extinct ground sloth Nothrotheriops shastensis. *Science 281 (5375)*, 402-406.

Poinar, H. N. & Stankiewicz, B. A., (1999). Protein preservation and DNA retrieval from ancient tissues. *Proceedings of the National Academy of Sciences of the United States of America 96 (15)*, 8426-8431.

Poulakakis, N., Parmakelis, A., Lymberakis, P., Mylonas, M., Zouros, E., Reese, D. S., Glaberman, S. & Caccone, A., (2006). Ancient DNA forces reconsideration of evolutionary history of Mediterranean pygmy elephantids. *Biology Letters 2 (3)*, 451-454.

Prager, E. M., Wilson, A. C., Lowenstein, J. M. & Sarich, V. M., (1980). Mammoth albumin. *Science 209 (4453)*, 287-289.

Pusch, C. M., Giddings, I. & Scholz, M., (1998). Repair of degraded duplex DNA from prehistoric samples using Escherichia coli DNA polymerase I and T4 DNA ligase. *Nucleic Acids Research 26 (3)*, 857-859.

Pusch, C. M., Kayademir, T., Prangenberg, K., Conard, N. J., Czarnetzki, A. & Blin, N., (2002). Documenting ancient DNA quality via alpha satellite amplification and assessment of clone sequence diversity. *Journal of Applied Genetics 43 (3)*, 351-364.

Radström, P., Knutsson, R., Wolffs, P., Lövenklev, M. & Löfström, C., (2004). Pre-PCR processing: strategies to generate PCR-compatible samples. *Molecular Biotechnology 26 (2)*, 133-146.

Ricaut, F. X., Keyser-Tracqui, C., Crubezy, E. & Ludes, B., (2005). STR-genotyping from human medieval tooth and bone samples. *Forensic Science International 151 (1)*, 31-35.

Richards, M. B., Sykes, B. C. & Hedges, R. E. M., (1995). Authenticating DNA Extracted From Ancient Skeletal Remains. *Journal of Archaeological Science 22 (2)*, 291-299.

Rohland, N. & Hofreiter, M., (2007). Comparison and optimization of ancient DNA extraction. *Biotechniques 42 (3)*, 343-352.

Saiki, R. K., Scharf, S., Faloona, F., Mullis, K. B., Horn, G. T., Erlich, H. A. & Arnheim, N., (1985). Enzymatic amplification of beta-globin genomic sequences and restriction site analysis for diagnosis of sickle cell anemia. *Science 230 (4732)*, 1350-1354.

Salamon, M., Tuross, N., Arensburg, B. & Weiner, S., (2005). Relatively well preserved DNA is present in the crystal aggregates of fossil bones. *Proceedings of the National Academy of Sciences of the United States of America 102 (39)*, 13783-13788.

Scholz, M., Giddings, I. & Pusch, C. M., (1998). A polymerase chain reaction inhibitor of ancient hard and soft tissue DNA extracts is determined as human collagen type I. *Anal Biochem 259 (2)*, 283-286.

Sidow, A., Wilson, A. C. & Pääbo, S., (1991). Bacterial DNA in Clarkia fossils. *Philosophical transactions of the Royal Society of London. Series B, Biological sciences 333 (1268)*, 429-432; discussion 432-423.

Smith, C. I., Chamberlain, A. T., Riley, M. S., Stringer, C. & Collins, M. J., (2003). The thermal history of human fossils and the likelihood of successful DNA amplification. *Journal of Human Evolution 45 (3)*, 203-217.

Smith, C. I., Nielsen-Marsh, C. M., Jans, M. M. E. & Collins, M. J., (2007). Bone diagenesis in the European Holocene I: patterns and mechanisms. *Journal of Archaeological Science 34 (9)*, 1485-1493.

Stiller, M., Green, R. E., Ronan, M., Simons, J. F., Du, L., He, W., Egholm, M., Rothberg, J. M., Keates, S. G., Ovodov, N. D., Antipina, E. E., Baryshnikov, G. F., Kuzmin, Y. V., Vasilevski, A. A., Wuenschell, G. E., Termini, J., Hofreiter, M., Jaenicke-Despres, V. & Pääbo, S., (2006). Patterns of nucleotide misincorporations during enzymatic amplification and direct large-scale sequencing of ancient DNA. *Proceedings of the National Academy of Sciences of the United States of America 103 (37)*, 13578-13584.

Sutlovic, D., Definis-Gojanovic, M., Andelinovic, S., Gugic, D. & Primorac, D., (2005). Taq polymerase reverses inhibition of quantitative real time polymerase chain reaction by humic acid. *Croatian Medical Journal 46 (4)*, 556-562.

Svintradze, D. V., Mrevlishvili, G. M., Metreveli, N., Jariashvili, K., Namicheishvili, L., Skopinska, J. & Sionkowska, A., (2008). Collagen-DNA complex. *Biomacromolecules 9 (1)*, 21-28.

Tuross, N., (1994). The biochemistry of ancient DNA in bone. *Experientia 50 (6)*, 530-535.

Walden, K. K. & Robertson, H. M., (1997). Ancient DNA from amber fossil bees? *Molecular Biology and Evolution 14 (10)*, 1075-1077.

Wang, H. L., Yan, Z. Y. & Jin, D. Y., (1997). Reanalysis of published DNA sequence amplified from cretaceous dinosaur egg fossil. *Molecular Biology and Evolution 14 (5)*, 589-591.

Weiner, S., Lowenstam, H. A. & Hood, L., (1976). Characterization of 80-million-year-old mollusk shell proteins. *Proceedings of the National Academy of Sciences of the United States of America 73 (8)*, 2541-2545.

Wilson, I. G., (1997). Inhibition and facilitation of nucleic acid amplification. *Applied and Environmental Microbiology 63 (10)*, 3741-3751.

Willerslev, E., Hansen, A. J. & Poinar, H. N., (2004). Isolation of nucleic acids and cultures from fossil ice and permafrost. *Trends in Ecology & Evolution 19 (3)*, 141-147.

Willerslev, E. & Cooper, A., (2005). Ancient DNA. *Proceedings. Biological Sciences 272 (1558)*, 3-16.

Woodward, S. R., King, M. J., Chiu, N. M., Kuchar, M. J. & Griggs, C. W., (1994a). Amplification of ancient nuclear DNA from teeth and soft tissues. *PCR Methods and Applications 3 (4)*, 244-247.

Woodward, S. R., Weyand, N. J. & Bunnell, M., (1994b). DNA sequence from Cretaceous period bone fragments. *Science 266 (5188)*, 1229-1232.

Yang, D. Y. & Watt, K., (2005). Contamination controls when preparing archaeological remains for ancient DNA analysis. *Journal of Archaeological Science 32 (3)*, 331-336.

Ye, J., Ji, A., Parra, E. J., Zheng, X., Jiang, C., Zhao, X., Hu, L. & Tu, Z., (2004). A simple and efficient method for extracting DNA from old and burned bone. *Journal of Forensic Sciences 49 (4)*, 754-759.

Yin, Z., Chen, H., Wang, Z., Zhang, Z., Zou, Y., Fang, X. & Wang, H., (1996). [Sequence analysis of the cytochrome b gene fragment in a dinosaur egg]. *Yi Chuan Xue Bao 23 (3)*, 190-195.

Zischler, H., Höss, M., Handt, O., von Haeseler, A., van der Kuyl, A. C. & Goudsmit, J., (1995). Detecting dinosaur DNA. *Science 268 (5214)*, 1192-1193; author reply 1194.

In: Forensic Genetics Research Progress
Editor: F. Gonzalez-Andrade

ISBN: 978-1-60876-198-2
© 2010 Nova Science Publishers, Inc.

*Chapter 9*

# FORENSIC MITOCHONDRIAL DNA ANALYSIS

*Luísa Pereira*[1,2,*], *Farida Alshamali*[3],
*Fabricio González-Andrade*[4-5,†]

[1]Instituto de Patologia e Imunologia Molecular da Universidade do Porto, Portugal
[2]Faculdade de Medicina da Universidade do Porto (IPATIMUP), Portugal
[3]Dubai Police Forensic Administration, Dubai, UAE
[4]Department of Medicine, Metropolitan Hospital, Av. Mariana de Jesús Oe8, Quito, Ecuador
[5]Forensic Genetics Laboratory, Forensic Medicine Department, University of Zaragoza, Calle Domingo Miral s/n, Zaragoza 50.009, Spain

## ABSTRACT

The introduction of mitochondrial DNA (mtDNA) investigation in forensic genetics allowed to obtaining results from ancient, residual and degraded samples, enlarging extensively the possibility of applying genetic analyses to difficult forensic cases. However, the particular characteristics of mtDNA brought some conceptual and statistical challenges to forensic genetics, namely: the uniparental (maternal) transmission implies lineage instead of individual characterization, so that mtDNA can be more informative in excluding rather than in including a suspect; the absence of recombination in mtDNA renders impossible to apply the product rule for estimation of match probabilities, so that evaluations are limited to the frequency of a certain haplotype in a database; most of mtDNA haplotypes are unique or very low frequent, implying that databases must have a considerable number of individuals in order to be informative; heterogeneity in mutation rates between mtDNA positions and heteroplasmy must be taken into account when evaluating if diverse haplotypes can come from the same individual. Typically, the mtDNA survey in forensic genetics is performed by sequencing two hypervariable regions in the control region or D-loop. Some databases, reporting

---

[*] E-mail: lpereira@ipatimup.pt
[•] E-mail: shamali@emirates.net.ae
[†] E-mail: fabriciogonzaleza@yahoo.es

haplotypes in diverse populations, are publically available for forensic purposes. Recently, information from other polymorphisms located in the coding region is being also added to forensic analyses, which allows to inferring more securely the haplogroup to which the haplotype belongs. This phylogenetic information can be very informative for quality purposes, helping in detecting possible mix-up of samples and in checking haplogroup defining polymorphisms. Lately, the mtDNA screening is being enlarged to the total control region (~1200bp), and in the near future to the complete molecule. Such amount of information, in such a short period of time, will challenge forensic genetics in maintaining its strict quality-control of sequences and in being efficient to updating online databases for match evaluation.

## THE MtDNA MOLECULE

The mitochondrial DNA (mtDNA) is a circular genome localized inside mitochondria, in a variable number of copies. In humans (Figure 1) it is about 16,569bp long and composed of two main regions: the coding and the control region. The coding region, extending from position 577 to 16123, bears the genes for 22 tRNAs, 2 rRNAs and 13 proteins of the oxidative phosphorylation cycle, as well as the origin of replication for the light chain. The control region or D-loop, located in the remaining ~1,200bp, contains the control regions for replication of the heavy chain and for translation, being some of these controls located in two regions having a higher mutation rate than the rest of the molecule, receiving the designation of hypervariable region I and II (abbreviated, HVI, HVSI or HVRI and HVII, HVSII or HVRII).

MtDNA is uniparentaly transmitted, by the maternal side: mothers pass mtDNA to daughters and sons, but in the next generation, only the daughters will transmit the mtDNA. It is not well known why mtDNA present in the sperm is not maintained in the egg, but maybe a chemical inhibition is involved. So, all maternal related individuals will share the mtDNA lineage.

MtDNA does not undergo recombination, being transmitted in block. Recently, there were some claims in the opposite, but were refuted or not confirmed in other individuals. This absence of recombination allows an easy reconstruction and dating of the phylogeny, explaining the huge success of mtDNA in the population genetic field, but renders ineffective the product rule so familiar in forensic genetics. It is therefore impossible to estimate the frequency of composite genotypes (such as HVRI and HVRII) from their individual frequencies, as it is done for autosomal markers.

The first population studies using mtDNA (Brown 1980; Cann et al. 1987) screened a few single nucleotide polymorphisms (SNPs) along the molecule by Restriction Fragment Length Polymorphism Analysis (RFLP), but soon after, in the early 1990's, the advent of PCR led to an extensive sequencing of HVRI. In forensic genetics, both HVRI and HVRII began to be typed, by using mainly primers described by Vigilant et al. (1989) or by Wilson et al. (1995).

The characterization of HVRI and RFLP diversity in worldwide populations led to the reconstruction of the mtDNA phylogenetic tree and to the definition of haplogroup, being a monophyletic group of sequences, hence sharing the same ancestral and set of polymorphisms (Torroni et al. 1993). The first haplogroups to be defined were Asian ones being observed in

America, receiving the designations of A, B, C and D. Following these, the Eurasian and sub-Saharan haplogroups received the remaining letters of the alphabet. Hierarchy inside a certain haplogroup is named by a number following the letter and so on (letter, number, letter, number). Sub-Saharan haplogroups were shown to be at the root of the human mtDNA phylogenetic tree, favoring the hypothesis of a unique origin for the modern humans, with the further verification that this origin was a recent one, around 200,000 years ago (Cann et al. 1987; see revision in Torroni et al. 2006). The Out-of-Africa migration, occurring between 80,000-60,000 years ago, was responsible for the settlement of the World, being all non-African mtDNA haplogroups derived from a unique typical East African haplogroup, designated L3 (Figure 2). Thus, sub-Saharan haplogroups include the most diverse ones: L0, L1, L2, L3, L4, L5, L6 and L7. The L3 out-of-Africa gave rise to two macro-haplogroups: N, which is more frequent in Eurasia; and M, more frequent in East Asia. The macro-haplogroup N comprises clades N1, N2, X and R, being this last one split in R0, JT and U (including K). M is divided in a multitude of haplogroups observed throughout East Asia, Southeast Asia and America.

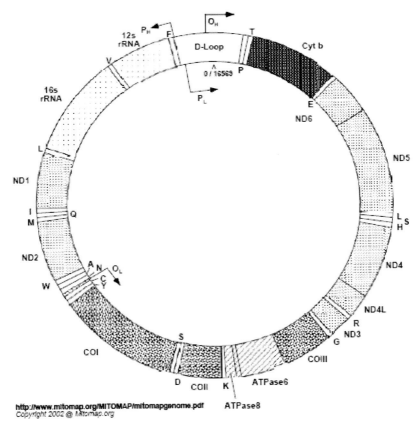

Figure 1. The map of the human mtDNA molecule, showing the D-Loop, the two rRNAs (12s rRNA and 16s rRNA), the 13 protein-coding genes (NADH dehydrogenases 1, 2, 3, 4, 4L, 5 and 6, cytochrome c oxidase I, II and III, cytochrome c oxidoreductase and ATP synthases 6 and 8), and the 22 tRNAs (represented by the first letter). The origins of replication of the two chains are represented ($O_H$ and $O_L$) as well as the strand-promoters for both chains ($P_H$ and $P_L$). Figure adapted from mitomap.org.

This high population structure, that is the existence of lineages characteristic from geographic regions, rendering the proportion of variance in diversity between population groups considerable, is in part due to the ¼ of mtDNA effective size when compared with autosomal markers. This lower effective size turns mtDNA much more sensitive to demographic phenomena such as founder effects, bottlenecks and genetic drift.

It would be tempting, in the forensic field, to assign an individual to a certain population group based on its mtDNA haplogroup. However, it should be stressed that mtDNA is only transmitted by the maternal side – while an individual can have a sub-Saharan mtDNA lineage, most of its nuclear genome can have a European constitution, and the individual present accordingly a European phenotype. For instance, the genetic composition just referred is observed in 10% of the autochthonous south Portuguese population (Pereira et al. 2004a).

## MtDNA Mutation Rate and Heterogeneity

The mutation rate in the control region is around 10 times higher than the one in the coding region (Vigilant et al. 1991). In 1996, Forster et al. estimated, more precisely, a rate of 1 substitution every 20,180 years for HVRI, between nucleotide positions 16090-16383. This mutation rate was used since then for the estimation of the Time for the Most Recent Common Ancestor (TMRCA) in the various haplogroups.

It was also shown around this time that the heterogeneity in mutation rates per position was higher for the HVRII when compared with HVRI, bearing many positions which are highly recurrent (as 150, 152 and 189) in long stretches of almost invariable positions (Meyer et al. 1999; Schneider and Excoffier 1999). These fast-evolving positions can mutate back and can appear in several haplogroup backgrounds (a condition known as homoplasy), being phylogenetically uninformative.

These mutation rates were being estimated by applying phylogenetic methods, and were shown to be lower than the estimates obtained when using genealogical inferences (analyzing mutations occurring along large familiar pedigrees; Howell et al. 1996). This uncertainty in the estimation of the mutation rates led to claims that they did not allow a safe reconstruction of phylogeny (Howell et al. 1996); a discussion ensued soon after, with opposite claims of a secure phylogenetic reconstruction by using mtDNA lineages (Macaulay et al. 1997). One explanation for the higher mutation rates when using genealogical inferences was that these were catching mutations in fast-evolving positions, which led to the over-estimation of the mutation rates. Although some arguments continued around this issue, this genome has been the main genetic tool used for inferences related with human migrations in the past.

A further support for its use came from the characterization of the complete molecule (the first population study was published by Ingman et al. 2000, for 53 worldwide samples), which showed the robustness of previous phylogenetic inferences. Surprisingly, some of the nucleotide positions located in the coding region showed also to be highly recurrent, as for instance 709, 3010 and 15301 (Freitas and Pereira 2008).

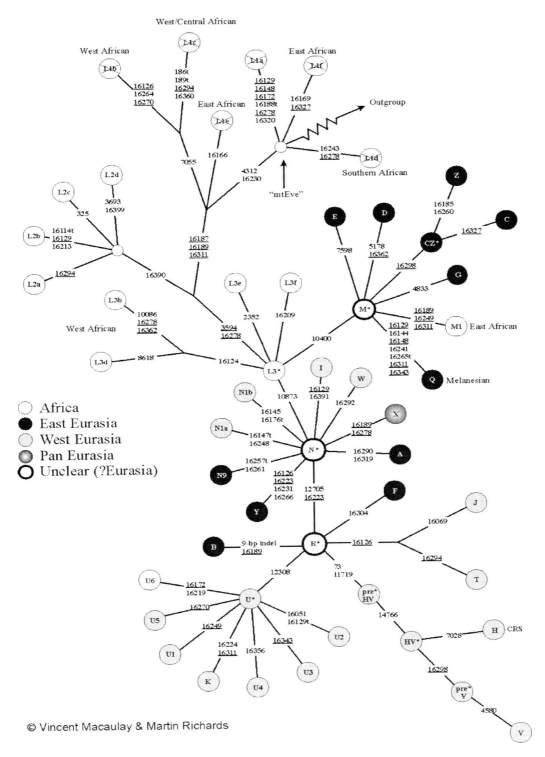

Figure 2. The human mtDNA worldwide phylogenetic tree based on HVRI and some RFLP diversities.

Forensic genetics must be, nonetheless, aware of this heterogeneity in mutation rates between positions, as they affect the evaluation of a match. Ultimately, the mutation rate for a certain position involved in a match evaluation should be taken into consideration. Unfortunately, there is still a lot of uncertainty around the estimation of mutation rates per position, for the human mtDNA. There are some tables reporting some values, but most are unapdated (see a sum up of these in Salas et al. 2007). The increasing publication of many complete human mtDNA sequences will soon resolve this situation.

## ISSUES RELATED WITH NOMENCLATURE

The first complete human mtDNA sequence was published by Anderson et al. (1981), being known as Cambridge Reference Sequence or CRS. Later on, Andrews et al. (1999) revised the CRS, correcting some of the previous errors, except insertions and deletions which would imply an alteration of the numbering; this new revised CRS, or rCRS, should be the one used as the human mtDNA reference sequence, versus which all the other sequences must be compared to. This sequence is deposited in GenBank with the Accession Number NC_000021.

This comparison versus a unique sequence for each species is very important in phylogenetic and forensic fields. Otherwise, data from diverse publications, each using a different reference sequence, would not be directly comparable. This confounding comparison versus several reference sequences was occurring for the dog mtDNA (Pereira et al. 2004b), a species that has gained an increasing interest in the forensic field.

Other nomenclature issues are also very important for standardization of mtDNA sequence report, such as the edition of the alignment in a homopolymeric track (a stretch of the same base). Different nomenclature criteria could misleadingly create diverse sequences. For instance, a track of 5 C's can be derived from one of 4 C's by deletion of a C in the first position, or in the second and so on. A few nomenclature rules were established in order to standardize these substitutions (Wilson et al. 2002a,b) – in the case referred, it was established that the substitution should be considered at the 3' end of the track and insertions referred as 15534.1C if the base inserted is a C (or X.2C if there is insertion of 2 Cs), while deletion coded as so (e.g., 15938del).

Concerning the recording of substitutions, for simplicity reasons, a haplotype can be described as being 15627-15639T/A-15814 or 15627-15639A-15814, where numbers without letters denote traansitions (15627 refers the A to G transition and 15814 the C to T), while transversions (as in the case of 15639) are explicitly indicated (or by just the new base).

There are other cases where the alignment of a certain gap can be interpreted in different ways, conducting to potentially miscoded variation. Wilson et al. (2002a) recommend an alignment approach that is based on a phylogenetic context using differential weighting of transitions, transversions and indels. Basically, they proved that most variants could be characterized if the following three recommendations are followed:

(1) Characterise profiles using the least number of differences from the reference sequence.

(2) If there is more than one way to maintain the same number of differences relatively to the reference, differences should be prioritised in the following manner:
   (a) indels
   (b) transitions
   (c) transversions
(3) Indels should be placed 3' with respect to the light strand. Insertions and deletions should be combined in situations where the same number of differences to the reference sequence is maintained.

For instance, when aligning the following haplotype F1 versus the reference:

F1 AAACCCTCCCCCTATG
Ref AAACCCTTCTCCCCTCCCCTATG

One possible alignment is:

F1 AAACCCT--------CCCCCTATG
Ref AAACCCTTCTCCCCTCCCC–TATG

that is: 15523del-15524del-15525del-15526del-15527del-15528del-15529del-15530del-15534.1C, where the combination of the insertion with the deletions is supported by phylogeny, since all the remaining F haplotypes have this insertion in comparison with the reference. But according to the first of the above rules, the following alignment must be considered

F1 AAACCCTC-------CCCCTATG
Ref AAACCCTTCTCCCCTCCCCTATG

that is: 15523-15524del-15525del-15526del-15527del-15528del-15529del-15530del, being the transition at position 15523 also supported by phylogeny.

Bandelt and Parson (2008) argued that a binary comparison does not solve all the problems, being bound to produce artificial alignments. Instead, they suggest a phylogenetic approach for multiple alignment and resulting notation, indicating the following rules:

- (Phylogenetic law) Sequences should be aligned with regard to the current knowledge of the phylogeny. In the case of multiple equally plausible solutions, one should strive for maximum (weighted) parsimony. Variants flanking long C tracts, however, are subject to extra conventions in view of extensive length heteroplasmy.
- (C tract conventions) The long C tracts of HVRI and HVRII should always be scored with 16189C and 310C, respectively, so that phylogenetically subsequent interruptions by novel C to T changes are encoded by the corresponding transition. Length variation of the short A tract preceding 16184 should be notated in terms of transversions.
- (Indel scoring) Indels should be placed 3' with respect to the light strand unless the phylogeny suggests otherwise.

## HETEROPLASMY

As there are many copies of mtDNA per mitochondrion and many mitochondria per cell, this genome is most of the times the only one recovered from residual and degraded samples, very common on the forensic routine. This explains the success of mtDNA in forensic casework related with some recent human calamities, such as the Asian tsunami in 2004 (Deng et al. 2005).

However, not all the mtDNA copies present in an individual are perfectly equal. As the mtDNA mutation rate is high, along life the mtDNA molecules will accumulate mutations, differing from the main dominant inherited molecule. Individuals are constituted by populations of diverse mtDNA molecules. This condition is known as heteroplasmy. For tissues which have a high replacement rate, such as blood, this issue is not problematic, as there is no time for accumulation of mutations in the mtDNA; but for tissues which have a low turnover (as cardiac muscle) or do not replace at all (as brain), the population of heteroplasmic molecules will increase with age.

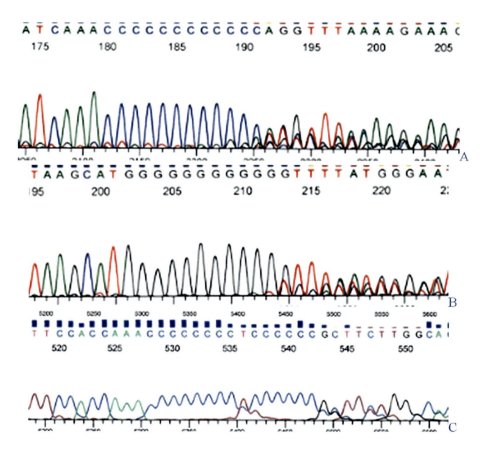

Figure 3. Length heteroplasmy in the region 16184-16193 in HVRI (A – forward and B- reverse senses) and 303-309 in HVRII.

In the forensic field, heteroplasmy is a very important issue when the samples consist in hairs collected in the crime scene, being this a very frequent occurrence. Each hair is a cell and its mitochondria passed through a severe bottleneck, so that the population of mitochondria present in one hair can be different from the other present in another hair. It was also shown that different shafts of the same hair can bear different populations of mtDNA (Brandstätter and Parson 2003).

Certain polymorphisms contribute extensively to heteroplasmy, as the indels in the homopolymeric tracks (for instance, the poly-C stretches in positions 303-309 and 310-315 in HVRII; and dinucleotides CAs between positions 514-523). These locations are highly prone to mutations due to slippage of the DNA polymerase, a condition known as length heteroplasmy (Figure 3).

When evaluating a match between the mtDNA from a suspect and a hair left in the crime scene, the possibility of heteroplasmy must be taken into account: it is possible that sequences differing in one position can still belong to the same individual, especially if it is a highly recurrent position. So, heterogeneity in mutation rates between positions is very important for the evaluation of heteroplasmy. Another issue which can contribute important information for the evaluation of heteroplasmy is phylogeny – heteroplasmy cannot erase one haplogroup and affiliate the sample in another haplogroup.

## WHEN ENVIRONMENT MIMICS MUTATION AND POSITIONS PRONE TO LAB HOTSPOTTING

Some old and degraded samples can still bear organic material enabling its molecular analyses; most probably, the mtDNA is the best preserved molecule or at least, due to the high number of copies per cell, the most frequent.

By the end of the 90's, there was a huge boom of publications reporting ancient mtDNA sequences. GenBank displayed even the mtDNA sequence of a dinosaur, which latter was shown to be a fragment of human mtDNA inserted in the nuclear genome (NUMTs; to be explained bellow). However, a natural limitation for ancient mtDNA studies was reported, due to DNA being postmortem degraded: calculations of deamination and depurination kinetics for the four nucleotides led to the estimation that under physiological salt conditions, neutral pH, and an ambient temperature of 15°C, 100,000 years is a likely limit of time beyond which DNA will be un-retrieved (Lindahl 1993).

These observations with ancient DNA can be valuable in the field of forensic genetics, where in some cases the only material available consists in very badly preserved bones. The biochemical modifications occurring in bones are analogous to those seen *in vivo*, and act through both the cross-linking and fragmentation of the molecule's chemical backbone and the alteration of individual nucleotide bases, being subjected to the environmental conditions (reviewed in Gilbert 2006). DNA fragmentation can be due to the effect of radiation or to the hydrolytic cleavage of diester bonds in the phosphate sugar backbone or the glycosidic bonds joining the bases to the sugars. DNA fragmentation will render amplification by PCR very difficult, especially if the fragments to amplify have around 300bp, as is typical in routine casework. In order to deal with this, some mini-sets of primers have been designed for highly degraded samples (Alonso et al. 2003; Eichmann and Parson 2008). With respect to the point base alterations, the most common damage-driven changes observed are the four transitions (C/T; G/A; T/C; A/G), mimicking the *in vivo* mutations and misleading the haplotyping identification.

Curiously, it was observed that lab processing of samples can also "induce" mutations. Brandstätter et al. (2005) analyzed 5,400 pairs of mtDNA control region electropherograms, from extant samples, for the light and heavy strands. These samples were typed with diverse chemistries and run in diverse automated sequencers. The authors were able to identify "phantom mutations", which are systematic artifacts generated in the course of the sequencing process, being the amount of these artifacts dependent on the sort of automated sequencer, the sequencing chemistry employed and other lab-specific factors. Further analysis of more than 30,000 published HVRI sequences confirmed some potential hotspots for phantom mutations, especially for variation at positions 16085 and 16197.

This propensity for hotspot under lab techniques and under postmortem modifications must also be taken into account in match evaluation and in phylogeny reconstructions.

## NUMTs AND CONTAMINATION

mtDNA only codes for 13 proteins of the oxidative phosporylation chain, which is composed of many more proteins. It is estimated that 80% of the mitochondrial proteins are coded by the nuclear DNA. Most probably, these proteins were once coded by the mtDNA, but genes coding them migrated, at some point, to the nucleus, being then lost from the mtDNA. These migrations of mtDNA fragments to the nuclear DNA do happen along time, and if they become successfully integrated in the nuclear DNA they receive the name of NUMTs – nuclear mitochondrial DNA sequences. When comparing the human and chimpanzee nuclear genomes, Mishmar et al. (2004) found a NUMT which is absent in the chimpanzee, showing that its insertion into the nuclear DNA occurred only in the line leading to *Homo sapiens*, being thus a very recent event. These authors accounted for a total of 247 NUMTs in the human genome.

Could these NUMTs be an additional source of contamination in routine forensic mtDNA analyses? In order to evaluate this possibility, Goios et al. (2006) analyzed the possibility of primer annealing for one of the most used HVRI and HVRII sets of primers in forensic genetics (the ones described by Wilson et al. 1995) in 19 of the 247 known human NUMTs bearing hypervariable regions. Their conclusion was that there is no possibility of HVRI and HVRII primer annealing in the NUMTs containing the hypervariable regions due to considerable mismatches between the primers and the complement region in the 19 NUMTs.

As it is now current to screen additional information from the coding region even in forensic investigations, these authors (Goios et al. 2008) conducted further analyses by focusing on a NUMT which bears a 97% homology to a segment of the mtDNA between positions 3914 and 9755. They designed two specific sets of primers for the mtDNA and for the nuclear DNA sequence by identifying regions with at least two mismatches between both genomes; these set of primers defined a segment of around 240bp which presented two SNPs allowing to distinguishing between mtDNA and nuclear segments. Amplifications with both sets of primers were performed along a range of annealing temperature and in several tissues (blood, hairs, buccal swabs and differential lyses of semen). Conclusions were that there was no risk of routine mis-amplification of nuclear fragments, being the opposite true: mtDNA mis-amplification by using nuclear specific primers at low temperatures. Some caution must, nevertheless, be taken into account when analyzing samples with very low number of mtDNA copies (as in the sperm).

## MTDNA DATABASES

mtDNA databases are essential tools for frequency estimations of mtDNA sequences, a basic step in the evaluation of a match.

When the first data on population mtDNA databases began to be analyzed, it was found that most haplotypes were unique. Pereira et al. (2004a) performed several empirical tests of the effect of sample size ($n$=50, 100, 200, 300 and 400) on the estimation of relevant parameters (such as haplotype diversity, number of different haplotypes, nucleotide diversity and number of polymorphic positions) in an enlarged mtDNA database ($n$=549) for the Portuguese population. While haplotype and nucleotide diversities did not vary significantly with sample size, the numbers of haplotypes and polymorphic positions raised continuously inside the tested interval. When using these data to extrapolate saturation curves (Figure 4), it was found that a sample size of 1,000 individuals is required for practical saturation of the number of haplotypes for HVRI (defined as the point where a sample size increase of 100 individuals corresponds to an increment in the diversity measure below 5%). For HVRII the same level is reached at $n$=900 and $n$=1,300 is needed when both regions are analyzed simultaneously. Consequently, the typical sample sizes of around 100 individuals are inadequate for both anthropological and forensic purposes.

Besides the issue of considerable sample sizes, in order to have an informative database, there is the issue of the high population structure. As already referred, a considerable proportion of genetic diversity is observed between populations when analyzing mtDNA, in opposition to when screening nuclear markers. This demands that question sample and control population must be geographically matched, even at a micro-geographic scale, when evaluating a mtDNA match (Pereira et al. 2005). A statistical significant bias can be committed when the frequency of a haplotype detected in a French casework is calculated in a Spanish mtDNA database.

Although there are many HVRI datasets published for most worldwide populations, in population genetic surveys, these cannot be all directly used in forensic evaluations. In fact, quality criteria in forensic investigations are very strict, implying that databases should pass a strong-quality control before its use. Errors and phantom mutations were detected in many population and clinical genetic studies (e.g. Salas et al. 2005), rendering these datasets inadequate for forensic applications.

One of the largest first databases with forensic purposes was designed by the FBI (Monson et al. 2002). But even in this case, a few errors were reported (Bandelt et al. 2004), namely mix-up of samples between HVRI and HVRII haplotypes, which are usually typed independently. These errors were corrected afterwards (Budowle and Polanskey 2005).

Salas, Bandelt and co-authors have published many examples of errors in datasets, aiming to call the attention of the forensic and clinical genetic fields to the amount of errors committed when reporting mtDNA sequences and its implications when included in databases (e.g. Salas et al. 2005). These authors also showed how phylogenetics can work as a quality control of mtDNA databases (Salas et al. 2007). Haplogroups are defined by motifs, or in other words, certain nucleotides at certain positions along the mtDNA molecule; hierarchy and absence of recombination renders that new mutations can appear additionally to the basic motif, but this cannot be erased, except for some defining mutations which can be located in fast-evolving positions (being prone to back-mutations). This phylogenetic analysis makes it possible to detect some mix-up of samples if, for instance, for a certain sample the indicated HVRI haplotype belongs to haplogroup J while its HVRII haplotype belongs to haplogroup X; most probably there were two different samples instead of one analyzed in the independent HVRI and HVRII screenings.

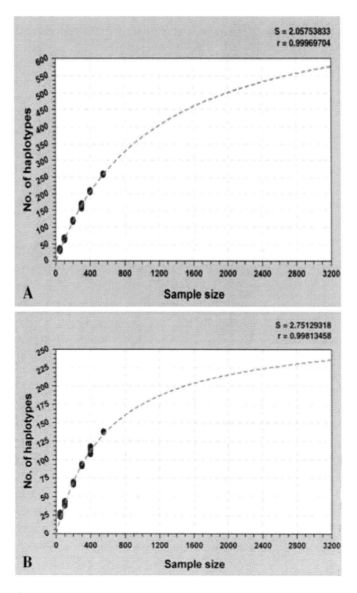

Figure 4. (Continued).

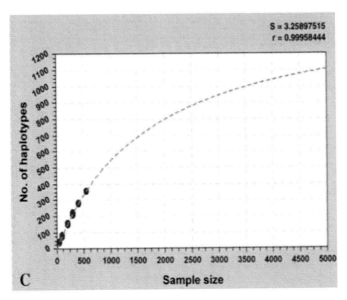

Figure 4. Sample sizes and number of haplotypes: regression curves for HVRI (*A*), HVRII (*B*) and HVRI+HVRII (**C**). *S* standard error, *r* correlation coefficient. All curves are of the form y=ax/(b+x), and coefficients were a=775.77 and b=1098.72 for HVRI, a=279.50 and b=588.64 for HVRII, a=1493.22 and b=1742.11 for HVRI+HVRII. (From Pereira et al. 2004a).

Taking these recommendations into account, several years were necessary for the development of a mtDNA database called EMPOP (EDNAP mtDNA Population Database), which meets forensic standards (Parson and Dür 2007). This database is available online at http://www.empop.org, and established a concept for mtDNA data generation, analysis, transfer and quality control (exemplified in Brandstätter et al. 2007). To help in the difficulty of detecting errors, the database displays software based on quasi-median network analysis for visualizing mtDNA data tables and thus pinpointing sequencing, interpretation and transcription errors. The first release launched on 16 October 2006 contained an effective of 5173. Most of these sequences were carefully screened for quality (a total of 4527), but the database also contains published databases (n=646).

## EVALUATION OF A MATCH

All the issues described so far make evaluation of a match for mtDNA haplotypes not an easy task to perform. The Scientific Working Group on DNA Analysis Methods (SWGDAM) published some guidelines for mtDNA nucleotide sequence interpretation, which although simplistic can work as a point of departure (SWGDAM 2003). These guidelines are to report:

*Exclusion* - If there are two or more nucleotide differences between the questioned and known samples

*Inconclusive* - If there is one nucleotide difference between the questioned and known samples

*Cannot Exclude* - If the sequences from questioned and known samples under comparison have a common base at each position or a common length variant in the HVRII C-stretch

*Weight of Evidence* - The mtDNA profile of a reference sample and an evidence sample that cannot be excluded as potentially originating from the same source can be searched in a population database.

One should bear in mind that there are many additional issues which must be taken into account when evaluating a match, namely:

- type of tissue of questioned and known samples, which influences dramatically the occurrence of heteroplasmy
- if heteroplasmy is under consideration, relative proportions of the two bases in forward and reverse senses must be compared
- type of polymorphism, knowing that indels are more recurrent and hence more prone to heteroplasmy; then transitions are more frequent than transversions; and the variable relative mutation rates between positions
- haplogroup affiliation: questioned and known samples must belong to the same haplogroup
- database must be reliable in terms of quality control of sequences, effective size and geographic matching.

The issue of an objective approach to match evaluation for mtDNA haplotypes is far from being resolved. It will continue to be a field of intense debate between forensic experts, which, most dangerously, can be perceived as a weakness by judges and lawyers. No matter the difficulties in interpreting mtDNA evidences, for sure superior to the autosomal ones, its power of information for resolving difficult forensic casework is not under question.

## THE PRESENT AND THE FUTURE

With the development of sequencing techniques, leading to faster, cheaper and easier typing, the sequencing of the hypervariable regions became complemented by screening some SNPs in the coding region. In particular, the description of minisequencing or SNaPshot allowed the design of multiplexes for several mtDNA SNPs. Some of the SNaPshots focused in sub-characterising the most frequent Eurasian haplogroup H (Quintáns et al. 2004; Brandstätter et al. 2006), other tried to sub-characterise all the Eurasian HVRI+HVRII haplotypes attaining a considerable frequency (Vallone et al. 2004), while still other aimed to help on the affiliation of samples in the main Eurasian haplogroups (Parson et al. 2008). As these SNPs are located in the coding region, a lower recurrence rate was expected. Nevertheless, several population data on complete mtDNA sequences and reconstructed phylogenies showed that some positions in the coding region can also be highly recurrent (as 3010, one of the positions defining a sub-haplogroup of H, called H1). But it is a fact that the combination of HVRI+HVRII+SNaPshot can increase considerable the power of discrimination between haplotypes (see Pereira et al. 2006 for the increase in resolution when screening 8 informative SNPs for sub-characterisation of haplogroup H in an extensive European dataset).

Other authors are performing the typing of the control region (~1,200bp) in forensic applications. Besides the hypervariable regions I and II, this region contains the highly recurrent position 16519, totally uninformative phylogenetically but conferring a high capacity of discrimination between haplotypes. However, the gain with the extension from HVRI+HVRII to the total control region is not so considerable as the segment between both hypervariable segments is among the most conserved ones in the mtDNA genome. Nevertheless, there are technical protocols for its typing in the forensic field (Brandstätter et al. 2004; Alshamali et al. 2008) and worldwide databases are being developed (Irwin et al. 2007).

There is no doubt that the desirable situation would be to sequence the complete mtDNA molecule, in order to obtain the maximum resolution. Parsons and Coble (2001) reported that of 31 individuals with the most common HVRI+HVRII haplotype, only three still matched after complete mtDNA sequencing, with similar high discrimination being seen for other common haplotypes. Technically, the complete mtDNA sequencing is easily accessible for normal-quality samples, being currently applied in population genetic studies. The first population study based on complete mtDNA sequences was published for a worldwide sample composed of 53 individuals (Ingman et al. 2000). By the end of August 2008, there were 5,140 complete human mtDNA genomes published in GenBank (revised in Pereira et al. 2009), amounting to around 85,164,660bp. Such amount of information poses serious problems on the maintenance of the strict forensic quality control criteria: when will it be possible to launch a forensic online database for complete mtDNA genomes scrutinized by the high-quality criteria? How many haplotypes would be there? How long would it take to update it?

Most of the complete mtDNA genomes screened in population genetic studies are being obtained by sequencing only one strand of the molecule, which is not adequate to forensic applications. In order to deal with this necessity to sequencing both strands, Fendt et al. (2009) published a protocol for high quality and reliable sequencing of full mtDNA genomes, consisting in: (1) amplifying two overlapping PCR-fragments comprising each about 8500 bases in length; and (2) then performing sequencing reactions with a set of 96 primers that can be applied to a (manual) 96 well-based technology, which results in at least double strand sequence coverage of the entire coding region.

Other challenges relate with the application of novel technologies rather than the typical automatic sequencing and mini-sequencing, in order to resolve difficult cases. One example is the development of mass spectrometry assays for resolving mixtures of mtDNA sequences (Hall et al. 2005). This technology can also be used to resolve heteroplasmy quantification.

## CONCLUSION

The inclusion of mtDNA analyses in forensic casework enlarged considerably the resolution of difficult cases through genetic evidence. These more than 20 years of application have shown that there are some technological challenges, namely related with heteroplasmy, admixture of samples and postmortem alterations. However, the highest difficulties relate with interpretation of data and evaluation of a mtDNA match. Experience has proved that a forensic investigator, when evaluating mtDNA evidence for the resolution of a forensic casework, must be aware of population genetics discoveries on the field of mtDNA. To do otherwise is equivalent to apply a poor scientific evaluation of the genetic proofs. Knowledge on phylogeography is essential for quality control of sequences; consideration of heterogeneous mutation rates between positions is basic for match evaluation; a sense of high population structure is fundamental on the calculation of the frequency of a haplotype in a reference database.

In the impossibility of deciding if it is preferable to have big databases containing a few errors or a very limited one in terms of sample size but of high quality, forensic genetics will pursuit in applying its high quality-control standards. This is, in our opinion, the biggest challenge faced now by forensic genetics: construct and maintain reliable and updated databases for complete mtDNA genomes under the restrictive forensic quality criteria. A lesson can be taken from the high quality HVRI+HVRII/control region EMPOP database: it took many years to be released and it was not updated since 16 October 2006. We must be more efficient in terms of bioinformatics sustained on phylogeographic knowledge. Otherwise so much information available will only contribute noise to our capacity of resolving forensic casework through mtDNA genetic evidences.

## COMPETING INTERESTS

The authors declare that they have no competing interests. The authors alone are responsible for the content and writing of the paper.

## REFERENCES

Alonso A, Martin P, Albarrán C, García P, Primorac D, García O, Fernández de Simón L, García-Hirschfeld J, Sancho M, Fernández-Piqueras J (2003) Specific quantification of human genomes from low copy number DNA samples in forensic and ancient DNA studies. *Croat Med J.* 44:273-280.

Alshamali F, Brandstätter A, Zimmermann B, Parson W (2008) Mitochondrial DNA control region variation in Dubai, United Arab Emirates. *Forensic Sci Int Genet.* 2:e9-10.

Anderson S, Bankier AT, Barrell BG, de Bruijn MH, Coulson AR, Drouin J, Eperon IC, Nierlich DP, Roe BA, Sanger F, Schreier PH, Smith AJ, Staden R, Young IG (1981) Sequence and organization of the human mitochondrial genome. *Nature.* 290:457-465.

Andrews RM, Kubacka I, Chinnery PF, Lightowlers RN, Turnbull DM, Howell N (1999) Reanalysis and revision of the Cambridge reference sequence for human mitochondrial DNA. *Nat Genet.* 23:147.

Bandelt HJ, Salas A, Bravi C (2004) Problems in FBI mtDNA database. *Science.* 305:1402-1404.

Bandelt HJ, Parson W (2008) Consistent treatment of length variants in the human mtDNA control region: a reappraisal. *Int J Legal Med.* 122:11-21.

Brandstätter A, Parson W (2003) Mitochondrial DNA heteroplasmy or artefacts - a matter of the amplification strategy? *Int J Legal Med.* 117:180-184.

Brandstätter A, Peterson CT, Irwin JA, Mpoke S, Koech DK, Parson W, Parsons TJ (2004) Mitochondrial DNA control region sequences from Nairobi (Kenya): inferring phylogenetic parameters for the establishment of a forensic database. *Int J Legal Med.* 118:294-306.

Brandstätter A, Sänger T, Lutz-Bonengel S, Parson W, Béraud-Colomb E, Wen B, Kong QP, Bravi CM, Bandelt HJ (2005) Phantom mutation hotspots in human mitochondrial DNA. *Electrophoresis.* 26:3414-3429.

Brandstätter A, Salas A, Niederstätter H, Gassner C, Carracedo A, Parson W (2006) Dissection of mitochondrial superhaplogroup H using coding region SNPs. *Electrophoresis.* 27:2541-2550.

Brandstätter A, Niederstätter H, Pavlic M, Grubwieser P, Parson W (2007) Generating population data for the EMPOP database - an overview of the mtDNA sequencing and data evaluation processes considering 273 Austrian control region sequences as example. *Forensic Sci Int.* 166:164-175.

Brown WM (1980) Polymorphism in mitochondrial DNA of humans as revealed by restriction endonuclease analysis. *Proc Natl Acad Sci U S A.* 77:3605-3609.

Budowle B, Polanskey D (2005) FBI mtDNA database: a cogent perspective. *Science.* 307:845-847.

Cann RL, Stoneking M, Wilson AC (1987) Mitochondrial DNA and human evolution. *Nature.* 325:31-36.

Deng YJ, Li YZ, Yu XG, Li L, Wu DY, Zhou J, Man TY, Yang G, Yan JW, Cai DQ, Wang J, Yang HM, Li SB, Yu J (2005) Preliminary DNA identification for the tsunami victims in Thailand. *Genomics Proteomics Bioinformatics.* 3:143-157.

Eichmann C, Parson W (2008) 'Mitominis': multiplex PCR analysis of reduced size amplicons for compound sequence analysis of the entire mtDNA control region in highly degraded samples. *Int J Legal Med.* 122:385-388.

Fendt L, Zimmermann B, Daniaux M, Parson W (2009) Sequencing strategy for the whole mitochondrial genome resulting in high quality sequences. *BMC Genomics.* 10:139.

Forster P, Harding R, Torroni A, Bandelt HJ (1996) Origin and evolution of Native American mtDNA variation: a reappraisal. *Am J Hum Genet.* 59:935-945.

Freitas F, Pereira L (2008) Heterogeneity in coding mtDNA mutation rates: implications in forensic genetics. *Forensic Sci Int: Genetics. Supplementary Series* 1: 274-276.

Gilbert MTP (2006) Postmortem damage of mitochondrial DNA. In Bandelt H-J, Macaulay V, Richards M (Eds) Human mitochondrial DNA and the evolution of *Homo sapiens. Nucleic Acids and Molecular Biology.* 18: 91-115. Springer Verlag. Berlin; Heildelberg.

Goios A, Amorim A, Pereira L (2006) Mitochondrial DNA pseudogenes in the nuclear genome as possible sources of contamination. *International Congress Series* 1288:697-699.

Goios A, Prieto L, Amorim A, Pereira L (2008) Specificity of mtDNA-directed PCR-influence of NUclear MTDNA insertion (NUMT) contamination in routine samples and techniques. *Int J Legal Med.* 122:341-345.

Hall TA, Budowle B, Jiang Y, Blyn L, Eshoo M, Sannes-Lowery KA, Sampath R, Drader JJ, Hannis JC, Harrell P, Samant V, White N, Ecker DJ, Hofstadler SA (2005) Base composition analysis of human mitochondrial DNA using electrospray ionization mass spectrometry: a novel tool for the identification and differentiation of humans. *Anal Biochem.* 344:53-69.

Howell N, Kubacka I, Mackey DA (1996) How rapidly does the human mitochondrial genome evolve? *Am J Hum Genet.* 59:501-509.

Ingman M, Kaessmann H, Pääbo S, Gyllensten U (2000) Mitochondrial genome variation and the origin of modern humans. *Nature.* 408:708-713.

Irwin JA, Saunier JL, Strouss KM, Sturk KA, Diegoli TM, Just RS, Coble MD, Parson W, Parsons TJ (2007) Development and expansion of high-quality control region databases to improve forensic mtDNA evidence interpretation. *Forensic Sci Int Genet* 1:154-157.

Lindahl T (1983) Instability and decay of the primary structure of DNA. Nature 362:709-715.

Macaulay VA, Richards MB, Forster P, Bendall KE, Watson E, Sykes B, Bandelt HJ (1997) mtDNA mutation rates--no need to panic. *Am J Hum Genet.* 61:983-990.

Meyer S, Weiss G, von Haeseler A (1999) Pattern of nucleotide substitution and rate heterogeneity in the hypervariable regions I and II of human mtDNA. *Genetics.* 152:1103-1110.

Mishmar D, Ruiz-Pesini E, Brandon M, Wallace DC (2004) Mitochondrial DNA-like sequences in the nucleus (NUMTs): insights into our African origins and the mechanism of foreign DNA integration. *Hum Mutat.* 23:125-133.

Monson KL, Miller KWP, Wilson MR, DiZinno JA, Budowle B (2002) The mtDNA population database: an integrated software and database resource for forensic comparison. *Forensic Sciences Communications.* 4.

Parson W, Dür A (2007) EMPOP-a forensic mtDNA database. *Forensic Sci Int Genet.* 1:88-92.

Parson W, Fendt L, Ballard D, Børsting C, Brinkmann B, Carracedo A, Carvalho M, Coble MD, Real FC, Desmyter S, Dupuy BM, Harrison C, Hohoff C, Just R, Krämer T, Morling N, Salas A, Schmitter H, Schneider PM, Sonntag ML, Vallone PM, Brandstätter A (2008) Identification of West Eurasian mitochondrial haplogroups by mtDNA SNP screening: results of the 2006-2007 EDNAP collaborative exercise. *Forensic Sci Int Genet.* 2:61-68.

Parsons TJ, Coble MD (2001) Increasing the forensic discrimination of mitochondrial DNA testing through analysis of the entire mitochondrial DNA genome. *Croat Med J.* 42:304-309.

Pereira L, Cunha C, Amorim A (2004a) Predicting sampling saturation of mtDNA haplotypes: an application to an enlarged Portuguese database. *Int J Legal Med.* 118:132-136.

Pereira L, Van Asch B, Amorim A (2004b) Standardisation of nomenclature for dog mtDNA D-loop: a prerequisite for launching a *Canis familiaris* database. *Forensic Sci Int.* 141:99-108.

Pereira L, Gonçalves J, Goios A, Rocha T, Amorim A (2005) Human mtDNA haplogroups and reduced male fertility: real association or hidden population substructuring. *Int J Androl.* 28:241-247.

Pereira L, Richards M, Goios A, Alonso A, Albarrán C, Garcia O, Behar DM, Gölge M, Hatina J, Al-Gazali L, Bradley DG, Macaulay V, Amorim A (2006) Evaluating the forensic informativeness of mtDNA haplogroup H sub-typing on a Eurasian scale. *Forensic Sci Int.* 159:43-50.

Pereira L, Freitas F, Fernandes V, Pereira JB, Costa MD, Costa S, Máximo V, Macaulay V, Rocha R, Samuels DC (2009) The diversity present in 5140 human mitochondrial genomes. *Am J Hum Genet* 58:1-13.

Quintáns B, Alvarez-Iglesias V, Salas A, Phillips C, Lareu MV, Carracedo A (2004) Typing of mitochondrial DNA coding region SNPs of forensic and anthropological interest using SNaPshot minisequencing. *Forensic Sci Int.* 140:251-257.

Salas A, Carracedo A, Macaulay V, Richards M, Bandelt HJ (2005) A practical guide to mitochondrial DNA error prevention in clinical, forensic, and population genetics. *Biochem Biophys Res Commun.* 335:891-899.

Salas A, Bandelt HJ, Macaulay V, Richards MB (2007) Phylogeographic investigations: the role of trees in forensic genetics. *Forensic Sci Int.* 168:1-13.

Schneider S, Excoffier L (1999) Estimation of past demographic parameters from the distribution of pairwise differences when the mutation rates vary among sites: application to human mitochondrial DNA. *Genetics.* 152:1079-1089.

SWGDAM (2003) Guidelines for mitochondrial DNA (mtDNA) nucleotide sequence interpretation. *Forensic Sci. Commun.* 5:2.

Torroni A, Schurr TG, Cabell MF, Brown MD, Neel JV, Larsen M, Smith DG, Vullo CM, Wallace DC. (1993) Asian affinities and continental radiation of the four founding Native American mtDNAs. *Am J Hum Genet.* 53:563-590.

Torroni A, Achilli A, Macaulay V, Richards M, Bandelt HJ. (2006) Harvesting the fruit of the human mtDNA tree. Trends Genet. 22:339-345.

Vallone PM, Just RS, Coble MD, Butler JM, Parsons TJ (2004) A multiplex allele-specific primer extension assay for forensically informative SNPs distributed throughout the mitochondrial genome. *Int J Legal Med.* 118:147-157.

Vigilant L, Pennington R, Harpending H, Kocher TD, Wilson AC (1989) Mitochondrial DNA sequences in single hairs from a southern African population. *Proc Natl Acad Sci* U S A. 86:9350-9354.

Vigilant L, Stoneking M, Harpending H, Hawkes K, Wilson AC (1991) African populations and the evolution of human mitochondrial DNA. *Science.* 253:1503-1507.

Wilson MR, DiZinno JA, Polanskey D, Replogle J, Budowle B (1995) Validation of mitochondrial DNA sequencing for forensic casework analysis. *Int J Legal Med.* 108:68-74.

Wilson MR, Allard MW, Monson K, Miller KW, Budowle B (2002a) Recommendations for consistent treatment of length variants in the human mitochondrial DNA control region. *Forensic Sci Int.* 129:35-42.

Wilson MR, Allard MW, Monson K, Miller KW, Budowle B (2002b) Further discussion of the consistent treatment of length variants in the human mitochondrial DNA control region. *Forensic Sci. Commun.* 4: 4.

In: Forensic Genetics Research Progress
Editor: F. Gonzalez-Andrade

ISBN: 978-1-60876-198-2
© 2010 Nova Science Publishers, Inc.

*Chapter 10*

# SNPs TECHNOLOGIES IN FORENSIC GENETICS: APPROACH AND APPLICATIONS

## *Anna Barbaro*[*]

Department of Forensic Genetics, SIMEF, Reggio Calabria, Italy and Instituto de Medicina Legal, Univeristy of Santiago de Compostela, Spain

### ABSTRACT

Single Nucleotide Polymorphisms (SNPs) represent the most common form of natural genetic variation in the human genome (approximately 90%) and are considered the major genetic source to phenotypic variability that differentiate individuals. Because SNPs occur frequently throughout the genome and tend to be relatively stable genetically, they serve as excellent biological markers for identification of genes in parts of the genome that may have some relation to a specific disease and even have influence on response to drug regimens.

In the last years the interest to SNPs is increased because they show a range of characteristics that make them well suited even to forensic analysis, including: abundance in the genome, Low mutation rates, reduced amplicon sizes (ability to analyze degraded DNA), relatively simple multiplex assays, potential for automation.

Single nucleotide polymorphisms may have in the near future a fundamental role in forensics, not only in specialized applications such as phylogeographical or ancestry studies (mtDNA, Y-SNPs) but also for the potential applications of autosomal SNPs either in the prediction of phenotypic traits than in real forensic caseworks applications.

Even if it is not likely that SNPs typing will totally replace STRs as the principal method for human identification, however new SNPs genotyping methods, chemistries and platforms are continuously being developed and considerable researches are still undergone to establish adequate scientific foundations for these applications.

---

[*] E-mail: simef_dna@tiscali.it

## INTRODUCTION

A single-nucleotide polymorphism (SNP) is a a single base change in a DNA sequence. It occurs when a single nucleotide (A, T, C, or G) in the genome is replaced by any of the other three bases and the DNA sequence differs between individuals of a species or between paired chromosomes in an individual. (An example: in the DNA sequence AGCT, a SNP occurs when the G base changes to a C, and the sequence becomes ACCT)A variation is considered to be a SNP, if it occurs in at least 1% of the population.

SNPs occur with a very high frequency, with estimates ranging from about 1 in 1000 bases to 1 in 100 to 300 bases along the 3-billion-base human genome: about 10 million SNPs exist in human populations that represent about 90% of all human genetic variation.

The rate of SNPs varies some along human chromosomes: the Y chromosome, such as the X chromosome, has less genetic variation than autosomes because the number of chromosomes ( effective population size) is fewer than for autosomes.

The most common type of SNPs has alleles A and G in a strand while in the opposite has alleles T and C. So an A/G SNP can also be described as a T/C SNP, depending upon strand orientation. It has been estimated that the distribution of the types of SNPs in human genome could be the following: 63 % A/G (and T/C), 17 % A/C (and T/G), 8 % CG, 4 % AT and 8% insertion/deletions [1]. Even if a SNP could theoretically have three or four alleles, almost all common SNPs have only two alleles: the minor allele is the one showed the lowest frequency at a locus analyzed in a particular population. There are variations between human populations, so an SNP allele that is common in one geographical or ethnic group may be much rarer in another.

A set of associated SNP alleles in a particular region of a chromosome is defined "haplotype". Almost most regions show only a few common haplotypes, with a frequency of at least 5%, which account for most of the variation from person to person in a population. Even if a chromosome region may contain many SNPs, only a few tag SNPs can provide most of the useful information about the pattern of genetic variation in that region.

SNPs are also evolutionarily stable, not changing much from a generation to another: it makes them easier to follow in population studies

SNPs may be found within coding or non-coding regions of genes, or in the intergenic regions between genes and in both nuclear and mitochondrial DNA. But only about 3 - 5 % of a person's DNA sequence codes for proteins, so most SNPs are found outside of the coding sequences.

SNPs within a coding sequence not always change the amino acid sequence of the protein, due to degeneracy of the genetic code. A SNP in which both forms lead to the same polypeptide sequence is called synonymous (a silent mutation) while if a different polypeptide sequence is produced, it's termed nonsynonymous.

A nonsynonymous change may either be missense or nonsense: a missense change produces a different amino acid while a nonsense change results in a premature stop codon. All that could alter the protein, which in turn could influence a person's health.

Single nucleotide polymorphisms that are not in protein-coding regions may have consequences for gene splicing, transcription factor binding, or the sequence of non-coding RNA.

Although more than 99% of human DNA sequences are the same, variations in DNA sequence can predispose people to disease or influence their response to disease, environmental factors (such as bacteria, viruses, toxins, and chemicals) drugs and therapies. [2], [3].

The abundance of SNPs and the ease with which they can be measured make these genetic variations useful for biomedical research and for developing pharmaceutical products or medical diagnostics.

Single nucleotide polymorphisms within a gene region have often been studied to evaluate their effect on phenotype. Although a single base pair change can produce a phenotypic change, however a phenotype is often influenced by the presence of multiple polymorphisms and their relative positions within a given region. This means that it is essential to study the haplotype, or the combination of multiple SNPs alleles on each chromosome in order to associate genomic changes with a particular phenotype. [4]

SNP markers are preferred over microsatellite markers for association studies because of their abundance along the human genome (SNPs with minor allele frequency > 10% occur in 1 of every 600 bp) [5], the low mutation rate and the potential to high-throughput genotyping.

Different genotyping applications require screening of different numbers of SNPs.

The determination of a single SNP can be sufficient to screen for the presence of a Mendelian disease even if to accurately evaluate whether mutations within a class of genes contribute to a disease, hundreds to thousands of SNPs must be studied in association studies.

In fact the number of SNPs required for genomewide association studies depends on the LD pattern. Recent studies [6],[7],[8,],[9],[10] have shown that the human genome can be partitioned into discrete blocks of high LD and relatively limited haplotype diversity, separated by shorter regions of low LD. One of the practical implications of this observation is that only a small fraction of all the single-nucleotide polymorphisms (SNPs) (referred as "tag SNPs") is sufficient to capture most of haplotype structure of the human genome in each block.

So it can be extremely useful for association studies in which it is not necessary to genotype all SNPs since it permits significantly to reduce genotyping effort. [11]

As a general rule, the greater is the number of polymorphic DNA markers, the greater is the statistical likelihood of finding significant correlations.

Many efforts in both the public (Human Genome Project) as well as the private (The SNP Consortium) sectors have been made underway to generate high-density SNPs maps that could provide the framework for research studies designed to identify genes involved in the physiology of multigenic diseases, as well as diagnostic markers or responsible of different individual response to drug or pharmaceuticals.

## SNPS RESEARCH PROJECT

In the past years, several research groups worked to create SNP maps of the human genome. Among these were the U.S. Human Genome Project (HGP) and a group of companies called the SNP Consortium.

The U.S. Human Genome Project was a 13-year effort coordinated by the U.S. Department of Energy (DOE) and the National Institutes of Health (NIH) with the aim to discover all the estimated 20,000-25,000 human genes and make them accessible for further biological study. [12]

The project begun in October 1990 and originally was planned to last 15 years, but rapid technological advances accelerated the completion date to 2003.

In 1998, as a part of the last five years research plans, the DOE and NIH established the following goals about Human Genome Sequence Variation:

- Develop technologies for rapid, large-scale identification and/or scoring of single nucleotide polymorphisms and other DNA sequence variants.
- Identify common variants in the coding regions of the majority of identified genes during this five-year period.
- Create a SNP map of at least 100,000 markers.
- Develop the intellectual foundations for studies of sequence variation.
- Create public resources of DNA samples and cell lines.
- (http://www.ornl.gov/sci/techresources/Human_Genome/hg5yp/goal.shtml)

The initial aim was briefly reached and widely exceeded since in February 2003 were mapped 3.7 million human SNPs. All data informations are stored in a public database accessible as a common resource for scientits. The SNP Consortium (TSC) was established in april 1999 under the leading of Arthur L. Holden as a collaboration of ten large pharmaceutical companies and the U.K. Wellcome Trust philanthropy . The goal was to discover in two years 300,000 SNPs and to produce a public widely accepted, high-quality SNPs map resource. [13]

The international member companies APBiotech, AstraZeneca Group PLC, Aventis, Bayer Group AG, Bristol-Myers Squibb Co., F. Hoffmann-La Roche, Glaxo Wellcome PLC, IBM, Motorola, Novartis AG, Pfizer Inc., Searle, and SmithKline Beecham PLC contributed at least $30 million to the consortium while the Wellcome Trust gave around $14 million. Laboratories funded by these companies to identify SNPs are located at the Whitehead Institute, Sanger Centre, Washington University (St. Louis), and Stanford University. Data management and analysis take place at Cold Spring Harbor Laboratory.

The final results largely exceeded the initial purpose and a high-density map with 1.8 million SNPs was created. Now that the first phase of the TSC project is essentially complete, the current goal is to determine the of the allele frequency/genotype frequency of certain SNPs in the major world populations.

A public website (http://snp.cshl.org), maintained at Cold Spring Harbor Laboratory, was established to make all TSC project data available to the research community, to provide information about the project itself and also to improve existing data browsing and searching facilities. [14]

The mapping of the human genome has made possible to develop a haplotype map in order to better define human SNP variability. The haplotype map or "HapMap" (www.hapmap.org) is a powerful tool that allow researchers to find genes and genetic variations that affect health and disease. The International HapMap Project is a multi-country effort started on October 2002 as a collaboration among scientists from public and private organizations in six countries (Canada, China, Japan, Nigeria, United States, United Kingdom).

The goal of the project is to compare the genetic sequences of different individuals to identify the common patterns of genetic variation in humans. This includes the chromosome regions with sets of strongly associated SNPs, the haplotypes in those regions, the SNPs that tag them, the identification of regions where associations among SNPs are weak.

All of the information generated by the Project are released into the public domain, in order to help researchers in finding genes that affect health, disease, and individual responses to therapeutic drugs and environmental factors.( http://snp.cshl.org/downloads/index.html.en)

In the initial phase of the Project, were analyzed genetic data from four populations with African, Asian, and European ancestry, from a total of 270 samples. The project is now in the 3th phase and contains genotypes data from 1301 individuals (including the original 270 samples used in Phase I and II of the International HapMap Projec) from 11 populations. (http://www.broad.mit.edu/~debakker/p3.html)

In the initial project for developing the HapMap, samples had to be genotyped for at least 1 million SNPs across the human genome. Since many chromosome regions show too few SNPs, and many SNPs were too rare to be useful, additional SNPs were required to develop the HapMap.

Approximately 1.3 million SNPs were genotyped in Phase I of the project, in Phase II a further 2.1 million SNPs were successfully genotyped on the same individuals, by october 2007 more than 3 millions SNPs were found and discovery still continues. [15]

Genotyping quality was assessed by using duplicate samples, since all centers genotyped a standard set of SNPs and checked some of the genotypes produced by other centers.

The Project initially (by about June of 2004) produced a map of 600,000 SNPs evenly spaced across the genome, which is a density of one SNP every 5000 bases, but the increased quantity of identified SNPs in the second phase generated a resulting HapMap with a density of around 1 SNP per kilobase and it has been estimated to contain approximately 25–35% of all the 9–10 million common SNPs in the assembled human genome.

## SNPs AND DISEASES

Most common diseases, such as diabetes, cancer, heart disease, depression, asthma are affected by many genes and environmental factors. Unrelated people share for about the 99.9% the same DNA sequences but the remaining 0.1% is important because it contains the genetic variants that could influence people response to common diseases risk or to pharmaceuticals.

Researchers have found that only rarely a SNP may be responsible for a disease, most of them do not cause diseases but they can help to determine the likelihood that someone will develop a particular illness. [16]

In fact if a SNP is frequently found close to a particular gene, it can act as a marker for that gene, helping the identification of multiple genes associated with illness. These associations are generally difficult to establish with conventional methods because a single altered gene may give only a small contribution to a particular disease.

To create a genetic test that will screen for a disease in which the disease-causing gene has already been identified, scientists collect blood samples and analyze their DNA for SNP patterns. Next, researchers compare these patterns to patterns.

In "association study" SNPs patterns from a group of individuals affected by the disease are analyzed and compared with the ones obtained by analyzing the DNA from a group of individuals not affected by the disease. This is performed to detect differences between the SNP patterns of the two groups, to evaluate which pattern is most likely associated with the disease-causing gene.

A good example of SNPs involved in a disease development is the apolipoprotein E (ApoE), one of the genes associated with Alzheimer's disease. ApoE contains two SNPs that result in three possible alleles for this gene: E2, E3, and E4. Each allele differs by one DNA base, and the protein product of each gene differs by one amino acid. Each person inherits one maternal copy of ApoE and one paternal copy of ApoE. A person who has at least one E4 allele will have a greater chance of developing Alzheimer's disease. This because the change of one amino acid in the E4 protein alters its structure and function, making disease development more likely. On the contrary E2 allele reduces the risk that a person develop Alzheimer's.

SNPs obviously are not the unique indicators of disease development. In fact has been showed that an individual with two E4 alleles may never develop Alzheimer's, while another one who has two E2 alleles may develop the disease. ApoE is just one gene that has been linked to Alzheimer's, but like most common chronic disorders even Alzheimer's has a polygenic nature. This obviously makes genetic testing for these disorders so complicated.

Since SNPs can be gene markers, SNP profiles can be also used to evaluate risk factors associated with complex diseases such as cancer. For example, if examining the SNP profiles from many individuals, including colon cancer patients, within the many different profiles is found a small subset of SNPs that is only present in colon cancer patient, this means that those SNPs are associated only with colon cancer. In this case SNPs may be considered markers for colon cancer genes. In another case if analyzing a random population of 100 people, 80% have SNPA and the remaining 20% have SNP B, while in another 100 people population with cancer 60% have SNPA and the remaining 40% have SNP B, this indicate that neither SNP A nor SNP B causes cancer. But a person who has SNP B is at a higher risk to develop cancer than a person with SNP A.

(http://nci.nih.gov/cancertopics/understandingcancer/geneticvariation)

## SNPs and Response to Drug Therapy

Since some individuals respond well to a specific drug treatment, while others have minimal or no response, SNPs may also be involved in different patients response to the same drug.

Many proteins are involved in drug transportation throughout the body, absorption into tissues, metabolism and excretion. If a person has SNPs in any one or more of these proteins, they may alter the time of the body exposure to active forms of the drug or any of its products.

So by studying SNP profiles in different groups of individuals who respond or not to a specific drug treatment, a correlations can emerge between certain SNPs and patients specific responses to a treatment (e.g. cancer treatment): this means that in a future a SNP profile can be used to advise a patient about any treatment options.

## SNPs and Susceptibility to Lung Cancer

It has been showed that when an individual smokes cigarettes, precarcinogens in the tobacco enter to lungs and placein the fat-soluble area of the cells. Some proteins bind them converting the precarcinogens into carcinogens. Detoxifying proteins quickly make carcinogens water-soluble, allowing in this way their elimination into the urine, before they damage the cell.

Because of SNPs, a person can have a very active carcinogen-making protein, or a slow one, or an intermediate type. A very active binding protein can "grab" more precarcinogen than usual or can convert precarcinogen into the carcinogen very fast. In both cases, the lungs are exposed to many carcinogens that damage the cells and leading to cancer. On the contrary, if the SNPs result in a slow carcinogen-making protein, fewer carcinogens are accumulated into lungs and so the chance of cancer is reduced.

SNPs can also have influence in the activity of detoxifying enzymes that prepare carcinogens for elimination from the body. SNPs that produce a very active forms of detoxifying enzymes remove the carcinogens quickly from the body, while SNPs that result in slow detoxifying enzymes permit carcinogens to remain in the body for a longer time, allowing more time for damage.

## TYPING METHODOLOGIES

In the years a variety of procedures useful for the molecular genotyping of SNPs have been described [17],[18],[19],[20] and among them those that discriminate alleles via hybridization (allele-specific PCR [21], DNA microarrays [22], Taqman [23] or via enzymatic (RFLP) [24], oligonucleotide ligation assay (OLA)[25],[26] and pyrosequencing [27].

## 1. Allele Specific Hybridization

Allele specific oligonucleotide hybridization (ASO) is a procedure widely used and based on distinguishing between two DNA targets that differ at one nucleotide position by hybridization. An ASO is an oligonucleotide of 15-21 bases in length, specifically designed to detect a difference of as little as 1 base in the target's genetic sequence, that makes it specific for only one of the alleles tested.

The length of the ASO probe, the strand to which it is complimentary and the stringency (temperature and ionic strength) of the reaction conditions under which the probe bind to the target sequence, play a fundamental role in the specificity of the SNPs assay. A part from the temperature and ionic strength of the reaction conditions, the thermal stability of an ASO probe hybrid is due to a large extent on the nucleotide sequence flanking a tested SNP.

In general two allele-specific probes are designed with the polymorphic base in a central position in the probe sequence. Under special optimized assay conditions, synthetic ASO probes only anneal to their complementary target DNA sequences in the sample if they are perfectly matched, with a single base-pair mismatch sufficient to prevent formation of a stable probe-target complex: so only the perfectly matched probe-target hybrids are stable while other hybrids with one-base mismatch are unstable.

PCR-amplified products can be applied to nylon filters or to a plate as a series of "dot blots" to which ASO probes are hybridized. Otherwise can also be used a reverse approach where the probes are fixed to a membrane support or in a microtiter plate format.

After hybridization, the duplex ASO probe- target DNA can be detected labbeling ASO probe with a radioactive, enzymatic, or fluorescent tag.

Simultaneous genotyping of multiple SNPs by ASO hybridization is unfortunately restricted by the poor specificity of ASO to discriminate between SNP genotypes when analyzing large genomes.

For example in the past years has been developed a procedure called (PCR-ELISA ASO typing) that provided a highly sensitive and quantitative detection of HLA regions.

This method was a combination of PCR amplification with ASO hybridization in a microtiter plate format using a colorimetric ELISA-based detection.

DNA template was amplified by PCR with the incorporation of digoxigenin-11-dUTP.

PCR products were analyzed in a microtiter plate format by alkaline denaturation and hybridization to biotinylated allele-specific capture probes bound to streptavidin-coated plates. The hybridized DNA was detected by ELISA, using anti-digoxigenin horseradish peroxidase conjugate and the colorimetric substrate 2,2'-azino-di-(3-ethylbenzthiazolinsulfonate). [28]

An application of ASO regards DNA microarrays that are generally used to measure changes in expression levels, to detect SNPs or for genotyping mutant genomes.

They consist of glass slides with spots of attached DNA fragments that act as probes for specific sequences in a sample.

The intrinsic property of allele-specific hybridization makes difficult the design of multiplexed ASO microarrays for genotyping any SNP. However Affimetrix developed a system (GeneChip) where this problem is solved by selecting the SNPs included in the panels on the basis of their assay performance and by interrogating each SNP with 40 different ASO probes.

The arrays are built to have 4 sets of 10 ASO probes (total 40 probes), corresponding to both strands of the tested SNP alleles: so there are matched and mismatched probes for each SNP position and for other 4 more nucleotide positions flanking the SNP of interest.

All this results in very large microarrays for highly multiplexed genotyping. The genotypes are than assigned on the basis of the joint fluorescence patterns generated by the 40 hybridization reactions for each SNP using special mathematical algorithms developed for this application. [29]

## *1.1.*

The TaqMan ® (Applied Biosystems) assay is based on the 5' nuclease activity of Taq polymerase that cleaves the oligonucleotide probes hybridized to the target DNA, generating a fluorescent signal. In the assay are used two TaqMan probes that have different fluorescent dyes (VIC and FAM) attached to the 5' end and a not fluorescent quencher attached to the 3' end. During the PCR annealing step, the TaqMan1 each probe hybridize to the complementary DNA sequence: one probe anneals to the wild-type allele and the other to the variant allele. When the probes are intact, the proximity of the reporter dye to the quencher dye, results in suppression of the reporter fluorescence by Förster-type energy transfer [30].

In the the extension step the polymerase cleaves only probes that are bound to the amplified target sequence: the cleavage separates the reporter dye from the quencher dye, producing an increase in fluorescence of the reporter dye. Mismatch probes are displaced without fragmentation.

Because the quencher does not fluoresce,the detection systems can measure reporter dye contributions more accurately. The fluorescence signal generated by PCR amplification indicates which alleles are present in the sample: this permits a genotype of a sample is determined by measuring the signal intensity of the two different dyes by a Real-time PCR instrument.

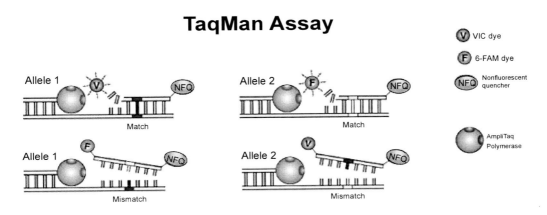

Figure 1. Eexample of TaqMan Assay by Applied Biosystems.

TaqMan SNP Genotyping Assays are the world's largest collection of single-tube, ready-to-use SNP assays available since it contains 4.5 million genome-wide SNPs providing unprecedented marker coverage.

*1.2.*

The Roche LightCycler® (https://www.roche-applied-science.com/lightcycler-online) is a real-time thermal cycler that permits a rapid detection and quantification of Polymerase Chain Reaction amplified products.

In the most innovative system PCR occurs in specially designed glass capillaries, which have an optimal surface-to-volume ratio to ensure rapid equilibration between the air and the reaction components.

Since any typical amplification cycle requires only 30 to 60 seconds than an amplification reaction with 30 cycles is usually complete in about 30 minutes.

Products are detected using two sequence specific oligonucleotides that hybridize adjacent to one another on the DNA target: one probe is labelled with fluorescein at its 3' end while the other one carries at 5' a CT Red label. One of the probes is arranged with the polymorphic SNP base in a central position.

When the oligonucleotides are bound to DNA, the two fluorescence dyes are placed in proximity to each other. Fluorescein is excited and emits green fluorescent light that excites the adjacent LC Red which subsequently emits fluorescent light.

Fluorescence Resonance Energy Transfer (FRET) is based on the transfer of energy from one fluorescent molecule (fluorescein at 470 nm) to another adjacent fluorescent molecule (e.g., LightCycler Red 640). [31]

FRET is highly dependent on the distance between the two dye molecules: in fact only if both molecules are within a space of 1–5 nucleotides, thus the energy transfer occurs at a high enough efficiency.

The light emitted by the tC Red molecule is measured at 640 nm and the increasing amount of fluorescence is proportional to the increasing amount of DNA generated during the PCR process.

The technique is highly sensitive and permits to obtain reliable and reproducible results even when working with low copy number target DNA. [32]

Many SNPs can be simultaneously genotyped combining the use of the different fluorescent labels with the design of probes that at different melting temperatures match the mutant and hav a mismatch with the wild type.

## 2. Primer Extension

Primer extension reation is based on the ability of DNA polymerase to incorporate specific deoxyribonucleotides complementary to the sequence of the template DNA.

### 2.1. Minisequencing or Single Nucleotide Primer Extension

This method was described the first time by Pastinen in 1997. It permits the identification of the specific mutations without sequencing the entire PCR product, even if maintaining the same qualitative characteristics of a sequence analysis.

The minisequencing method has proven to be extremely efficient, as compared to sequence analysis and very sensitive since it can be powerful performed on low quality PCR products.

In fact the elevated sensitivity explains the higher success rate can be obtained compared to sequence analysis since are obtained informative results with as little as 1 ng of PCR product.

While with traditional sequencing mutation analysis often fails when it is performed on scarce PCR products. [33]

However non-interpretable results after minisequencing can be observed because of the presence of background extra-peaks due to not-optimal purification of PCR products leading to incomplete removal of some PCR reagents, such as primers and dNTP.

This because minisequencing is designed as a primer-driven reaction: in this procedure the polymorphic base is determined by the addition, made by a DNA polymerase, of a ddNTP complementary to the base tested. The DNA polymerase can promote the allele-specific extension only if the primers have a perfect match with the DNA template .

So minisequencing is strongly sensitive to the presence of residual primers: PCR primers that have not been removed can participate in the primer extension reaction and simulate informations coming from the real minisequencing extension primer. [34]

Data interpretation require a computer-assisted mutation analysis, allowing exact base identity determination and computer assisted visualization of the specific mutation(s), thus facilitating data interpretation and management, and reducing sources of error.

The main benefit of minisequencing is the use of an analysis protocol based on a common procedure for all mutations analysed. Another useful feature is that different mutation sites can be investigated simultaneously in a multiplex reaction, even if they are placed in different regions of a gene.

In multiplex reactions, different primers are placed in a single tube reaction format and products are analysed in a single electrophoresis run. Obviously to avoid overlapping and to be able to distinguish different loci by the corresponding sizes of the final products (spatial separation of peaks), the primers referring to the different mutation sites are designed so to differ significantly in size. [35]

*2.1.1.*

The most known commercial system based on minisequencing reaction, followed by electrophoresis and laser fluorescence detection is the SNaPshotTM kit produced by Applied Biosystems. (www.appliedbiosystems.com)

The SNaPshot chemistry is based on the dideoxy single-base extension of one or more unlabeled oligonucleotide primers . An unlabelled primer is positioned with the 3' end at the base immediately upstream to the SNP site. Each primer binds to a complementary template in the presence of fluorescently labeled ddNTPs and the polymerase extends the primer by one nucleotide, adding to its 3´ end a single ddNTP that has assigned only one specific fluorescent dye.

The fluorescent dyes assigned to the individual ddNTPs are the following ones: A (dR6G= Green), C (dTAMRA™ Black), G (dR110 Blue), T -U (dROX™ Red).

The result is marker fragments for the different SNP alleles that are all the same in length, but will vary by color.

SNaPshot multiplexing can be achieved by adding a tail at the 5' end of the unlabeled SNaPshot primers with varying lengths of non –complementary oligonucleotide sequences that serve as a mobility modifier. The resulting products can then be separated by capillary electrophoresis in an automated DNA sequencer in the presence of a fifth-orange dye-labeled size standard (generally LIZ120). The alleles of each single marker appear as different coloured peaks around the same size in the electropherogram window. The size of the different allele peaks will vary slightly due to differences in molecular weight of the dyes.

Applied Biosystems recommends limiting SNP marker size to between 20 and 105 bp. Loci less than 36 bp should be spaced a minimum of 6 bp apart, while loci greater than 36 bp should be spaced 4 bp apart.

According to the manufacturer's protocol, The SNaPshot Multiplex kit can investigate up to 10 SNP markers simultaneously by using primers of different lengths, but larger multiplexes have been developed.

Minisequencing by SNaPshot is at the moment the most popular procedure in forensic laboratories, because the method is simple, low cost, and the detection is performed on the same automatic capillary electrophoresis instruments that are commonly used for STRs analysis.

*2.1.2.*

Microarrays are also suitable for genotyping SNPs with minisequencing: the analysis can be performed on the chip surface or in solution.

In the first case the reaction, also known as arrayed primer extension (APEX), is performed on a two-dimensional arrayed series of oligonucleotides (up to 6000 known 25-mer oligos) immobilized at 5' end on a coated glass surface (DNA chip), by a covalent bond to a chemical matrix.

DNA sample is amplified with primers flanking the SNP to be identified and the primers are extended by a DNA polymerase with 4 colour- fluorescently labelled ddNTPs. A complementary fragment of PCR amplified DNAproduct is annealed to oligos. Covalent bonds between oligo and dye terminator allow the slides to be stringently washed in order to improve the ratio signal/noise before the microarray is scanned to measure fluorescence.

The total time required for the analysis, including sample preparation, is less than four hours.

Main advantages of APEX-based genotyping ( http://www.asperbio.com/APEX.htm) are the ability to analyze hundreds to thousands of SNPs /mutations in a single reaction and that arrays can be designed to be either locus or disease-specific.

The second method is based on minisequencing in solution prior to hybridisation to universal tag-arrays. In particular single base extension reaction is performed in solution using minisequencing primers with a unique sequence tag at the 5' end so that each SNP has a distinct identifying tag.

PCR product of the multiplex minisequencing reaction is than bound to the reverse complementary sequences of the tags arrayed onto the chip.

The advancement of technologies to assess human genetic variation in a high-throughput, combined with the low costs per data point offer significative advantages for SNP genotyping on a large scale and in fact are in development microarray systems for highly multiplexed genotyping as a potential for genome-wide SNP genotyping.

The robustness of the multiplexed microarray-based SNP genotyping systems is determined by the reaction principles applied for SNP allele distinction and the microarray formats used. Moreover special software are required for designing probes and primer for the assays, and also algorithms for assigning the genotypes. In fact to achieve relative concentration independence and minimal cross-hybridization, SNPs of multiple databases are scanned to design the probes and each SNP on the array is than interrogated with different probes.

The main problem of microarrays detection is that the reproducibility and validation is difficult and time consuming. Even though at the present the number of markers is limited, however when fully developed, microarray analysis could provide a promising system for efficient sensitive SNP analysis also of forensic samples. [36]

Nanogen Inc. (www.nanogen.com) developed a microarray technology based on the use of microelectronic chip for fast and accurate SNP genotyping . [37]

In fact, the combination of microfabrication, chemistry and molecular biology have allowed the generation of microarrays that permit rapid and miniaturized multiplex analysis of DNA samples.

Nanogen's microchips are made by standard semiconductor and have around1cm in size with 25-site, 100-site or 400-site arrays .[38]

The test sites are clustered in the center of the array surrounded by some counter electrodes, while a platinum wire connects each individual site and their respective counter electrode in the pad chips. This allows the microinsulation of these sites and provides equal access to the molecules in an overlaying electrolyte solution. A flow cell on top of the array serves as a chamber for electronics, washing and optical window. The cartridge also contains multiple valves and interconnected channels leading to the flow cell for sample application and washing.

An agarose permeation layer, on the top of the chip, serves as an interface between the electrodes and the solution and prevent damaging of electrochemical reactions on top of the active electrode.

Two different formats for SNP assays are available: in the capture down format, probes are loaded to the desired site by electronically activating the electrode positive charged and the counter electrodes with a negative charge. The electric field strength generated by this configuration drives the DNA molecules, negatively charged, to migrate over the positively sites.

Streptavidin molecules anchored in the agarose permeation layer electronically bind biotinylated capture probes to individual or multiple pads on the array.

The PCR products must be accurately purified after amplification because the presence of salt will strongly inhibit the microarray hybridization. Then the denatured amplicons are electronically hybridized to the captured probes on site. The Nanogen technology requires that a mixture of reporter oligos complementary to both wild type or SNP variant alleles and respectively labeled with different Cy3 or Cy5 dyes, is hybridized to the target. The universal reporting system utilizes a non-labeled SNP-specific discriminator oligonucleotide combined with a universal recognition sequence complementary to one of the two reporter probes.

This permits a rapid electronic hybridization of the target DNA to capture probes and passive hybridisation of fluorescently labelled reporter probes. [39]

In the amplicon down format, biotinylated amplicon DNA is initially bound to the sites on the pad and oligo probes are hybridized to the anchored amplicon.

The microelectronic chip has greater flexibility (using the same DNA chip format for different SNP genotyping assays) than other microarray/chip methods, which are limited to genotyping of a standard predesigned set of SNPs and allows simultaneous use of a wide variety of probes of different lengths and chemical compositions on the same chip.

The microelectronic assay also allow the use of different optimized stringency conditions for each site of the chip, while, on standard microarray chips, common reaction and stringency conditions have to be applied to all sites. [40]

The main expense of genotyping by the microelectronic chip is the chip itself (72% of cost of supplies), but it can be reduced by maximizing the number of SNPs typed per chip, an element that also contribute to high throughput. In addition the cost can be further reduced by using previously used microelectronic chips for detection of new SNPs in other genes without loss of accuracy.

SNP detection by microelectronic chips is comparable to RFLP analysis in terms of throughput, accuracy, and cost-effectiveness, but unfortunately it has also some limitations (high purchase price and lower amenability to automation), that must be evaluated before any routine purpose. [41]

*2.1.3.*

The Matrix assisted laser desorption/ionization time-of-flight (MALDI-TOF) mass spectrometry is the most reproducible method for SNPs analysis: it measures the molecular weight of DNA products formed in a minisequencing reaction.

It represents the most direct method of detection in comparison with other procedures that on the contrary permits the identitfication of the products by monitoring the fluorescence emitted by labelled molecules.

The MassEXTEND,Sequenom assay use ddNTP with dNTPs during the extension reaction in order to increase mass differences between the alleles of a SNP. If the minisequencing products have non overlapping mass, the assay can be multiplexing.

In a first PCR reaction, a primer is annealed to the targeted DNA immediately upstream of the interest SNP site. After the PCR, remaining nucleotides are deactivated by SAP treatment. The single base primer Subsequently the extension reaction step is performed: MassExtend Primers, DNA polymerase, dNTPs, ddNTPs are added to samples plate in order to produce allele-specific primer extension product generally 1-4 bases longer than the original primer.

The common primer that identifies both SNPs alleles is hybridized to the polymorhic site, dNTPs are incorporated until a specific ddNTP is added and the reaction terminates. Since the termination point and the number of nucleotides is sequence specific, the mass of the extension product is used to clearly identify SNPs variants and is extended by a single base in the presence of all four ddNTPs. The base at the SNP site is identified by the mass added onto the primer.

Each addition of a nucleotide to the primer extension product increases the mass depending on the nucleotide added.

An aliquot of an amplified sample is spotted from the microplate onto a matrix on the surface of a Spectrochip (able to load 384 samples) that is than placed into the MassArray Analyzer.

The matrix containing DNA products are hit with a pulse produced by from a laser beam in a process known as "desorption". So the energy from the laser beam is transferred to the matrix and it is vaporized. As result a small amount of the DNA product is expelled into a flight tube where an electrical field pulse is applied and charged DNA is accelerated towards a detector.

The electrical field pulse and collision of the DNA product with the detector is referred to as "the time of flight". This is a very precise measure of the molecular weight of the DNA products, since the molecular mass is directly correlated with time of flight: lighter molecules fly faster and reach the detector quicker than heavier molecules. Specific software converts the time of flight into an exact mass.

The Mass ARRAY system is able to detect any sample changes or modifications since it has a resolution as small as three Daltons. The smallest mass difference is between ddA and ddT: 9 Da. With automated features, it analyzes data and assigns a confidence level to samples as spectra are acquired.

Sequenom MassARRAY® Platform (www.sequenom.com) provides an ideal balance of multiplexing and throughput that enables researchers to make a fine-mapping and SNP validation studies, or any routine applications that employ focused SNP panels. [42], [43]

One limitation of MALDI-TOF analysis is the purity of the sample required by the assay and the salts effect that could render it more difficult to accurately measure the peak masses due to the presence of Na, Mg and K adducts.

MALDI-TOF seem to be suitable for forensic purposes, and there are also some works in those directions even if this technology, in contrast with SNaPshot, require an expensive dedicated equipment and the multiplex capability of MALDI-TOF is lower than with other minisequencing technologies. [44]

*2.1.4.*

Fluorescence polarization can be used for detecting any allelic discrimination product only if the initial and the final molecules have different sizes.

FP is a technique that measures the vertical and horizontal components of the fluorescence emission produced WHEN a fluorescent molecule is excited by plane polarized light.

The degree of fluorescence polarization, under constant temperature and solvent viscosity, is proportional to the molecular weight of the dye molecule and the polarization values are inversely related to the speed of molecular rotation, by monitoring the FP of is possible to detect significant changes in the molecular weight of the molecule.

This means that any genotyping method in which the product of the allelic discrimination reaction is larger or smaller than the starting fluorescent molecule can use FP as a detection method.

Since in a minisequencing reaction the incorporation of a fluorescent terminator into a primer oligonucleotide increases its polarization, FP is therefore an excellent detection mechanism for SNPs genotyping assays. [45]

Perkin Elmer Life Sciences (www.perkinelmer.com) developed a novel assay, the AcycloPrime™-FP SNP Detection Kit based on fluorescence polarization (FP) detection. The system permits to determine the base at an SNP location in an amplified DNA sample by a modification of Template-directed Dye terminator incorporation.

Following PCR amplification of the sequence containing the SNP of interest, after excess of primer and dNTPs removing , a thermostable DNA polymerase adds one of two fluorescent terminators to a primer that ends immediately upstream of the SNP site. This increases around 10- fold the molecular weight of the fluorophore and the terminator(s) added are identified by their increased FP representing the original allele(s) present in the tested sample. The assay is commonly performed as a singleplex.[46]

## 2.2. PYROSEQUENCING

An alternative approach also based on a sequencing-by-synthesis method, is Pyrosequencing™ that is an established genetic analysis method based on the principle of sequencing by synthesis.

It permits to obtain sequence information within minutes and for that is an ideal choice for genetic analysis in clinical research.

Pyrosequencing method was developed by Biotage, a global company focused on life sciences. (www.biotage.com) whose Biosystems Unit has been recently acquired by Qiagen .

This technology uses an enzyme cascade system, consisting of four enzymes and specific substrates, to produce light .

In the first step of the procedure a sequencing primer is hybridized to an amplified DNA template, in single strand and than incubated with some enzymes (DNA polymerase, luciferase, apyrase ATP sulfurylase,) and substrates (adenosine 5´ phosphosulfate (APS) and luciferin)

In a second step, a deoxynucleotide triphosphate (dNTP) is added to the reaction and DNA polymerase catalyzes the incorporation of the dNTP into the DNA strand, if it is complementary to the base in the template strand. Each incorporation event is accompanied by release of pyrophosphate (PPi) in a quantity equimolar to the amount of incorporated nucleotide.

In a third step the ATP sulfurylase, in the presence of adenosine 5´ phosphosulfate, transforms PPi into ATP that favorits the luciferase-mediated conversion of luciferin to oxyluciferin. This event produces visible light in an amount proportional to the one of ATP. If the added nucleotide is not complementary to the next base in the template no light will be generated. The light intensity is proportional to the number of incorporated nucleotides.

The light produced in the luciferase-catalyzed reaction can be detected by a CCD (charge coupled device) camera and observed as a peak in a pyrogram™. The final light signal is proportional to the number of nucleotides incorporated during the reaction.

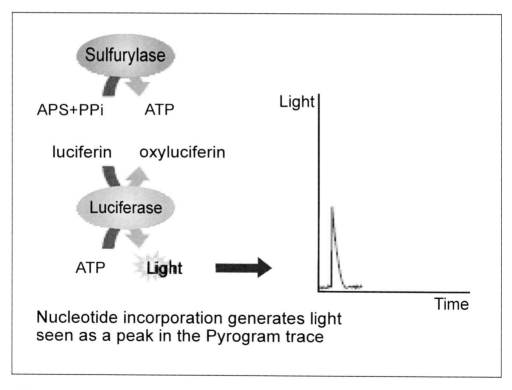

(http://www.pyrosequencing.com/graphics/3019.pdf)

In step 4 the apyrase enzyme continuously degrades unincorporated dNTPs and excess ATP, as the degradation proceeds, another new dNTP is added. Than, in the final step , as the process continues by adding dNTPs one at a time, the complementary DNA strand is built up and the resulting nucleotide sequence can be determined from the signal peak in the Pyrogram® graphic.

Limiting factors of pyrosequencing procedure are the DNA template preparation, the low multiplex capability and the low suitability to automation, because several steps need to be performed before the detection. On the contrary, the main advantage seems to be the ability to quantify the contribution of each allele, that is a very useful tool in the analysis of mixtures profiles.

Pyrosequencing technology, being a direct DNA sequencing technique, gives unambiguous genotyping results: it provides rapid real-time determination of 20–30 bp of target DNA: not only SNP alleles are determined but also the adjacent base sequences as a control, which serves as a valuable internal control, obtained for each sample. [47]

Moreover Pyrosequencing method is highly sensitive for SNP typing and this may be suitable to analyse low-quantity DNA samples since it has been demonstrated the ability to obtain by this procedure reliable results from as little as 8pg of DNA. [48]

## 2.3. OLIGONUCLEOTIDE LIGATION ASSAY (OLA)

OLA is a rapid, sensitive, and specific method for the detection of known single nucleotide polymorphisms (SNPs). This method is based on the ability of ligase to bind covalently two oligonucleotides (Capture and Reporter Oligos) when they hybridize next to one another to a complementary DNA target (PCR product).

The OLA assay requires that three probes were designed, one common and two allele specifics.

Generally, for each allele there are two capture probes that differ only in sequence at the last base at the 3' end: one is complementary to one allele, with the other allelic probe complementary to the alternative allele.

Allele discrimination occurs by the ability of DNA ligase to join perfectly matched probes, any 3' mismatch in the capture probe will prevent ligation.

The common probe contains universal PCR primer–binding sequences as and sequences complementary to ASO and LSO probes. It anneals to the target DNA immediately downstream of the SNP. The two allelic probes compete to anneal to the DNA target adjacent to the common probe. This generates a double stranded region where only the allelic probe perfectly complementary to target DNA is ligated to the common probe by the DNA ligase

All probes are designed to function under the same hybridization conditions: unligated probes and linkers and the genomic DNA are removed by enzymatic digestion (exonuclease).

Different assay formats have been developed for detecting the OLA products. Commonly PCR amplification of purified ligation products is performed using a single pair of PCR primers, one of which is biotinylated: amplified biotinylated products are than bound within wells of streptavidin-coated microtiter plates. Use of biotin on the common probe and a reporter group on the allelic specific probe allows for product capture and detection.

In other assays the biotin have been replaced with mobility modifiers and the allelic specific probes have been labelled with different fluorescent dyes. The mobility modifiers allow the precise regulation of the mobility of each ligation product regardless of oligonucleotide length

The use of mobility modifiers and fluorescent dyes allows this the ligation products to be discriminated by size and colour, enabling multiplexed OLA reactions.

In fact PCR products of this reaction can be separated electrophoretically under denatured conditions with fluorescent detection.

In the last years have been developed some technologies based on the specificity of ligases such as the SNPlex™ Genotyping System (Applied Biosystems) and the Illumina genotyping system (Illumina Inc.)

The SNPlex™ Genotyping System (www.appliedbiosystems.com) uses Oligonucleotide Ligation Assay/PCR technology for allelic discrimination and ligation product amplification by universal PCR. Amplification of ligated products is performed, using two universal primers, one of them labbelled with biotin. Than biotinylated duplex amplicons are bound to streptavidin-coated plates and converted in single-stranded products.

Genotype information is then decoded by an universal set of dye-labeled probe containing mobility modified fragments (Zipchute™ Mobility Modifiers). Each ZipChute probe hybridyze to the unique complementary sequences of the single-stranded amplicons.: so to analyze 48 SNPs, 96 different ZipCode sequences and 96 unique ZipChute probes are required.

The same set is used for every SNPlex™ pool, regardless of which SNPs are chosen, this permit a rapid and reproducible detection by capillary electrophoresis.The system is configured as a 48-plex per reaction but it could be increased to a 96-plex per reaction.

The SNPlex™ Genotyping System is well suited to perform a range of medium to large-scale genotyping studies such as linkage or fine mapping, disease association, population stratification quantitative trait loci analysis. [49]

Ilumina Inc. developed the GoldenGate Genotyping Assay (www.illumina.com) that became one of the main application for multiplexed genotyping assays during the International HapMap Project which used this method to identify more than 258,000,000 genotypes.

The first step in the GoldenGate Assay is DNA activation for binding to paramagnetic particles.

For each SNP locus there are three oligonucleotides: two are allele-specific oligos (ASO) while a third oligo is a locus-specific oligo (LSO) that hybridizes to several bases downstream from the SNP site.

All three oligonucleotide sequences contain universal PCR primer sites while only the LSO oligo contains a unique sequence that targets a particular micro bead type.

ASOs and LSOs oligos hybridize to the genomic DNA sample bound to paramagnetic particles.

The ligation products serve as the PCR templates for universal PCR primers; PCR products obtained are fluorescently labelled, with different colour being used for each allele of a SNP.

The single-stranded, dye-labeled PCR products are than hybridized to their complementary bead type through their unique sequences.

The detection system is based on the BeadArrayTM technology, which is based on fiberoptic substrates with randomly assembled arrays of beads.

After hybridization, the BeadXpress® Reader is used for microbead code identification and fluorescent signal detection. During scanning, a laser beam penetrates the microbead and generate a unique code image: each bead is a sensor for a specific DNA-sequence.

This system allows a rapid and highly specific detection of more than 1100 SNPs per assay.

Producing a high quality data that show a high degree of sample success, locus success, call rates, reproducibility in both 96 and 384 plex levels.

Table 1. Schematic review of SNPs main detection methods

| a. | b. Allele specific c. hybridization | d. Primer Extension | e. OLA |
|---|---|---|---|
| f. Fluorescence g. Electrophoresis | h. | i. X | j. X |
| k. Fluorescence l. Arrays | m. X | n. X | o. |
| p. Fluorescence Resonance Energy Transfer | q. X | r. X | s. X |
| t. Fluorescence u. Polarization | v. X | w. X | x. |
| y. z. Mass Spectrometry | aa. | bb. X | cc. X |
| dd. ee. Luminescence | ff. | gg. X | hh. |

# NON-AUTOSOMAL RELEVANT SNP CLASSES

## SNPs on Chromosome Y

Males have one X chromosome and one Y chromosome, that contains a gene which triggers the embryonic development as a male.

Since some years, Y chromosome analysis has became a common method for tracing human evolution through male lineages as well as application to male identification in forensic situations. In fact the ability to separate and identify the male component from evidences containing mixtures of male and female DNA is strongly useful in many forensic situations.

In fact, for example in case of sexual assault, the use of Y chromosome specific primers can improve the chances of detecting low levels of the perpretator's DNA in a high background of the female victim's DNA without any procedure for differential DNA extraction between male and female cells. Y chromosome analysis can also benefit paternity testing when a male offspring is in question: in fact since fathers pass their Y chromosome onto their sons unchanged (except for an occasional mutation), all males in a paternal lineage will possess a common Y chromosome haplotype. The lack of recombination along most of the Y-chromosome makes it a useful tool in difficult paternity analysis for reconstruction of male linage or application in kinship analysis, in human evolutionary studies and for assessing male migration patterns .

To assess the reliability of a database as representation of actual population haplotype frequencies, however the extent of structure among populations also needs to be considered in particular because Y chromosome haploid and paternal mode of inheritance makes it more sensitive to genetic drift than the autosomes.

Extensive studies are still performed to identify numerous single nucleotide polymorphisms (SNPs) on the Y chromosome. These SNPs are single base changes or insertion/deletions, which are slowly evolving in comparison with the short tandem repeat markers, which evolve more rapidly

The analysis of single nucleotide polymorphisms located within the male-specific region of the Y-chromosome (MSY) is widely used as a powerful tool for evolutionary studies and for measuring the variability between populations.

In fact due to the specific distribution of Y-haplogroups among populations, Y-SNP permit to infer the origin, evolution, and history of humans by tracing back male initiated patterns of migration from modern human populations. The non-random distribution of the Y chromosome lineages worldwide permits an accurate characterisation of haplogroups associated with specific geographic areas. [50],[51].

Even if the validation of the Y chromosome SNPs multiplexes described for forensic application is still in progress, however SNP typing could in a near future significantly contribute to forensic investigation by providing information on the ethnic origin of a male DNA sample and combined with STR markers, could be a powerful tool for mass disasters or terrorist attacks being able to identify people from various geographical areas involved. [52]

## SNPs on Chromosome X

The X-chromosome is present in a single copy in males, who inherit their one X-Chr from their mother, while female individuals receive one X from the mother and the other one from the father. So, female individuals fathered by the same man share their paternal Chromosome X. Female individuals fathered by the same man share their paternal Chromosome X.

X chromosome analysis have been proven to be useful in case of deficiency paternity testing and in effective mother-son kinship and father-daughter testing. [53]

Hence in case of deficiency paternity in which the mother is available for typing, the possible X alleles of the putative father can be determined and the paternal profile can be reconstructed.

The X-chromosome has features that make it a good source of information for population genetic studies. It has a lower recombination and mutation rate than autosomes and also a small population size that results in a faster genetic drift. As consequence the linkage disequilibrium (LD) and population structure in the X chromosome are stronger than in autosomes.

X chromosome polymorphisms reflect the history of females: following to recombination, X-chromosome markers in females provide a multilocus system, while the mtDNA and Y-chromosome are linked haplotypes.

X-chromosome SNPs markers can be used to complement the results obtained from STR markers since they show some advantages compared to STRs suc as the low mutation rate, the high number in the human genome and the ability to be typed also in partly degraded samples: all features that makes them particularly useful in forensic caseworks, complex kinship analysis or immigration case. [54],[55].

## Mitochondrial SNPs

Mitochondrial genome is highly polymorphic, making it useful for human identification.

The vast majority of the human genome is located within the nucleus of each cell, however also mithocondria which are placed in the cytoplasm, contain a small circular genome.

Human mt-DNA was first sequenced in 1981 in the laboratory of Frederick Sanger in Cambridge, England. The original sequence is the reference sequence to which new sequences are compared and is commonly known as the Anderson sequence or the Cambridge reference sequence.

Mt-DNA is useul to the forensic DNA community because it can be efficiently amplified from limited or severaly degraded biological material.

The likelihood of recovering mtDNA in small or degraded biological samples is greater than for nuclear DNA because mtDNA molecules are present in high copy number (hundreds to thousands) in each cell compared to the nuclear complement of two copies per cell. Therefore samples that lack sufficient nuclear DNA as shed hairs, old bones and in general scarce human remains, even if degraded by environmental insult or time, may provide enough material for typing the mtDNA locus. Unlike nuclear DNA, which is passed from both mother and father to the offspring, mtDNA is only maternally inherited so that in situations where an individual is not available for a direct comparison with a biological sample, any maternally related individual may provide a reference sample. Moreover it has a relatively infrequent mutation rate and it remains the same through many generations. Thus, mt-DNA analysis will not differentiate women that are in the same maternal lineage or children with the same mother. [56]

Since considerable effort and expense are required to obtain a full HVI (positions 16024–16365 ) and HVII (positions 73–340 ) mtDNA sequence so several mtDNA screening methods have been developed that permit rapid resolution of non-matching samples. Moreover the discrimination power of an mtDNA analysis is limited because common haplotypes exist in HVI/HVII mtDNA sequences that can reduce the ability to differentiate two unrelated samples.

In all this cases it can be useful the analysis of some coding region variations in addition to the non-coding polimorphysms. The sequence analysis of the coding region require more material than the one generally present in forensic samples and for that an alternative SNP analysis approach is possible in order to analyze SNPs polymorphisms within the hypervariable region as well as in the coding region. Even though the number of markers in the current system is limited, it can easily be extended to yield a greater power of discrimination. When fully developed, microarray analysis provides a promising system for efficient sensitive SNP analysis of forensic samples in the future.

The typing of mithocondrial SNP allows the differentiation between individuals possessing an identical HV1/HV2 sequence. [57], [58]

Multiplex SNP panels are in development to resolve mitotypes in some populations such as Caucasian, Hispanic, and African American.

For example a set of 11 SNPs has been selected by NIST reserachers for distinguishing individuals of the most common Caucasian HV1/HV2 mitotype.

The 11-plex assay probed SNPs located at positions 477, 3010, 4580, 4793, 5004, 7028, 7202, 10211, 12858, 14470 and 16519 in were incorporated in an allele-specific primer extension assay. for multiplex detection of these SNPs. Locus specific primers of varying lengths were employed in multiplex primer extension reactions. Extension primers binding 5' adjacent to the SNP site of interest were enzymatically extended using fluorescently labeled ddNTPs.

Resolution and detection of products were achieved by electrophoresis on a capillary sequencer The development of the mtSNP 11-plex assay is ian accurate method for typing sequence variant mtSNPs on a platform common to almost all forensic laboratories.

Currently are in developing additional multiplex SNP panels to resolve other common mitotypes such as Caucasian, Hispanic, and African American. [59],[60],[61]

Therefore, the forensic genetics fields have been increasingly interested in studying these polymorphisms, assembling information on genetic variation of human populations and their history and also using SNPs for individual identification purposes.

Coding region SNPs can fulfill a useful role for separating common HV1/HV2 mitochondrial DNA types and assays have been developed to reliably examine mtDNA coding region SNP variation

While Y-SNPs have limited utility for individualizing a sample, they may, depending on the population(s) of interest, be helpful in aiding estimations of ethnic origin

## FORENSIC APPLICATIONS

Since many years forensic laboratories commonly use short tandem repeats (STRs) as the standard DNA identification method , because they have been widely validated and some multiplexes are commercially available. Even if STRs represent the ideal approach for personal identification and paternity tests, however also SNPs could be a valuable tool for this application.

The primary advantage of using SNPs is that a higher recovery of information from degraded DNA samples is possible since a smaller target region is needed to be analysed.

In fact when working with degraded or scarce DNA samples, the analysis of autosomal single nucleotide polymorphisms (SNPs) might be more successful because only a single nucleotide needs to be measured instead of hundreds of nucleotides in length as with STRs.

Common STRs markers generally have a range in length between 150 and 450 bp, so they often fail to amplify in degraded DNA samples.

SNPs allow designing small PCR target sequences in order to obtain amplicon shorter in length than other markers and that enable efficient amplification of evidences from crime scenes or formalin-fixed paraffin-embedded tissues that contain often degraded DNA or Low Copy Number DNA (less than 100 pg DNA per sample).

Another advantage of SNPs is that they possess mutation rates approximately 100 thousand times lower than STR. Thus, since they're more stable in terms of inheritance, SNPs could aid parentage testing in complex cases or kinship analysis for example for identifying mass disaster victims .

Unfortunately several significant disadvantages exist with SNP markers when considered as a possible replacement for currently used STR loci.

First of all SNPs are not as polymorphic as STRs, so more SNPs are required to reach equivalent powers of discrimination or random match probabilities. To obtain a similar discrimination power than 13–15 STR loci commonly in use today in forensic identification, around 40–60 well balanced SNPs are necessary.

Moreover 15 STRs can be routinely amplified simultaneously in a single multiplex amplification reaction from minimal amounts of DNA sample using commercially available kits.

Multiplex PCR amplification of such a large number of SNPs has been only recently obtained and the commercialisation of robust assays with their use in routine practice will require a long time being more difficult than initially supposed.

In multiplex PCR, the number of undesired interactions between the PCR primers increases exponentially as the number of primers included in the reaction mixture increases. This interaction usually produces preferential amplification of unwanted 'primer-dimer' artifacts instead of the tested DNA templates. Moreover another problem that often occurs in a multiplex reaction are variations in PCR efficiency between the amplicons, due to sequences differences in the template.

The problem of multiplexing can be reduced by using PCR primers that are as similar as possible to one another, even if the multiplexing level that can be achieved not yet is able to reach the same capacity offered by present technologies for producing STRs multiplex.

Also the cost of examining more loci appear to be higher than with traditional STRs even if it seems that for high-throughput the cost of SNPs could be lower than the cost per STR using commercial kits.

Another problem is concerning data interpretation: in fact when attempting to analyse a greater number of loci, there is an increased complexity of data to be examined. In fact more loci mean also more peaks and the possibility to observe more artefacts. With so many loci being typed, an accurate data analysis could become very difficult and necessary requires the support of validated computer expert systems.

Assays with a larger number of loci are more sensitive to the quantity and integrity of the input DNA template in particular when working with low amount DNA so many loci may be lost during analyis. Unfortunately with limited amounts of starting material there may not be opportunities to do further attempts in order to recover missing loci.

Moreover failed loci on reference material samples may be different from those on the evidentiary sample leaving even less of an overlap of successfully typed loci for comparison purposes.

So if a few dozen or even hundreds of loci fail to produce a result on a sample, these data are excluded from the final analysis. In fact this type of data loss when attempting to perform a direct comparison between a suspect and evidence is unacceptable under the current paradigm of traditional sample matching performed with STR typing.

In addition great experience on STRs has been accumulated during the last 10 years. For instance mutations or polymorphisms in flanking regions are increasingly more known for STRs and can be a problem for SNPs since an extensive validation in population groups is required for an increased number of markers.

Another significant disadvantage of SNPs analysis is that the limited number of alleles per SNP locus (typically only 2) that can strongly affect the interpretation of mixture.

On the contrary since STRs are highly pholimorphic, a STR profile on the basis of the number of alleles observed at multiple loci can clearly suggest if there's one or more donor of a sample: this means that multiple contributors to a mixture can be identified because they have non-overlapping alleles.

Since the past years, a wide number of different SNP typing technologies have been developed based on various method, different chemistries and detection platforms.

Products of the allelic discrimination reactions can be detected with more than one method, and the same detection method can analyze products obtained with different reactions or assay formats.

Before SNPs markers can be introduced in routine forensic application a decision must be taken by the forensic community on the SNP markers to be employed and the detection system to be utilized, even if since technologies and validations are still in evolution it become quite difficult to decide on the best options available.

Most SNPs genotyping assays can be attributed to one of the following groups based on molecular mechanism: allele specific hybridisation, primer extension, invasive cleavage, oligonucleotide ligation and several detection methods (luminescence, fluorescence, mass measurement, etc.) are available for analysing the products of that type of reactions.

Reactions that occur in solution are more suitable for the automation because they do not require any separation or purification step after the allele discrimination reaction. Unfortunately they have a limited multiplex capability.

On the contrary reactions taking place on a solid support such as a bead, a glass slide, a chip, etc.. have greater multiplex capability but they're lessflexible because further manipulations are required before the automation.

These methods offer the capability of accurate genotyping, even if they all rely on standard PCR amplification of target sequences as the initial front-end step in generating material. Because of the nature of standard solution-based multiplexed PCR, which often can require extensive optimisation of primers and reaction conditions the inherent amplification requirement effectively limits the extent to which these varied platforms can be modified for highly multiplexed genotyping.

**Table 2. SNPs main features in forensic applications**

ii. Main Advantages
- Abundance in the genome
- Low mutation rates
- Reduced amplicon sizes (ability to analyze degraded DNA)
- Simple multiplex assays
- High-throughput genotyping
- Potential for phenotypic trait prediction

jj. Main Disadvantages
- Low polymorphism and discrimination power
- Requirement for large numbers of individual SNPs to be analized
- Difficulties with body fluid mixture detection and interpretation
- High analysis cost
- Uncertainty in reliability of multiplex-capable platforms

The ability to convert hundreds of PCR primer-pairs into a single-tube, multiplexed reaction producing specific, robust products from a complex genomic DNA template would greatly reduce the requirements for large-scale, population-based SNP genotyping. [62]

The SNPforID Consortium (www.SNPforID.org) is a research group having as partners:

- Institute of Legal Medicine, Johannes Gutenberg University Mainz, Germany
- Institute of Legal Medicine, University of Santiago de Compostela, Spain
- Institute of Forensic Medicine, University of Copenhagen, Denmark
- Institute of Cell and Molecular Sciences, Queen Mary, University of London, UK
- Institute of Legal Medicine, Medical University Innsbruck, Austria

The consortium main objectives are:

- Selection of 50 SNPs suitable for the identification of persons of unknown ethnic origin, and determination of population genetic frequencies in major ethnic groups.
- Development of a highly efficient DNA amplification strategy for the simultaneous analysis of up to 50 independent SNPs in a single assay.
- Assessment of high-throughput DNA typing platforms for reliable and accurate multiplex SNP typing.
- Investigation of the efficiency of multiplex high-throughput SNP typing using different microarray technologies in forensic casework.

All data generated by the SNPforID consortium are available online on the SNPforID browser that is a public accessible database for searching and review SNPs allele frequencies of the studied markers from all the available populations used by SNPforID.

Validated panels of SNPs for a variety of forensic applications have been generated with the browser concentrating on the single-tube identification SNP set comprising 52 markers. The web tool has been designed to favorite the combination of populations in groupings, the comparison between populations individually or amongst groupings or with equivalent HapMap data. [63]

SNPs may play a useful role in several forensic applications such as [64]:

a) Individual Identity test— SNPs for individualization
b) Lineage test, family reconstruction - sets of linked SNPs useful as haplotype markers to identify missing persons through kinship analyses (Y-SNPs, mt-SNPs)
c) Ancestry study - informative SNPs for establishing high probability of a person geographical ancestry (AIMs)
d) Phenotypic identification – selected SNPs for establishing if an individual has a particular characteristic, such as skin color, hair color or eye color for investigative purpose (identikit)

## a) Identity Informative SNPs

SNPs selected for Identity-tests have the same function as the forensic STR loci: in fact they provide genetic information to differentiate people in order to exclude/include a suspect as a source of an evidentiary sample or to attribute/esclude the origin as a putative family member.

The best SNPs for identity testing are those that have the highest heterozygosity and low coefficient of inbreeding, because these charactheristics permit to reach high levels of power of discrimination even using fewer SNPs and also a fewer reference population data is required for statistical evaluations.

Many studies have been performed and are still in progress to select SNP panels useful for identity-kinship tests. [65]

Kidd et al. tested more than 90,000 candidate SNPs in a variety of populations (European Americans, African Americans, Chinese-Japanese).

These candidate SNPs were then reduced as a consequence of further evaluations and finally the result of the study was that 19 SNPs showing the required charateristics were identified. [66]

A 52 SNP-multiplex that amplifies 52 DNA fragments with 52 autosomal SNP loci in only one multiplex PCR was developed by the SNPforID consortium.

The 52 SNPs are detected in two separate single base extension (SBE) multiplex reactions with 29 and 23 SNPs, respectively, using SNaPshot kit and capillary electrophoresis. [67], [68].

Results obtained were really good and demonstrate that SNP typing with SBE, capillary electrophoresis and multicolour detection methods can be developed for forensic genetics.

## b) Lineage Informative SNPs

Lineage SNPs are placed on the Y chromosome or in mithocondrial DNA genome.

They show a lack of recombination and a low mutation rate, so they are e informative for evolutionary studies and kinship analyses, in particular in complex cases when the evidence and the reference sample are separated by several generations.

In fact the most useful forensic application of lineage SNPs is for missing person or mass disaster identifications, even if the success of analysis in kinship test is limited by the amount of DNA in samples,the number of family members available for comparison, and the characteristics of the used genetic markers.

In fact the lineage markers,currently available have a limited power of discrimination.

Coble et al. selected for lineage forensic applications 59 that have been sub-divided into 8 different multiplex panels targeting 18 specific common Caucasian HVI/HVII types. [69]

However other studies are in progress to select more SNPs either on Ychromosome and mt-DNA than on the autosomes that all together may serve as lineage-based markers. [70]

## c) Ancestry Informative SNPs

In all cases where no suspects are available for a comparison with an evidentiary sample or not match is found against a DNA database , it may be useful, for investigative purpose, to define the genetic biogeographical ancestry of a perpetrator.

Forensic STR loci are powerful identity markers, but they are poor informative as ancestry markers because of the high degree of allele-sharing among different populations.

Y chromosome and mtDNA markers used for evolutionary purposes may give some informations also about the genetic ancestry even they're not good candidates for ancestry studies because of their uniparental inheritance (haplotypes) and limited representation of the human genome.

Ancestry informative markers (AIMs) are SNPs that reveal ancestral origin of a sample donor but not identify directly physical characteristics.

They are distributed throughout all the human genome and show different frequencies in different populations [71].

Tests that infer the ancestral origin of a DNA sample may have a considerable potential in the development of forensic tools that can assist crime investigation. [72],[73]

Since this method is based on the correlation of phenotypic expression with certain elements of population ancestry structure, thus it strongly requires the assessment of the genetic variation that correlates with specific populations and the development of specific databases to quantify AIMs.

Moreover a complex statistical classification algorithm based on maximum likelihood, is required to predict ancestral origin from the profiles obtained.

A reliable forensic test for assigning the most likely ancestry can be achieved from multiplexed assays by choosing SNPs that exhibit significative allele frequency differences between population so to characterize sequences of DNA that are more prevalent in people from one continent than another.

In this perspective multiplexes have been developed by DNAPrint® Genomics(www.dnaprint.com):

- *EurasianDNA* 1.0 breaks the European ancestry into 4 groups, Northwestern European, Southeastern European, Middle Eastern and South Asian.
- *EuropeanDNA* 2.0 analyzes 1,349 AIMs elucidates European sub-ancestry in particular in Southeastern European , Iberian, Basque, Continental European Northeastern Europea groups

The test is based on the study recently published from Dr. Mark Shriver's laboratory at the Pennsylvania State University. (Bauchet et al). In this large study, 11,071 autosomal SNPs, found on Chromosomes 1-22,were genotyped by chips technology in 12 populations of continental Europeans and Eurasians and were identified predominant axes of population structure not only along a North-South axis, but also along a West-East axis. [74]

## d) Phenotype Informative SNPs

SNPs can be taken into consideration as DNA markers for phenotypic traits (eye colour, hair, skin,etc) that enable a genetic prediction of appearance for investigative purpose to identify the perpetrator of a crime. They also may have value in anthropology studies for the reconstruction of unknown human remains. AIMs provide useful information regarding the likely appearance of a suspect connexed only with biogeographic ancestry, so they can be indirect measures of the phenotype of an individual.

Studies are performed to determine the genetic polymorphisms,simple and complex, responsible for these different phenotypic traits, SNPs in a number of pigmentation genes have been associated with various human hair, skin, and eye color phenotypes.

This requires an assessment of a set of SNPs that strongly affects a specific phenotype as well as development of databases to relate these variants to the specific traits [75].

To date most work on phenotype SNPs has concentrated on pigmentation, since the genetic basis of hair, skin and eye colour is well understood from animal model studies.

Thus, they have very limited value for describing the physical appearance of an individual and the informative value must be taken into consideration on a case-by case basis. DNA markers that describe phenotypic traits would enable a more precise genetic prediction of appearance for investigative leads to identify the perpetrator of a crime. They also may be of value in anthropology studies for the facial reconstruction of unknown human remains (i.e., the skull).

DNA evidence left by a perpretor at a crime scene or on a victim's body can be analyzed to obtain physical informations about the donor in order to construct a physical portrait of the person, giving an high improvement to the investigation.

The most obvious descriptors of an individual's appearance are coloring, height, and facial features, which are all highly heritable It should therefore be possible to determine responsible for different phenotypic traits variation. [76].

A rapid forensic screening assay was developed for 12 MC1R variants for the red hair phenotype: individuals that do not carry the variants typically do not have red hair, approximately 84% of red heads are detectable with this panel. [77]

Two genes SLC45A2 and SLC24A5 have been demonstrated to be associated in the determination of human pigmentation phenotype, while it seems that another one SLC24A4 is related with hair and eye color. [78]

The F374L polymorphism in the SLC45A28 (also called MATP) gene shows highly statistically significant associations with dark hair, skin, and eye pigmentation [79]

**Table 3. Schematic review of SNPs main forensic applications**

| kk. | ll. Autosomal SNPS | mm.   Y-SNPs – X-SNPs | nn.   Mt-SNPs |
|---|---|---|---|
| oo.   Identity test pp. | qq.   X | rr. X | ss. |
| tt. Lineage test uu. | vv. | ww.   X | xx.   X |
| yy.   Ancestry study zz. | aaa.   X | bbb.   X | ccc.   X |
| ddd.   Phenotypic identification | eee.   X | fff. | ggg. |

Moreover other genes such as the P (OCA2) gene, the TYRP1 (tyrosinase-related protein 1 gene) and DCT (dopachrome tautomerase) appears to be associated with eye color. [80], [81], [82]

In addition Relative hand skill (HSR) is a trait of potential use as a physical characteristic in forensic analysis. Relation seems to be exist between handedness (HSR) and CAPG gene:

the test for hand skill can simply predict that a person is right handed and only for ~80–82% of all right handed individuals [83], [84].

Even if the genetic mechanisms that underlie physical characteristic traits are fully described, their real applicability on the field of forensic genetics will be strongly influenced by the ability to create a mangeable test system with a practical number of SNPs. Such test will then need to be validated by the international forensic community and their use shown to be applicable across a wide number of jurisdictions. [85]

## CONCLUSION

Forensic Laboratories often deal with a common problem concerning the genetic identification of degraded biological samples such as the ones collected from crime scenes or mass disaster that may have been exposed to harsh environmental conditions (sunlight, humidity, etc.) that damage DNA structure, by randomly breaking the molecule into smaller pieces.

In addition, some PCR inhibitors can be present in a sample and to be co-extracted with DNA interfering with the ability to obtain a full DNA profile from a biological evidence.

To overcome these problems new markers has been selected in the last years, in order to recover as more information as possible from smaller regions of DNA, which are more likely to be intact following DNA damage. These include miniSTRs and single nucleotide polymorphisms (SNPs).

In particular the interest in SNPs is rising because of their abundance in the human genome and because they show some characteristics that make them especially appropriated to forensic studies.

SNPs can be detected in short amplicons (less than 150bp) that is really useful for the analysis of degraded samples; moreover they show a low mutation rate, that is relevant for the paternity investigations and finally they can be adapted to automation with high throughput.

In addition they could be useful for population studies in order to estimate the allele frequencies of the SNPs selected, for increasing the power of kinship test or family reconstruction analysis and also for creating criminal DNA databases.

Unfortunately SNPs are less informative for identity testing than STR, because most of them have only two alleles. This means more SNPs are required to reach the same level of discrimination obtained with 13-15 STR loci. This involves the necessity to produce multiplexes with a large panel of SNPs that obviously require for typing far more DNA than the one needed for several multiplex STR systems.

In the last years biotechnology companies are making big efforts in developing new strategies for SNP typing: this rapid technological progress makes difficult to choose the appropriate method for specific applications.

Probably, different technologies are to be used for forensic casework since it is often difficult to collect adequate amounts of DNA from scarce samples, and in paternity testing or for DNA databases where the DNA quality/quantity is much less critical.

In general, all technologies that have limited multiplexing capability should be excluded as candidates for routine forensic analysis either because of the limited quantity of DNA available from evidences, than because the number of markers must be as large as possible to yield a significative power of discrimination.

Furthermore, it is possible to make differences between autosomal-SNPs and Y-chromosome and mitochondrial SNPs regarding the number of markers that it is necessary to analyze per sample and the strategy of the analysis. The level of throughput and the multiplex requirements are not the same for both applications and also the appropriate technology could be different for different types

In fact some applications use a few SNPs in a large sample size, other ones require the analysis of a large number of markers in a limited number of samples, finally there are other applications that need large number of both SNPs and samples. In general for forensic applications a medium throughput is enough for criminal casework and paternity test while a high throughput is necessary for DNA databases.

For example MALDI-TOF MS analysis might be a useful future tool in routine analysis of SNPs in forensic, genealogical and other applications, because it's time-saving and cost-efficient. However in comparison with other sequencing methods, the MALDI-TOF MS technology is not only always similar reliable and the multiplex capability is lower. Moreover it requires high-purity samples for genotyping that increase time consume for analysis and sample-processing costs .

Although other DNA microarray systems can simultaneously detect many SNPs in an individual, genotyping is limited because of the need to use predefined sets of SNPs, the low accuracy of heterozygous samples and the high cost. Aother problem of microarrays detection is that the reproducibility and validation is quite difficult.

Pyrosequencing has a very low multiplex capability and it's not suitable to automatation, even if it permit the quantification of the contribution for each allele, a very useful tool in the analysis of mixed samples.

On the contrary, OLA application has a very high, multiplex capability but unfortunately, since the reaction is performed directly on genomic DNA, it requires an high amount of DNA not always available from forensic samples.Procedures based on FRET detection (such as LightCycler, TaqMan ) perform amplification and allelic discrimination in the same reaction, thus this avoids further manipulation steps and favourits the automation and the high throughput of the process., However they show a limited multiplexing capability. As a consequence, these technologies can be useful for validating candidate SNPs or for setting DNA databases, but not for routine application in forensic casework.

NanoChip platform appears as a sensitive and accurate method that permits a rapid multiplex analysis from limited samples under high throughput conditions. So it's a suitable technology for SNP multiplex typing that can be evaluated for forensic casework, even if high purchase price and lower amenability to automation must be evaluated.

Actually, for routine application minisequencing by SNaPshot analysis seems to be the best choice method in forensic laboratories in terms of cost and efficiency, because of the high multiplex capacity, the sensitivity of the system, the ability to perform detection on an automatic capillary electrophoresis instrument, without the requirement of any special platform.

SNP typing could be useful to help investigators with obtained from the biological evidence left at the crime scene. Personal identification seems likely to be the first application of SNPs in routine caseworks, followed by the lineage based family reconstructions.

Moreover the ability to perform genetic typing of biological traces collected at the crime scene, in order to obtain information about a donor's physical characteristics, is a very attractive prospect for forensic analysis and it could potentially offer a powerful new tool for crime scene investigations.

In fact Predicting ancestry or phenotypic characteristics, such as hair, skin or eye colour, is another role that SNPs may play: obviously this more specialized applications will require considerably more research and development efforts to provide reliable predictions about a persons.

Before the introduction in routine casework analysis, it will be relevant for the forensic community, to establish which SNP markers/platforms may be useful for catching up the procedure to a level acceptable for forensic application and than to validate selected SNP panels with sufficient analysis repeat rates.

However, since the expertise in STR typing is more than decennal and all forensic databases are well-established on STR loci, thus it is unlikely that SNPs will replace STR loci as the primary forensic markers for human forensic identification.[86].

It's favorable that once validated for forensic applications, SNPs may be used as a supplementary battery of forensic markers, while retaining STRs as the primary set of markers for forensic DNA analysis.

## COMPETING INTERESTS

The author declares that they have no competing interests. The author alone is responsible for the content and writing of the paper.

## REFERENCES

[1] Miller, R.D., P. Taillon-Miller, and P.Y. Kwok. (2001) Regions of Low Single-Nucleotide Polymorphism Incidence in Human and Orangutan Xq: Deserts and Recent Coalescences. *Genomics* 71: 78-88.

[2] Third International Meeting on Single Nucleotide Polymorphism and Complex Genome Analysis (2000). *Eur. J. Hum. Genet.* 9, 316-18.

[3] Weiner MP, Hudson TJ (2002) Introduction to SNPs: Discovery of Markers for Disease. *BioTechniques* 2002 Jun;Suppl:4-7, 10, 12-3.

[4] Michael H. Shapero, Kerstin K. Leuther, Anhthu Nguyen, et al. (2001). SNP Genotyping by Multiplexed Solid-Phase Amplification and Fluorescent Minisequencing. *Genome Res.* 2001 11: 1926-1934.

[5] Wang N, Akey JM, Zhang K, Chakraborty R, Jin L (2002). Distribution of recombination crossovers and the origin of haplotype blocks: the interplay of population history, recombination and mutation. *Am J Hum Genet* 71:1227–1234.

[6] Daly MJ, Rioux JD, Schaffner SF, Hudson TJ, Lander ES (2001). High-resolution haplotype structure in the human genome. *Nat Genet* 29:229–232.

[7] Johnson GCL, Esposito L, Barratt BJ, Smith AN, Heward J, Di Genova G, Ueda H, Cordell HJ, Eaves IA, Dudbridge F, Twells RCJ, Payne F, Hughes W, Nutland S,

Stevens H, Carr P, Tuomilehto-Wolf E, Tuomilehto J, Gough SCL, Clayton DG, Todd JA (2001) Haplotype tagging for the identification of common disease genes. *Nat Genet* 29:233–237.

[8] Patil N, Berno AJ, Hinds DA, Barrett WA, Doshi JM, Hacker CR, Kautzer CR, Lee DH, Marjoribanks C, McDonough DP, Nguyen BTN, Norris MC, Sheehan JB, Shen N, Stern D, Stokowski RP, Thomas DJ, Trulson MO, Vyas KR, Frazer KA, Fodor SPA, Cox DR (2001). Blocks of limited haplotype diversity revealed by high-resolution scanning of human chromosome 21. *Science* 294:1719–1723.

[9] Dawson, E., Abecasis, C.R., Bumpstead, S., Chen, Y., Hunt, S., Beare, D.M., Pabial, J., Dibling, T., Tinsley, E., Kirby, S., et al. 2002. A first-generation linkage disequilibrium map of human chromosome 22. *Nature* 418: 544–548.

[10] Gabriel SB, Schaffner SF, Nguyen H, Moore JM, Roy J, Blumenstiel B, Higgins J, DeFelice M, Lochner A, Faggart M, Liu-Cordero SN, Rotimi C, Adeyemo A, Cooper R, Ward R, Lander ES, Daly MJ, Altshuler D (2002). The structure of haplotype blocks in the human genome. *Science* 296:2225–2229.

[11] James D. Hurley, Linda J. Engle, Jesse T. Davis, Adam M. Welsh, and John E. Landers (2004) A simple, bead-based approach for multi-SNP molecular haplotyping. *Nucleic Acids Res.* 2004; 32(22): e186.

[12] International_Human_Genome_Sequencing_Consortium. 2001. Initial sequencing and analysis of the human genome. *Nature* 409: 860-921.

[13] the SNP Consortium Website: Past, Present, and Future. 2003. *Nucleic Acids Research* 31(1), 124-27.

[14] The International HapMap Consortium (2007). A second generation human haplotype - map of over 3.1 million SNPs - Vol 449,18 October 2007, doi:10.1038/nature06258

[15] The_International_SNP_Map_Working_Group.(2001)A map of human genome sequence variation containing 1.42 million single nucleotide polymorphisms. *Nature* 409: 928-933.

[16] Chakravarti, A. (2001) Single Nucleotide Polymorphisms: …To a Future of Genetic Medicine. *Nature,* Volume 409, Issue 6822, pp. 822-823 (2001).

[17] Landegren, U., Nilsson, M., and Kwok, P. Y. (1998) Reading Bits of Genetic Information - Methods for Single Nucleotide Polymorphism Analysis, *Genome Research,* 8: 769-776.

[18] Shi M.M.(2001) Enabling large-scale pharmacogenetic studies by high-throughput mutation detection and genotyping technologies. *Clin. Chem.* 47:164–17.

[19] Sobrino B, Brion M., Carracedo A.(2005) SNPs in forensic genetics: a review on SNP typing methodologies. *Forensic Science International* 154 (2005) 181–194.

[20] M. H. Shapero, K. K. Leuther, A. Nguyen, M. Scott and K. W. Jones SNP Genotyping by Multiplexed Solid-Phase Amplification and Fluorescent Minisequencing. *Genome Res.* 2001. 11: 1926-1934.

[21] Liu Q., Thorland E.C., Heit J.A., Sommer S.S. (1997) Overlapping PCR for bidirectional PCR amplification of specific alleles: A rapid one-tube method for simultaneously differentiating homozygotes and heterozygotes. *Genome Res.* 7:389–398.

[22] Wang D.G., Fan J.B., Siao C.J., Berno A.,Young P., Sapolsky R., Ghandour G., Perkins N., Winchester E., Spencer J., (1998) Large-scale identification, mapping, and

genotyping of single-nucleotide polymorphisms in the human genome. *Science* 280:1077–1082.

[23] Livak K.J.(1999) Allelic discrimination using fluorogenic probes and the 5' nuclease assay. *Genet. Anal.* 14:143–149.

[24] Kan Y.W., Dozy A.M. (1978) Polymorphism of DNA sequence adjacent to human β-globin structural gene: Relationship to sickle mutation. *Proc. Natl. Acad. Sci.* 75:5631–5635.

[25] Grossman P.D., Bloch W., Brinson E., Chang C.C., Eggerding F.A., Fung S., Iovannisci D.M., Woo S., Winn-Deen E.S., Iovannisci D.A. (1994) High-density multiplex detection of nucleic acid sequences: Oligonucleotide ligation assay and sequence-coded separation. *Nucleic Acids Res.* 22:4527–4534.

[26] Iannone M.A., Taylor J.D., Chen J., Li M.S., Rivers P., Slentz-Kesler K.A., Weiner M.P. (2000) Multiplexed single nucleotide polymorphism genotyping by oligonucleotide ligation and flow cytometry. *Cytometry* 39:131–140.

[27] Alderborn A., Kristofferson A., Hammerling U. (2000) Determination of single-nucleotide polymorphisms by real-time pyrophosphate DNA sequencing. *Genome Res.* 10:1249–1258.

[28] J. C. Knight, W. McGuire, M. Mosobo Kortok and D. Kwiatkowski (1999). Accuracy of Genotyping of Single-Nucleotide Polymorphisms by PCR-ELISA Allele-specific Oligonucleotide Hybridization Typing and by Amplification Refractory Mutation System. *Clinical Chemistry.* 1999;45:1860-1863.

[29] Syvänen A.C. (2005)Toward genome-wide SNP genotyping. *Nature Genetics* 37, S5 - S10 (2005) doi:10.1038/ng1558.

[30] Förster T. (1948) Intermolecular energy migration and fluorescence. *Ann. Phys.* 2, 55–75. doi:10.1002/andp.19484370105.

[31] Lakowicz, J. R. (1983) *Principles of Fluorescence Spectroscopy,* pp. 258-305, Plenum Press, New York.

[32] Teo IA, Choi JW, Morlese J, Taylor G, Shaunak S (2002) LightCycler qPCR optimisation for low copy number target DNA. *J Immunol Methods,* 2002 Dec 1;270(1):119-33.

[33] Pastinen, T. Kurg, A., Metspalu, A., Peltonen, L. and SyvaÈnen, A.C. (1997). Minisequencing: a specifc tool for DNA analysis and diagnosis on oligonucleotide arrays. *Genome Res.,* 7, 606-614.

[34] SyvaÈnen, A.C. (1999) From gels to chips: ``minisequencing" primer extension for analysis of point mutations and single nucleotide polymorphisms. *Hum. Mutat.,* 13, 1-10.

[35] Bąbol-Pokora K. and Beren J. (2008) SNP-minisequencing as an excellent tool for analysing degraded DNA recovered from archival tissues *ActaBiochimicaPolonica* - Vol. 55 No. 4/2008, 815–819.

[36] Bogus M., Sobrino B., Bender K., Carracedo A., Schneider P.M., SNPforID Consortium (2006) Rapid microarray-based typing of forensic SNPs *International Congress Series* 1288 (2006) 37– 39.

[37] Feng L. and Nerenberg M. (1999) Electronic microarray for DNA analysis *Gene Ther Mol Biol* Vol 4, 183-191, 1999.

[38] Mahajan, S. (1993) *Handbook on semiconductors 3.* Moss, T. Ed.; North Holland, Amsterdam.

[39] Sosnowski, R. G., Tu, E., Butler, W. F., O'Connell, J. P., Heller, M. J., (1997) Rapid determination of single base mismatch mutations in DNA hybrids by direct electric field control. *Proc Natl Acad Sci* USA Feb 94, 1119-1123.

[40] Sethi A. A., Tybjærg-Hansen A., Værn Andersen R.,Nordestgaard B. G (2004). *Nanogen Microelectronic Chip for Large-Scale Genotyping Clinical Chemistry.* 2004;50:443-446.

[41] Balogh M.K., Bender K, Schneider P.M and SNPforID Consortium(2006). Application of Nanogen microarray technology for forensic SNP analysis. *SNPforID Consortium International Congress Series* 1288 (2006) 43– 45.

[42] Werner M, Sych M., Herbon N.,Illig T., König I.R., Wjst M. (2002). Large-scale determination of SNP allele frequencies in DNA pools using MALDI-TOF mass spectrometry *Human Mutation* Volume 20 Issue 1, 2002 Pages 57 – 64.

[43] C. Phillips, R. Fang, D. Ballard, M. Fondevila, C. Harrison, F. Hyland, E. Musgrave-Brown, C. Proff, E. Ramos-Luis, B. SobrinoEvaluation of the Genplex SNP typing system and a 49plex forensic marker panel. Forensic Science International: *Genetics,* Volume 1, Issue 2, Pages 180-185.

[44] Sobrino B. and Carracedo A. (2005) SNP Typing in Forensic Genetics. *Forensic DNA Typing Protocols* 1064-3745 (Print) Volume 297.

[45] Chen, X., Levine, L. and Kwok, P-Y (1999)Fluorescence polarization in homogeneous nucleic acid analysis.*Genome Res.* 9:492-498 (1999).

[46] Greene R.A., DiMeo J.J., Malone M.E., Swartwout S., Liu J.and Buzby P.R. (2001) A Novel Method for SNP Analysis Using Fluorescence Polarization. *PerkinElmer Life Sciences*, P10131 rev. 07/01.

[47] Nilsson TK, Johansson CA. (2004) A novel method for diagnosis of adult hypolactasia by genotyping of the -13910 C/T polymorphism with Pyrosequencing technology. *Scand. J. Gastroenterol.* 2004; 39:287–290.

[48] Harrison C., Musgrave-Brown E., Bender K., Carracedo A., Morling N., Schneider P.,Syndercombe-Court D.,the SNPforID Consortium (2006). A sensitive issue: Pyrosequencing as a valuable forensic SNP typing platform. *International Congress Series* 1288 (2006) 52–54.

[49] Andreas R. Tobler (2005). The SNPlex Genotyping System: A Flexible and Scalable Platform for SNP Genotyping. *J. Biomol Tech.* 2005 December; 16(4): 398–406.

[50] A. Blanco-Verea, M. Brion, E. Ramos-Luis, M.V. Lareu, A. Carracedo (2008). Forensic validation and implementation of Y-chromosome SNP multiplexes. Forensic Science International: *Genetics Supplement Series* 1 (2008) 181–183.

[51] M. Brion, J.J. Sanchez, K. Balogh, C. Thacker,A. Blanco-Verea a, C. Børsting b, B. Stradmann-Bellinghausen, M. Bogus, D. Syndercombe-Court, P.M. Schneider, A. Carracedo, N. Morling (2006) Analysis of 29 Y-chromosome SNPs in a single multiplex useful to predict the geographic origin of male lineages. *International Congress Series* 1288 (2006) 13– 15.

[52] Bouakaze C., Keyser C., Amory S., Crubézy E. and Ludes B.(2007). First successful assay of Y-SNP typing by SNaPshot minisequencing on ancient DNA. *International Journal of Legal Medicine,* Volume 121, Number 6,2007.

[53] PetkovskiE, Keyser-TracquiC,HienneR,LudesB (2005). SNPs and MALDI-TOF MS: Tools for DNA typing in forensic paternity testing and anthropology. *Journal of Forensic Sciences,* Volume 50, Issue 3, 2005.

[54] C. Tomàs, J.J. Sanchez, A. Barbaro, C. Brandt-Casadevall, A. Hernandez, M. Ben Dhiab, M.M. Ramon, N. Morling (2008)The Mediterranean basin: A population genetic study based on 25 X-chromosome SNPs. *Forensic Science International: Genetics Supplement Series August* 2008 (Vol. 1, Issue 1, Pages 170-172).

[55] Tomas C. Sanchez J.J., Barbaro A. , Brandt-Casadevall C., Hernandez A., Ben Dhiab M., Ramon M.and Morling N. (2008) X-chromosome SNP analyses in 11 human Mediterranean populations show a high overall genetic homogeneity except in Northwest Africans (Moroccans).*BMC Evolutionary Biology* 2008, 8:75.

[56] Kimberly A. Sturk, Michael D. Coble, Suzanne M. Barritt, Thomas J. Parsons 1, Rebecca S. Just (2008) The application of mtDNA SNPs to a forensic case. Forensic Science International: *Genetics Supplement Series* 1 (2008) 295–297.

[57] Kline, M.C., Vallone, P.M., Redman, J.W., Duewer, D.L., Calloway, C.D., and Butler, J.M. (2005) Mitochondrial DNA typing screens with control region and coding region SNPs. *J. Forensic Sci.* 50(2): 377-385.

[58] Just, R.S., Irwin, J.A., O'Callaghan, J.E., Saunier, J.L., Coble, M.D., Vallone, P.M., Butler, J.M., Barritt, S.M., and Parsons, T.J. (2004) Toward increased utility of mtDNA in forensic identifications. *Forensic Sci. Int.* 146S: S147-S149.

[59] Vallone, P.M., Just, R.S., Coble, M.D., Butler, J.M., and Parsons, T.J. (2004) A multiplex allele-specific primer extension assay for forensically informative SNPs distributed throughout the mitochondrial genome. *Int. J. Legal Med.* 118: 147-157.

[60] Coble, M.D., Just, R.S., O'Callaghan, J.E., Letmanyi, I.H., Peterson, C.T., Irwin, J.A., Parsons, T.J. (2004) Single nucleotide polymorphisms over the entire mtDNA genome that increase the power of forensic testing in Caucasians. *Int. J. Legal Med.* 118: 137-146.

[61] Allan F. McRae, Enda M. Byrne, Zhen Zhen Zhao, Grant W. Montgomery, and Peter M. Visscher (2008) Power and SNP tagging in whole mitochondrial genome association studies. *Genome Res.* 2008 June; 18(6): 911–917.

[62] Butler J.M., Coble M.D., Vallone P.M. (2007) STRs vs. SNPs: thoughts on the future of forensic DNA testing. *Forensic Sci Med Pathol* (2007) 3:200–205 201.

[63] Amigo J, Phillips C, Lareu M, Carracedo A.(2008) The SNPforID browser: an online tool for query and display of frequency data from the SNPforID project. *Int J Legal Med* 2008, 122(5):435-440.

[64] Budowle B, van Daal A.(2008) *Forensically relevant SNP classes BioTechniques* 44:603-610,2008 pp. 603–610.

[65] Costa G., Dario P., Lucas I. Ribeiro T., Espinheira R., Geada H. (2008) Autosomal SNPs in paternity investigation. *Forensic Science International: Genetics Supplement Series* 1 (2008) 507–509.

[66] Kidd, K.K., A.J. Pakstis, W.C. Speed, E.L. Grigorenko, S.L. Kajuna, N.J. Karoma, S.Kungulilo, J.J. Kim, et al. (2006). Developing a SNP panel for forensic identification of individuals. *Forensic Sci. Int.* 164:20-32.

[67] Sanchez, J.J., Phillips C., Børsting C., Balogh K., Bogus M., Fondevila M., Harrison C.D, Musgrave-Brown E., Salas A., Syndercombe-Court D., Schneider P., Carracedo A., Morling N. (2006). A multiplex assay with 52 singlenucleotide polymorphisms for human identification. *Electrophoresis* 27:1713-1724.

[68] J.J. Sanchez, C. Børsting, K. Balogh, B. Berger, M. Bogus, J.M. Butler, A. Carracedo D. Syndercombe-Court L.A. Dixon, B. Filipovi , M. Fondevila, P. Gill, C.D. Harrison,

C. Hohoff, R. Huell, B. Ludes, W. Parson, T.J. Parsons, E. Petkovski, C. Phillips, H. Schmitter, P.M. Schneider, P.M. Vallone, N. Morling (2008) *Forensic typing of autosomal SNPs with a 29 SNP-multiplex-Results of a collaborative EDNAP exercise FSI genetics* - Volume 2, Issue 3, Pages 176-183

[69] Coble, M.D., R.S. Just, J.E. O'Callaghan, I.H. Letmanyi, C.T. Peterson, J.A. Irwin, and T.J. Parsons (2004). Single nucleotide polymorphisms over the entire mtDNA genome that increase the power of forensic testing in Caucasians. *Int. J. Legal Med.* 118:137-146.

[70] Tishkoff, S.A. and B.C. Verrelli. (2003) Role of evolutionary history on haplotype block structure in the human genome: implications for disease mapping. *Curr. Opin. Genet. Dev.* 13:569-575.

[71] Shriver, M.D., M.W. Smith, L. Jin, A. Marcini, J.M. Akey, R. Deka, and R.E. Ferrell. (1997) Ethnic-affiliation estimation by use of population-specific DNA markers. *Am. J. Hum. Genet.* 60:957-964

[72] Frudakis, T., K. Venkateswarlu, M.J. Thomas, Z.Gaskin, S. Ginjupalli, S. Gunturi, V. Ponnuswamy, S. Natarajan, and P.K. Nachimuthu. (2003) A classifier for the SNP-based inference of ancestry. *J. Forensic Sci.* 48:771-782.

[73] Phillips C, Salas A, Sánchez JJ, Fondevila M, Gómez-Tato A, Alvarez-Dios J, Calaza M, de Cal MC, Ballard D, Lareu MV, Carracedo A , SNPforID Consortium. (2007) Inferring ancestral origin using a single multiplex assay of ancestry informative marker SNPs. *Forensic Sci Int Genet.* 2007 Dec;1(3-4):273-80.

[74] Bauchet M, McEvoy B, Pearson L, Quillen E, Sarkisian T, Hovhannesyan K, Deka R, Bradley D, Shriver M. (2007) Measuring European population stratification with microarray genotype data. *American Journal of Human Genetics* 80(5): 948-956.

[75]. Frudakis, T. N. (2007) *Molecular Photofitting: Predicting Ancestry and Phenotype from DNA*. Academic Press Publishers (Elsevier), Amsterdam, Netherlands. Edition - 2007-09-21

[76] Silventoinen, K., S. Sammalisto, M. Perola, D.I. Boomsma, B.K. Cornes, C. Davis, L. Dunkel, M. De Lange, et al. (2003). Heritability of adult body height: a comparative study of twin cohorts in eight countries. *Twin Res.* 6:399-408.

[77] Grimes, E.A., P.J. Noake, L. Dixon, and A. Urquhart. (2001). Sequence polymorphism in the human melanocortin 1 receptor gene as an indicator of the red hair phenotype. *Forensic Sci. Int.* 122:124-129.

[78] Sulem, P., D.F. Gudbjartsson, S.N. Stacey, A. Helgason, T. Rafnar, K.P. Magnusson, A. Manolescu, A. Karason, et al. (2007). Genetic determinants of hair, eye and skin pigmentation. *Nat. Genet.* 39:1443-1452.

[79] Graf, J., R. Hodgson, and A. van Daal. (2005). Single nucleotide polymorphisms in the MATP gene are associated with normal human pigmentation variation. *Hum. Mutat.* 25:278-284.

[80] Frudakis, T., M. Thomas, Z. Gaskin, K. Venkateswarlu, K.S. Chandra, S. Ginjupalli, S. Gunturi, S. Natrajan, et al. (2003). Sequences associated with human iris pigmentation. *Genetics* 165:2071-2083.

[81] Frudakis, T., T. Terravainen, and M. Thomas. (2007). Multilocus OCA2 genotypes specify human iris colors. *Hum. Genet.* 122:311-326.

[82] Eiberg, H., J. Troelsen, M. Nielsen, A. Mikkelsen, J. Mengel-From, K.W. Kjaer, and L. Hansen. (2008). Blue eye color in humans may be caused by a perfectly associated

founder mutation in a regulatory element located within the HERC2 gene inhibiting OCA2 expression. *Hum. Genet.* 123:117-187.

[83] Francks C., DeLisi L. E., Fisher S. E., Laval S. H., Rue J. E., (2003). Confirmatory evidence for linkage of relative hand skill to 2p12-q11, *American Journal of Human Genetics,* 72, 499–502.

[84] C. Phillips, A. Barbaro M.V. Lareu, A. Salas, A. Carracedo (2006) Initial study of candidate genes on chromosome two for relative hand skill. *International Congress Series Volume* 1288, April 2006, Pages 798-800.

[85] Sang Hong Lee, Julius H. J. van der Werf, Ben J. Hayes, Michael E. Goddard, and Peter M. Visscher (2008) *Predicting Unobserved Phenotypes for Complex Traits from Whole-Genome SNP Data PLoS Genet.* 2008 October; 4(10).

[86] Gill, P., D.J. Werrett, B. Budowle, and R. Guerrieri. (2004). An assessment of whether SNPs will replace STRs in national DNA database: joint considerations of the DNA working group of the European Network of Forensic Science Institutes (ENFSI) and the Scientific Working Group on DNA Analysis Methods (SWGDAM). *Sci. Justice* 44:51-53.

In: Forensic Genetics Research Progress
Editor: F. Gonzalez-Andrade

ISBN: 978-1-60876-198-2
© 2010 Nova Science Publishers, Inc.

*Chapter 11*

# STATISTICAL ASSESSMENT OF DNA PATERNITY TESTS IN UNCOMMON CASES: FROM THE ROUTINE TO THE EXTREME

*Iosif S. Tsybovsky, Nikolay N. Kuzub and Vera M. Veremeichyk*[*]

Center of Forensic Expertise and Criminalistics, Minsk, Belarus

## ABSTRACT

Nowadays, more and more paternity investigations using microsatellite information are carried out in the laboratories all over the world. Tests were proceeded almost equally due to the basis of DNA-analysis – commercial multiplex kits PowerPlex16 System and AmpFlSTR Identifiler, distributed by American companies Promega and Applied Biosystems. Nevertheless, the practice of using these test-systems in parentage and forensic laboratories, complexity of some expert cases (deficient paternity, reverse paternity determination, occurrence of mutations, etc) have specific moments and need being studied and discussed in forensic community. Presented herein is comparative analysis of the paternity investigation results in 394 trio cases (mother, child, alleged father) and 77 duo cases (child, alleged father). Totally 1336 samples collected during paternity testing case work were analyzed using two nonaplex kits, developed in our laboratory. These kits form the universal panel of 17 STR loci (plus amelogenin), compatible to CODIS and test-systems by Promega and Applied Biosystems. We have demonstrated advantages of using this universal panel of 17 loci for resolving cases of disputable paternity. It is established that absence of the biological sample of mother in routine paternity testing reduces the level of random match probability at more than 800 folds. Values of paternity statistics were obtained for all 4 studied test-systems (CODIS – 13 loci, PowerPlex16 System and AmpFlSTR Identifiler – 15 loci and our kits – 17 loci) and compared. Our results underlined the necessity of inclusion of the mother in a paternity investigation, increase the number of analyzed STR loci and examination of

---
[*] E-mail: veraveremeichik@gmail.com

more sets of genetic markers (Y- and X-chromosome, mtDNA) to match growing needs of routine expertise and clarify paternity in uncommon cases.

## INTRODUCTION

Since the mid-1980s, Deoxyribonucleic acid or DNA testing has been used for the purposes of human identification [1]. In recent years DNA analysis, being the most accurate form of testing, has become an important tool in forensic and civil casework [2, 3]. Shortly after establishment of RFLP technology, the PCR was presented, a method that enables the amplification of short polymorphic repeats of the DNA (STR) [4] and unambiguous scoring of DNA profiles, rapid processing and analysis [5-7]. It quickly led to a revolution in the forensic investigation of biological samples [8, 9] and in paternity analysis [10]. After development of multiplex PCR kits, most forensic and paternity cases are investigated using multiplex-PCRs with subsequent automatic fluorescent detection of the labeled PCR product [11]. Thus the rapid development of STR typing technology has increased its power in human identification providing objective evidence for a fair and swift resolution of civil and criminal cases.

The basis of paternity testing is the uniqueness of our individual DNA and the inheritance of that DNA from both of our biologic parents [12]. Most paternity investigations were carried out to prove paternity or exclude paternity when the identity of the biological father is under dispute, to support claims for inheritance, immigration and for peace in the family. Although in many cases the experts have reversed the investigation (reverse paternity) to identify a "child" of a "known" father when it was necessary, to identify a deceased individual for example etc.

There are many issues surrounding the accuracy of paternity testing to be considered by forensic scientists. As recently as 20 years ago, DNA parentage testing was performed using Red Blood Cell (RBC), serum protein testing, and Human Leukocyte Antigen (HLA) testing. Throughout the1980's and the early 1990's, it was appropriate for the state legislature to require a probability of paternity of 95.0% to 99.0% because the available tests were limited in their ability to exclude a falsely accused man from paternity. The definition of "appropriate" testing is in part determined by the development of technology. However, the advent of DNA technology in the late 1980's and the early 1990's has revolutionized parentage testing by dramatically increasing our ability to accurately exclude falsely accused men. In turn, when an accused man is not excluded following thorough paternity testing, his probability of paternity will typically be greater than 99.99999%, thereby removing any doubts of paternity.

In the perfect world, the laboratory would provide very extensive testing in all cases and would test to a level of certainty as high as possible, 99.9999999% or more. Currently, the technology is available to provide that level of certainty in every case. The application of STRs allows paternity testing even in so called deficiency cases, i.e. families in which father or mother are absent or – as it can be assumed for many cases - when for financial or private reasons only the child and putative father were investigated. Usually, the results are reliable; however, considerable problems may arise in paternity cases in which a relative (e.g. brother, father or son) of the putative father has to be taken in account as the biological father without the laboratory being aware of those circumstances [13,14]. The following types of cases are sometimes difficult to examine even with present multiplexes of 15 autosomal STRs loci: motherless paternity or fatherless maternity-deficiency cases; reverse paternity cases [15-17]; incest cases [18]; full sibling impersonating as parent/child [19]; cases involving mutational events and chromosomal abnormalities etc [20-22].

There are some recommendations given for the forensic community and mathematical considerations for resolving difficult cases [23-26]. Nevertheless, some of the commercially available test-systems have not been sufficient in the court in deficiency cases because of the risk carried of including the wrong person (false paternity inclusions). Allen et al. were reported it for SGM Plus and Identifiler [27]. In some specific cases, such as absence of one of the progenitors, these kits have not been sufficient to determine the right putative father [28, 14]. Even when the expert increased the number of loci examined [29], trying to exclude the possibility of finding mutation [30], most commercial multiplex systems may be insufficient in the presence of some exclusion, because of increasing risk of finding more mutations [31].

Recently, Thomson et al. [32] computer simulated the investigation of 10,000 nephew/uncle pairs; the authors calculated that, based on population allele proportions, in 63.4% of all cases, three or more mismatches would be found. Two mismatches were expected in 14.9%, one mismatch in 11.6%, and a complete match in 3.3% of the nephew/uncle pairs. The study of von Wurmb-Schwark et al. [31], based on the investigation of 15 STRs from 125 uncle/child pairs, led to similar results: three or more non-matching STRs were found in 68.8% of all cases; 16.8% showed two mismatches; 10.4% one mismatch; 4% a complete match. Thomson et al. postulated that their simulation resulted in low likelihood ratio (LR), which would merit further investigations, minimizing the risk to wrongly include the alleged parent. The Fung's group [33] also dealt with the problem of excluding relatives of the biological father from paternity. They found that, using AmpFlSTR Profiler Plus system, 9.7% of the alleged fathers in nephew/uncle and niece/uncle cases could not be excluded from fatherhood. Thus, at least in immigration cases, verbal predicates such as "practically proven" should be avoided or handled with great caution.

In some countries they have been established their so called National unidentified human remains databases for determination of kinship (first-degree) matches. During analysis of these databases there have been found that DNA profiles matched unrelated individuals along with known members of the families sharing one allele at all loci analyzed resulting in a false inclusion [34-37]. The fewer loci are used there are more chances of a false inclusion. Such a situation occurs in the isolation of DNA from degraded samples (human skeletal remains etc), when less than the optimal amount of DNA is present.

At the same time, the use of various reference population databases for the statistical calculations (paternity index, power of evidence, typical paternity index) has shown no significant differences in the results obtained in trio paternity studies [38]. Lee et al. reported that there may be mismatches which do not discarded a paternity, even in presence of 3 or more exclusions, being an extremely rare but not improbably incident [39].

Almost in every forensic laboratory experts deal with difficult cases mentioned above. A lot of studies performed to find the most acceptable guidelines to resolve these cases but neither the necessary nor the minimum number of autosomal STR loci has been clearly established [40]. There has only been showed that the greater the number and the types of markers analyzed, the greater the power of discrimination of the system used. Wenk et al.

established, that roughly 25 STR loci appear necessary to achieve 95% confidence to detect at least one genetic inconsistency indicative of non-parentage [41].

Short Tandem Repeat (STR) technology for performing DNA analysis for forensic purposes is currently being used by laboratories here in Belarus. There were some features in parentage testing in our country – experts from different laboratories are using different test-systems – PowerPlex16 (Promega) or Identifiler (Applied Biosystems). Various test-systems are being used in practice of resolving paternity cases in approximately equal proportions, what, on one side, promotes accumulation of large experience in both test-systems using. On other side, certain problems appeared to be in carrying out repeated expert analyses.

When an expert made repeated examinations on the basis of the test-system which differs from those used in primary research, he is able to compare only 13 loci which were equal for the both kits (loci from "COmbined DNA Index System" – CODIS) [42]. This fact automatically reduces the reliability of repeated researches results because an expert' conclusion reliability in DNA-analysis was defined by quantity of the loci investigated and their genetic characteristics. At the same time the level of expert' conclusion proof was the key moment defining the further practical importance of the expert's statement in the trial.

The purpose of our research was to create the universal panel of 17 loci providing practical compatibility of the test-systems PowerPlex16 and Identifiler for resolving paternity cases during the establishment of biological relationship (paternity). The comparative efficiency estimation of 17 loci panel with 15 loci sets of systems PowerPlex16 and Identifiler and 13 loci of CODIS were also provided.

## MATERIALS AND METHODS

### Materials

Buccal swabs were obtained from individuals requesting paternity tests in the Center of Forensic Expertise and Criminalistics from 2003 to 2008. Totally 1336 samples from real 471 cases were analyzed: 394 trio cases (mother, child, alleged father) and 77 duo cases (child, alleged father).

### DNA Extraction

The buccal swabs were treated with lysis buffer, containing SDS and proteinase K [43]. DNA purification were carried out by consecutive chromatography on calcium tartrate gel [44] and gel-filtration on polyvinyl carriers after phenol-chloroform extraction [45].

### PCR Amplification

To analyze allelic polymorphism of 17 STR-loci, D2S1338, D19S433, D3S1358, TH01, D21S11, D18S51, Penta E, D5S818, D13S317, D7S820, D16S539, CSF1PO, Penta D, vWA, D8S1179, TPOX and FGA, DNA amplification was performed by multiplexed polymerase chain reaction using two nonaplex test-systems developed in the laboratories on the basis of FL, TAMRA and JOE-labeled primers (Syntol, Russia).

Nonaplex I included loci TPOX, vWA, TH01, D3S1358, D19S133, FGA, CSF1PO, Penta E and amelogenin. The structure of nonaplex II included loci D2S1338, D5S818, D7S820, D8S1179, D13S317, D16S539, D18S51, D21S11 and Penta D. Working concentration of each of oligonucleotide primers were optimized experimentally. Primer sequences for loci vWA, TH01, D5S818, D13S317, D7S820, D16S539 and amelogenin corresponded to those described in [46], primer structure for loci TPOX, CSF1PO, D3S1358, D8S1179, D21S11 and FGA – to [47]. For loci D18S51, Penta E, Penta D, D2S1338 and D19S433 the structure of primers was optimized during the development of nonaplexes, taking into account compatibility with oligonucleotide structures of other loci.

PCR was performed using thermal cycler GeneAmp PCR System 9700 (Applied Biosystems, USA) in a 15 µl volume using 5-10 ng template DNA, 67 mM tris-HCl pH 8.6; 50 mM KCl; 0,01 % Tween 20; 1,5 mM MgCl$_2$; 0,2 mM of each dNTP and 0,075 µM of each primers one of which is modified by fluorescent label FL, TAMRA or JOE. Reaction of amplification was started by adding 0,75 unit of Taq DNA polymerase (Bion, Russia) after initial DNA denaturation at 95°C for 5 minutes. First 10 cycles were carry out in the following amplification conditions: 94°C for 1 min, 60°C for 1 min, 70°C for 1 min; subsequent 25 cycles: 92°C for 1 min, 60°C for 1 min, 69°C for 1 min, and the final extension of 60°C for 10 minute.

## DNA Fragment Analysis

PCR-amplified fragments were analyzed by capillary electrophoresis with the automatic DNA Sequencer MegaBACE 750 (Amersham Biosciences, USA) in a mode of genotyping: 1ul of each PCR product, 0.2ul ET550-R Size Standard and 11.8ul 0.1% Tween-20 (both from Amersham Biosciences, USA). Allele assignment was performed by comparison with commercially available ladders and determination of fragment sizes using MegaBACE Genetic Profiler v.2.2 software (Amersham Biosciences, USA).

## Statistical Analysis

Calculation of paternal signs random match probability (RMP), revealed in genotypes of the child and the prospective father, was made according to known methodical recommendations [48]. Under the formulas considering combinations of genotypes of mother and the child: $p_1\,(2-p_1)$ – for homozygotic and heterozygotic child's genotypes with only one allele sharing between child and mother; $p_1\,(2-p_1) + p_2\,(2-p_2) - 2\,p_1\,p_2$ – for heterozygotic child's genotypes with both alleles sharing between child and mother. $P_1$ and $p_2$ are values of population allele frequencies revealed at the child. During the calculation of random match probability for the results received in using the test-systems manufactured by the companies Promega and Applied Biosystems, the same tabular values of allele frequencies were used.

## RESULTS AND DISCUSSION

Modern test-systems gave the chance of simultaneous genotyping of 16 loci: 15 autosomal loci and a locus amelogenin (defining a sex). PCR products were analyzed using automated sequencers which allowed to register multichrome fluorescence of five (sequencers ABI Prism manufactured by Applied Biosystems) or four (sequencers MegaBACE manufactured by Amersham) spectrally distinguishable dyes.

Hexadecaplex AmpFlSTR Identifiler developed by the company Applied Biosystems in 2001 included 16 loci (CSF1PO, FGA, TPOX, TH01, VWA, D3S1358, D5S818, D7S820, D8S1179, D13S317, D16S539, D18S51, D21S11, D19S433, D2S1338 and amelogenin) and had identifying ability $1/2,1 \times 10^{17}$ [49].

Hexadecaplex PowerPlex16 System offered by the company Promega included 16 loci – CSF1PO, FGA, TPOX, TH01, VWA, D3S1358, D5S818, D7S820, D8S1179, D13S317, D16S539, D18S51, D21S11, Penta E, Penta D and amelogenin and had identifying ability $1/1,83 \times 10^{17}$ [50].

Thus, a basis of both test-systems makes 13 loci checked up by practice representing the American Combined DNA Index System – CODIS. What concerns the company Promega, there are two highly polymorphic pentanucleotide loci in addition: Penta E and Penta D [51]. Inclusion of loci with pentanucleotide tandems provides the PowerPlex16 test-system with certain advantages at work with forensic samples: during amplification of such kind of STR-loci there are no artifact PCR-products formed, such as stutters (slippery effect of Taq-polymerase) etc [52, 53]. As to discriminating ability of both test-systems the introduction in set structure Identifiler loci D19S433 and D2S1338 equalizes the possibilities of discussed test-systems that is caused by similar characteristics of polymorphism of pairs Penta E – D2S1338 and Penta D – D19S433 [47].

Universal panel from 17 autosomal loci (15 from test-system PowerPlex16 plus 2 loci – D19S433, D2S1338 from the set Identifiler) gives the chance to compare the efficiency of using the test-systems of various manufactures and expands possibilities of the practical expert analysis.

Results of comparative investigation of various sets of loci efficiency for the forensic problems solution at disputable paternity are shown in table 1 and figure 1.

The maximum and minimum values of paternal signs random match probability (RMP) are shown in table 1. The quantity of values which are in the same numerical range (figures in brackets) and values of the median are resulted. The median in this case reflects the level of similarity and distinctions more adequately than mean value.

From the data shown in table 1 it follows, that genotypes random match probabilities for the test-system Identifiler in general are 1,15-1,5 folds as more as for the test-system PowerPlex16 in case both with trios and duos. In 237 full family groups the results reliability were higher using the PowerPlex16; the Identifiler was more effective in 137 cases.

In case of repeated DNA-analyses using the set PowerPlex16 after the primary research performed with the kit Identifiler, the results of 13 loci investigation, which were equal for the both sets (CODIS loci) could only be comparable. Thus the RMP values received at research of the full families increased in 17,2 and 15,3 folds as compared with the results of the 15 loci analysis using full sets PowerPlex16 and Identifiler, accordingly.

## Table 1. Comparative efficiency of resolving disputable paternity with use of various sets of loci

| Number of loci analyzed | Trios (n=394) Value of random match probabilities ||| Duos (n=77) Value of random match probabilities |||
|---|---|---|---|---|---|---|
| | Max | Min | Median | Max | Min | Median |
| **CODIS**, 13 loci | $5,12*10^{-4}$ | $4,77*10^{-11}$ | $1,42*10^{-6}$ | $3,85*10^{-3}$ | $3,91*10^{-5}$ | $4,07*10^{-4}$ |
| **Identifiler**, 15 loci | $6,81*10^{-5}$ | $8,66*10^{-13}$ | $9,27*10^{-8}$ | $9,69*10^{-4}$ | $8,53*10^{-7}$ | $9,66*10^{-5}$ |
| **PowerPlex16**, 15 loci | $8,00*10^{-5}$ | $2,69*10^{-12}$ | $8,24*10^{-8}$ | $1,20*10^{-3}$ | $3,09*10^{-6}$ | $6,25*10^{-5}$ |
| **Universal panel**, 17 loci | $4,67*10^{-6}$ | $4,88*10^{-14}$ | $5,43*10^{-9}$ | $3,03*10^{-4}$ | $3,91*10^{-8}$ | $1,44*10^{-5}$ |

Adding two loci – D19S433 and D2S1338 – from the set Identifiler to the test-system PowerPlex16 raises the research efficiency in 15,2 folds (RMP decreases in 15,2 times). Adding two loci – Penta E and Penta D – from the set PowerPlex16 to the test-system Identifiler leads to increasing of reliability in 17,1 folds. At last, adding four additional loci (Penta E, Penta D, D19S433 and D2S1338) to 13 loci of CODIS results in reducing of RMP value in 261 folds. For all compared groups of loci the comparative analysis using median values are performed. Computed results show, that when comparing two expert evaluation results (repeated examination) carried out using the different commercial test-systems, the conclusions reliability will decrease more than in 200 folds.

In figure 1 there is a range distribution of genotypes random match probability values at the resolving disputable paternity in 394 full families (A) and 77 incomplete families (B). Figure 1A shows that both sets – PowerPlex16 and Identifiler – reveal the similar distribution of random match probability values. Thus the maximum of values for the both systems 10 times differs from the values received for 17 loci panel. Maxima of random match probability values for 13 loci of CODIS and for 17 loci of the universal panel differ not less than in two orders.

While working with deficiency cases it appeared to be the following picture shown in table 1. The full range of loci raises the resolving paternity analysis efficiency in 28 folds as compared with 13 loci of CODIS; in 4,34 folds as compared with the set PowerPlex16 and in 6,71 folds – as compared with Identifiler. Range distribution of RMP values in paternity cases in 77 incomplete families is shown in figure 1B.

Particular interest for the forensic community is the comparative estimation of median random match probability values for all 4 represented analyzed groups of the loci obtained from full (3 persons) and incomplete (without mother) families.

It is established, that in the absence of the mother's sample RMP has increased: for 13 loci of CODIS – in 285 folds; for hexadecaplexes PowerPlex16 and Identifiler – in 750 and 1040 folds; for the universal panel of 17 loci – in 2650 folds. The data obtained once again confirmed, when resolving the disputable paternity, it was recommended to avoid motherless cases when it is impossible to differentiate child's alleles on "motherly" and "fatherly" by the origin.

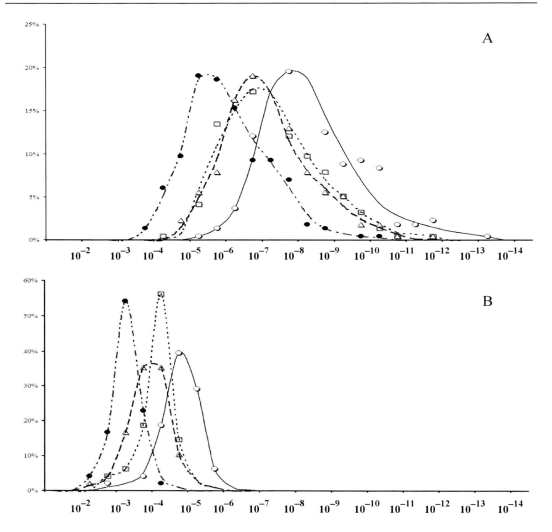

Figure 1. Range distribution of genotypes random match probability values at the disputable paternity in 394 full families (A) and 77 incomplete families (B). An ordinate axis shows the quantity of the revealed values (in percents), an abscissa axis – a range of random match probability values. Designations: —○— – universal panel of 17 loci; ·□·· – PowerPlex16; ·△— – Identifiler; —●·  – CODIS loci.

There is another factor effecting on the genotypic results reliability level besides of ones described above. This is the number of loci having complete heterozygotic genotype sharing between the child and the mother. The loci having both alleles completely coincide in child's and mother's genotypes are uninformative for paternity testing because they don't allow to reveal unequivocally "fatherly" allele of the child. Moreover, such kind of loci can carry the information about possible exclusion of paternity (the "latent" paternity exclusion). Expert practice shows, that in some cases the number of loci, "hiding" the information, can reach 5-7 out of 15-17 investigated (30-40 %). Having such high share of uninformative loci the standard research of 15 loci can appear to be insufficient for the formulation of an expert conclusion and it will be necessary to perform deeper analysis.

**Table 2. Influence of "uncertain" loci number on the reliability of the paternity testing**

| Number of loci analyzed | Number of families with both alleles sharing in child and mother in several loci ||||||||  For all 394 families |
|---|---|---|---|---|---|---|---|---|---|
| | Number of sharing loci |||||||| |
| | 7 | 6 | 5 | 4 | 3 | 2 | 1 | 0 | |
| CODIS, 13 loci | 0 (0,0%) | 5 (1,3%) | 16 (4,1%) | 40 (10,2%) | 83 (21,1%) | 105 (26,6%) | 96 (24,4%) | 49 (12,4%) | |
| Identifiler, 15 loci | 1 (0,3%) | 11 (2,8%) | 22 (5,6%) | 50 (12,7%) | 87 (22,1%) | 92 (23,4%) | 96 (24,4%) | 35 (8,9%) | |
| PowerPlex16, 15 loci | 0 (0,0%) | 10 (2,5%) | 21 (5,3%) | 59 (15,0%) | 72 (18,3%) | 118 (29,9%) | 75 (19,0%) | 39 (9,9%) | |
| Universal panel, 17 loci | 3 (0,8%) | 15 (3,8%) | 29 (7,4%) | 63 (16,0%) | 81 (20,6%) | 101 (25,6%) | 74 (18,8%) | 28 (7,1%) | |
| RMP Median | $3,5 \cdot 10^{-7}$ | $6,2 \cdot 10^{-8}$ | $4,0 \cdot 10^{-8}$ | $2,2 \cdot 10^{-8}$ | $4,8 \cdot 10^{-9}$ | $5,1 \cdot 10^{-9}$ | $7,3 \cdot 10^{-10}$ | $1,0 \cdot 10^{-9}$ | $5,4 \cdot 10^{-9}$ |

The table shows, that the increase of number of loci sharing between heterozygotic child's and mother's genotypes from 1 to 5 poorly influences on the random match probability value (an estimation on the median). At simultaneous revealing of 6 loci with identical genotypes at mother and the child the average RMP values increase almost at 60 folds. Apparently, in this case the level of RMP value is defined by the ratio of two factors: 1) the number of "fatherly" alleles with low frequency of occurrence ("rare" alleles) and 2) the number of sharing loci between mother's and child's genotypes. Presence of "rare" alleles decrease the random match probability. Its influence is more significant and "will neutralize" in high degree the negative effect of the second factor – the number of "uncertain" loci with sharing alleles.

Low level of reliability in paternity analysis in deficiency cases, using a standard set of loci, forces to expand the panel of loci analyzed (additional autosomal loci, STR-loci of Y- and X-chromosomes etc). Our results show that even using the universal panel of 17 loci the random match probability was lower $10^{-5}$ only in 32 cases out of 77. Thus the maximum level of conclusions reliability was 99,999996% (minimum RMP level was $3,9*10^{-8}$, corresponding to possibility of revealing of a required genotype with frequency 1: 25600000).

## CONCLUSION

During the comparative analysis of the data from real paternity cases it was shown, that the genotypes random match probability (RMP) for the test-system Identifiler is higher on the average in 1,15-1,5 times than for the test-system PowerPlex16 in both types of cases: for full families and for motherless ones. The universal created panel from 17 loci provides the practical compatibility of test-systems PowerPlex16 and Identifiler for the solution of disputable paternity, increases the expert researches efficiency and expands possibilities of the practical expert analysis.

It was shown, that the increase of number of loci sharing between heterozygotic child's and mother's genotypes from 1 to 5 poorly influenced on the random match probability value. In typical paternity testing, when the biological sample of mother is absent, the level of expert conclusion reliability decreased in 750-1040 folds. Low level of reliability in paternity analysis in deficiency cases, using a standard set of loci, urged to expand the panel of loci analyzed with involving of other groups of genetic DNA-markers besides autosomal ones.

Increase the number of loci analyzed is necessary for revealing the mutations connected with change of the tandem numbers in the allele structure.

Expert practice showed, that the combination of sets PowerPlex16 and Identifiler was required in cases of mutations in primer-binding sites – the problems of "null"-allele (pseudo-homozygosity). As far as the primers nucleotide structure is different in mentioned above test-systems, the same mutation in such kind of sites can appear in different ways.

Prompt growth of urban population and megapolis formation highly demand the proper level of expert conclusions reliability concerning these cities inhabitants. Paternity testing in deficiency cases requires increase the number of loci investigated because the rising of conclusions reliability level for this category of cases for now is not a scientific problem and is defined exclusively by technological and economic components. The expansion of loci investigated panel is especially important in missing persons cases, when it is necessary to carry out the indirect identification of biological traces and remains through biological relationship when the samples only from the one of parents are accessible for analysis.

## COMPETING INTERESTS

The authors declare that they have no competing interests. The authors alone are responsible for the content and writing of the paper.

## REFERENCES

[1] Jeffreys, AJ; Wilson, V; Thein, SL. Individual-specific "fingerprints" of human DNA. *Nature,* 1985 316, 76–79.

[2] Alonso, A; Andelinovic, S; Martin, P; Sutlovic, D; Erceg, I; Huffin, E; de Simon, LF; Albarran, C; Definis-Cojanovic, M; Fernandez-Rodriquez, A; Garcia, P; Drmic, I; Rezie, B; Kuret, S; Sancho, M; Primorac, D. DNA typing from skeletal remains: evaluation of multiplex and megaplex STR systems on DNA isolated from bones and teeth samples. *Croat Med J,* 2001 42, 260-266.

[3] von Wurmb-Schwark, N; Harbeck, M; Wiesbrock, U; Schroeder, I; Ritz-Timme, S; Oehmichen, M. Extraction and amplification of nuclear and mitochondrial DNA from ancient and artificially aged bones. *Legal Med,* 2003 5, 169-172.

[4] Mullis, K; Faloona, F; Scharf, S; Saiki, R; Horn, G; Erlich, H. Specific enzymatic amplification of DNA in vitro: the polymerase chain reaction. *Cold Spring Harb Symp Quant Biol,* 1986 51, 263-273.

[5] Butler, JM. *Forensic DNA Typing: Biology and Technology Behind STR Markers.* Academic Press: San Diego; 2001.

[6] Butler, JM. Short tandem repeat typing technologies used in human identity testing. *Biotechniques,* 2007 43, 2-5.

[7] Butler, JM. Genetics and genomics of core short tandem repeat loci used in human identity testing. *J Forensic Sci,* 2006 51, 253-265.

[8] Jeffreys, AJ; Allen, MJ; Hagelberg, E; Sonnberg, A. Identification of the skeletal remains of Josef Mengele by DNA analysis. *Forensic Sci Int,* 1992 56, 65-76.

[9] Higuchi, R; von Beroldingen, CH; Sensabaugh, GF; Erlich, HA. DNA typing from single hair. *Nature,* 1988 332, 543-546.

[10] Skawronska, M; Koc-Zorawska, E; Pepinski, W; Janica, J; Niemcunowicz-Janica, A. DNA based paternity testing in Department of Forensic Medicine, Medical Academy of Bialystok, Poland. *Rocz Akad Med Bialymst,* 2002 47, 287-293.

[11] Buse, EL; Putinier, JC; Hong, M; Yap, A; Hartmann, JM. Performance evaluation of two multiplexes used in fluorescent short tandem repeat DNA analysis. *J Forensic Sci,* 2003 48, 1-10.

[12] Baird, ML. Use of DNA identification for forensic and paternity analysis. *J Clin Lab Anal,* 1996 10, 350–358.

[13] Coletti, AB; Lancia, MB; Massetti, SB; Dobosz, SB; Carnevali, EB; Bacci MB. Considerations on a motherless paternity case with two related fathers: Possible pitfalls. *Forensic Sci Int Genet,* 2008 1(1), 505-506.

[14] Gonzalez-Andrade, F; Sanchez, D; Penacino, G; Jarreta BM. Two fathers for the same child: A deficient paternity case of false inclusion with autosomic STRs. *Forensic Sci Int Genet,* 2009 3(2), 138-140.

[15] Mixich, F; Ioana, M; Mixich, VA. Paternity analysis in special fatherless cases without direct testing of alleged father. *Forensic Sci Int.* 2004 146, Suppl:S159-61.

[16] Pretty, IA; Hildebrand, DP. The forensic and investigative significance of reverse paternity testing with absent maternal sample. *Am J Forensic Med Pathol,* 2005 26(4), 340-342.

[17] Gornik, I; Marcikic, M; Kubat, M; Primorac, D; Lauc, G. The identification of war victims by reverse paternity is associated with significant risks of false inclusion. *Int J Legal Med,* 2002 116(5), 255-257.

[18] Robino, C; Barilaro, MR; Gino, S; Chiarle, R; Palestro, G; Torre, C. Incestuous paternity detected by STR-typing of chorionic villi isolated from archival formalin-fixed paraffin-embedded abortion material using laser microdissection *J Forensic Sci,* 2006 51(1), 90-92.

[19] Fung, WK; Wong, DM; Hu, YQ. Full sibling impersonating parent/child prove most difficult to discredit with DNA profiling alone. *Transfusion,* 2004 44, 1513-1515.

[20] Bein, G; Driller, B; Schurmann, M. Schneider, PM; Kirchner, H. Pseudo-exclusion from paternity due to maternal uniparental disomy 16. *Int J Legal Med,* 1998 111(6), 328-330.

[21] Gunn, PR; Trueman, K; Stapleton, P; Klarkowski, DB. DNA analysis in disputed parentage: the occurrence of two apparently false exclusion of paternity, both at short tandem repeat (STR) loci, in the one child. *Electrophoresis,* 1997 18, 1650-1652.

[22] Chan, V; Chan, TP; Lau, K; Todd, D; Chan, TK. False non-paternity in a family for prenatal diagnosis of beta-thalassaemia. *Prenat Diagn,* 1993 13, 977-982.

[23] Gjertson, DW; Brenner, CH; Baur, MP; Carracedo, A; Guidet, F; Luque JA; Lessig, R; Mayr WR; Pascali, VL; Prinz, M; Schneider, PM; Morling, M. ISFG: Recommendations on biostatistics in paternity testing, *Forensic Sci Int Genet,* 2007 1(3), 223-231.

[24] Morling, N.; Allen, RW; Carracedo, A; Geada, H; Guidet, F; Hallenberg, C; Martin, W; Mayr, WR; Olaisen, B; Pascali, VL; Schneider, PM. Paternity testing commission of the international society of forensic genetics: recommendations on genetic investigations in paternity cases. *Forensic Sci Int,* 2002 129(3), 148-157.

[25] Chakraborty, R; Jin, L; Zhong, Y. Paternity evaluation in cases lacking a mother and nondetectable alleles. *Int J Legal Med,* 1994 107, 127-131.

[26] Brenner, CH. A note on paternity computation in cases lacking a mother. *Transfusion,* 1993 33, 51-54.

[27] Allen, RW; Fu, J; Reid, TM; Baird, M. Considerations for the interpretation of STR results in cases of questioned half-sibship. *Transfusion,* 2007 47(3), 515-519.

[28] Wenk. RE; Houtz, T; Chiafari, FA Maternal typing and test sufficiency in parentage analyses. *Transfusion,* 2006 46(2), 199-203.

[29] Hou, JY; Tang, H; Liu, YC; Hou, YP. How many markers are enough for motherless cases of parentage testing. *Forensic Sci Int Genet,* 2008 1(1), 649-651.

[30] Junge, A; Brinkmann, B; Fimmers, R; Madea, B. Mutations or exclusion: an unusual case in paternity testing. *Int J Legal Med,* 2006 120(6), 360-363.

[31] von Wurmb-Schwark, N; Mályusz, V; Simeoni, E; Lignitz, E; Poetsch, M. Possible pitfalls in motherless paternity analysis with related putative fathers. *Forensic Sci Int,* 2006 159(2-3), 92-97.

[32] Thomson, JA; Ayres, KL; Pilotti, V; Barret, MN; Walker, JIH; Debenham, PG. Analysis of disputed single-parent/child and sibling relationships using 16 STR loci. *Int J Legal Med,* 2001 115, 128-134.

[33] Fung, WK; Chung, YK; Wong, DM. Power of exclusion revisited: probability of excluding relatives of the true father from paternity. *Int J Legal Med,* 2002 116, 64-67.

[34] De Ungria, MC; Frani, AM; Magno, MM; Tabbada, KA; Calacal, GC; Delfin, FC; Halos, SC. Evaluating DNA tests of motherless cases using a Philippine genetic database. *Transfusion,* 2002 42, 954-957.

[35] Gornik, I; Marcikic, M; Kubat, M; Primorac, D; Lauc, G.The identification of war victims by reverse paternity is associated with significant risks of false inclusion. *Int J Legal Med,* 2002 116, 255-257.

[36] Presciuttini, S; Ciampini, F; Alu, M; Cerri, N; Dobosz, M; Domenici, R; Peloso, G; Pelotti, S; Piccinini, A; Ponzano, E; Ricci, U; Tagliabracci, A; Baley-Wilson, JE; De Stefano, F; Pascali, V. Allele sharing in first-degree and unrelated pairs of individuals in the Ge. F.I. AmpFlSTR Profiler Plus database. *Forensic Sci Int,* 2003 131, 85-89.

[37] Pu, CE and Linacre, A. CPI distribution and cut-off value for duo paternity building. In: *Proceedings of the 58th Annual Meeting of the American Academy of Forensic Sciences*; Seattle; WA; USA; 2006; 172-173.

[38] Moroni, R; Gasbarra, D; Arjas, E; Lukka, M; Ulmanen, I. Effects of reference population and number of STR markers on paternity testing. *Forensic Sci Int Genet. Supplement Series,* 2008 1(1), 654-655.

[39] Lee, HS; Lee, JW; Han, GR; Hwang, JJ. Motherless case in paternity testing. *Forensic Sci Int,* 2000 114(2), 57-65.

[40] Poetsch, M; Ludcke, C; Repenning, A; Fischer, L; Malyusz, V; Simeoni, E; Lignitz, E; Oehmichen, M; von Wurmb-Schwark, N. The problem of single parent/child paternity analysis - practical results involving 336 children and 348 unrelated men. *Forensic Sci Int,* 2006 159(2-3), 98-103.

[41] Wenk, RE; Gjertson, DW; Chiafari, FA; Houtz, T. The specific power of parentage exclusion in a child's blood relatives. *Transfusion,* 2005 45(3), 440-444.

[42] Miller, KWP; Brown BL; Budowle, B. The Combined DNA Index System. *Progress in Forensic Genetics* 9. In: *Proceedings from the 19th International Congress Series.* 2003 1239, 617-620.

[43] *PCR-based typing protocols.* Washington; DC: FBI Laboratory; 1994.

[44] Akhrem, AA; Drozhdenyuk, AP. Calcium Tartrate Gel. *Analytical Biochemistry,* 1989 179, 86-89.

[45] Sambrook, J; Fritsch, EF; Maniatis, T. *Molecular Cloning. A Laboratory Manual.* 2nd ed. Cold Spring Harbor, New York: Cold Spring Harbor Laboratory Press; 1989.

[46] Masibay, A; Mozer, TJ; Sprecher, CA. Promega Corporation reveals primer sequences in its testing kits. *J Forensic Sci,* 2000 45(6), 1360-1362.

[47] Butler, JM; Shen, Y; McCord, BR. The development of reduced size STR amplicons as tools for analysis of degraded DNA. *J Forensic Sci,* 2003 48(5), 1054-1064.

[48] Perepechina, IO; Grishechkin SA. *Likelihood calculations in DNA-dactyloscopy: Methodical recommendations.* Moscow: EKC of the Ministry of Internal Affairs of Russia; 1996.

[49] *GenePrint PowerPlex ™ 16 System. Technical Manual.* Promega; 2000.

[50] *AmpFlSTR Identifiler ™ PCR Amplification Kit. User's Manual.* Applied Biosystems; 2005.

[51] Bhoopat, T; Steger, HF. STR loci Penta D and Penta E: data from a Northern Thai population sample. *Leg Med (Tokyo),* 2004 6(3), 174-177.

[52] Shlotterer, C; Tautz, D. Slippage synthesis of simple sequence DNA. *Nucl Acids Res,* 1992 20, 211-215.

[53] Bacher, J; Schumm, JW. Development of highly polymorphic pentanucleotide tandem repeat loci with low stutter. *Profiles in DNA,* 1998 2(2), 3-6.

In: Forensic Genetics Research Progress
Editor: F. Gonzalez-Andrade

ISBN: 978-1-60876-198-2
© 2010 Nova Science Publishers, Inc.

*Chapter 12*

# MtDNA ANALYSIS FOR GENETIC IDENTIFICATION OF FORENSICALLY IMPORTANT INSECTS

### *Adriano Tagliabracci*[*] *and Federica Alessandrini*
Institute of Legal Medicine, Università Politecnica delle Marche, Via Conca 71, 60126 Ancona, Italy

## ABSTRACT

The determination of the time of death (post-mortem interval, PMI) has been the major topic of forensic entomologist. The method is based on the link of developmental stages of arthropods, particularly blowfly larvae, to their age. The major advantage against the standard forensic pathological methods for the determination of the early post-mortem interval is that arthropods can represent an accurate measure even in the later stages of the post-mortem interval when the classical methods fail.

Insect species have different developmental lifecycle timings and therefore, to utilise the correct developmental information, species need to be accurately identified. The misidentification of a specimen could produce a PMI estimate that, depending on the species and temperature, could be off by more than a week.

A technical difficulty faced by a forensic entomologist is that it is often difficult or impossible to identify the species of a maggot using classical methods. They require specialized taxonomic knowledge and although identification keys are available, only a few experts are able to identify the larvae of forensically important insects to species level. In addiction, differentiation at larval stages using morphological criteria is still not possible for some groups of insects. Definitive identification may be achieved by rearing larvae to adults but this can be time consuming and require larvae to be collected live and kept in conditions suitable for continued development.

Based on the above disadvantages of the morphological identification process, a forensic entomological investigation can benefit from molecular genotyping methods. There are several reports on the use of DNA techniques for identification of forensically important flies carried out on immatures insects stages and adult flies. As with so much

---
[*] E-mail: a.tagliabracci@univpm.it

of animal molecular systematics, mtDNA has played a leading role in insect genomic studies. High copy number, haploidy, and the availability of conserved mtDNA primers for more than a decade made it easy to obtain mtDNA sequence data from many previously unstudied insect species. The result was an explosive growth in mtDNA sequence data. Most forensic insect species-diagnostic papers focused on some portion of the genes for cytochrome *c* oxidase subunits one and two (COI+II). Coincidentally, the 5 end of COI is also the site of the proposed universal animal DNA barcode.

Suggested targets other than COI+II included randomly amplified polymorphic DNA (RAPDs), the gene for 28S ribosomal RNA, the ribosomal internal transcribed spacer regions, and NADH dehydrogenase subunit 5. Some authors have included more than one locus in a single analysis. However, there is no single agreed-upon locus for DNA-based identification of forensic insects, and it is not clear that there could be.

## INTRODUCTION

A corpse present a temporary and progressively changing habitat and food source for a variety of organisms, ranging from microbes like bacteria and fungi, to vertebrate scavengers. Out of these, arthropod fauna comprises the major element and insects are important agents in the biological breakdown of corpses. These creatures dominate the terrestrial and fresh water carrion fauna.

For many years the worms crawling in the eyes, nose, and other orifices and wounds on dead bodies were considered just another disgusting element of decay, something to be rinsed away as soon as the corpse was placed on the table for autopsy. While blood spatter analysis, ballistics, firearm examination, bite-marks, gunpowder residue chemistry, and other elements of scientific criminology were studied and refined, the insects associated with death scenes were largely ignored (Catts and Haskell 1990).

Entomology is derived from the Greek words *entomon* (insect) and *logos* (word, reason), meaning the study of insects. Forensic entomology is the name given to any aspect of the study of insects and their arthropod counterparts that interacts with legal matters (Hall and Doisy 1993). Lord and Stevenson (1986) divided the field of forensic entomology into three areas: urban entomology, stored product entomology and medico-criminal entomology (also referred to as medico-legal entomology).

Urban entomology refers mainly to controversies involving insects and related animals that affect manmade structures and other aspects of the human environment; stored product entomology involves disputes over arthropods infesting stored commodities such as cereals and other kitchen products. Medico-criminal entomology is the use of the insects, and their arthropod relatives that inhabit decomposing remains to aid legal investigations in case of murder, suicide and rape, but also physical abuse and contraband trafficking.

Information obtained from medico-criminal entomology is typically used to determine time of death, by estimating the developmental stages of arthropods recovered on the corpse. This estimate is often referred as post mortem interval (PMI), but the term colonization interval would be more appropriate, because the corpse may have been stored previously under conditions that restricted access to insects (i.e. rainy, very cold or well sealed environments).

Evaluation and interpretation of entomological evidence at a crime scene can address other complicated issues in addition to time of death, including: season of death, geographic location of death, movement or storage of the remains following death, location of specific sites of trauma on the body, sexual molestation and use of drugs (Haskell 1997, Erzinçlioglu 2003).

## BRIEF HISTORY OF FORENSIC ENTOMOLOGY

The concept of forensic entomology dates back to at least the 1300s but only in the last 30 years has it been systematically explored as a feasible source for evidence in criminal investigations. In history there have been several accounts of vague applications and experimentation of this science.

Insects were first used in a forensic context in thirteenth century in China. A farmer had been killed in a rice field with a sharp weapon. All the suspects were called together and were told to place their sickles

on the ground. No obvious evidence could be seen, but one sickle attracted numerous blowflies, apparently because of invisible traces of blood on the blade. The owner of the sickle, when confronted with this entomological evidence, confessed to the killing. During medieval times, the correlation between maggots on a cadaver and the oviposition of adult flies was not recognized. The idea of the spontaneous development of life emerging from pure matter prevailed. By the seventeenth century, the metamorphosis of insects had become more commonly understood. In 1668, experiments performed by Francesco Redi with rotting meat yielded the observation that the development of blow flies later produced maggots. Up until that time, it was believed that insects such as maggots developed from the rotten meat itself.

The first modern forensic entomology report to include an estimation of PMI was provided by the French physician Bergeret in 1855. He used insects to determine the time of death of an infant, whose body was hidden behind a plastered mantle in a house. His investigations subsequently proved that the guilty party was not the present occupants of the house but the previous owners, based on the presence of insects on the dead body.

At the end of 1800s Jean Pierre Mégnin, an army veterinarian, published many articles and books on various subjects including the book "La Faune des Cadavres" in which he exposed the theory of predictable waves, or successions of insects onto corpses and focused on larval and adult forms of a number of families of insects recovered on the corpse. Mégnin's work and study of the larval and adult forms of insect families found in cadavers sparked the interest of future entomologists and encouraged more research in the link between arthropods and the deceased, and thereby helped to establish the scientific discipline of forensic entomology. In the following years, issues such as grave fauna, the skeletonizing of corpses, or modification or corpses caused by insects were explored, but data concerning the biology, ecology and succession of necrophagous insects were not applied to determine postmortem interval in Europe. Leclercq and Nuorteva were among the first to use forensic entomology for the determination of the postmortem interval in Europe. At the beginning of the 21$^{st}$ century, forensic entomology is recognized in many countries as an important forensic tool (Goff 1991, Greenberg 1991, Anderson 1995, Introna 1998, Amendt 2004).

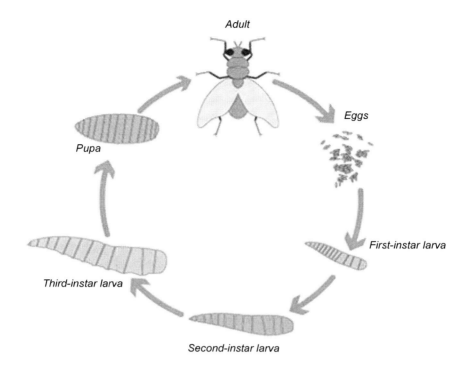

Figure 1. Life cycle of forensically important flies.

## GENERAL ENTOMOLOGY AND INSECT BIOLOGY

Insects are the most numerous and diverse organism on the planet. They inhabit almost all terrestrial habitats and most aquatic ones, with the exception of salt water. Two major groups are attracted to cadavers and provided the majority of information for forensic investigations: the flies (Diptera) and the beetles (Coleoptera).

Although a bewildering array of shapes, sizes and colors, insects have evolved from a common ancestral form. Insect's body is segmented and present three functional regions, the head, the thorax and the abdomen. Each of these regions has specialized external and internal structures that perform certain functions. The head is the area deputated to sensory perception and the point of ingestion. Internally it contains the brain. Externally features are eyes, antennae and mouthparts, important characters used for the identification of insects. Insects have a pair of multifaceted compound eyes; the shape of the compound eyes and their location are features sometimes used in identification. Antennae are often the most noticeable appendages on the insect head. They vary in shapes and sizes, and are one of the key taxonomic features to identify insects down to family level.

Insect antennae are sensory organs, covered with chemical receptors to evaluate the environment. Flies have very different antennae from beetles. The three most important groups of flies attracted to human remains (blow flies, flesh flies and house flies) have an antenna type called aristate, composed of three large segments, the outermost of which has a long, thin hair (arista) protruding from it. The antennae of this flies are very small and difficult to see with the naked eye and need to be observed with a microscope. On the contrary beetles antennae are usually long and composed of 10-20 segments. Other significant characters of the head are the mouthparts, whose shape and morphology are indicative of the type of food the adult insect consumes. Fly larvae have paired, hardened mouth hooks that tear and cut into the carrion upon which they feed. These mouth hooks often have a distinctive shape and can be used in the identification of fly larva species.

The thorax, located directly behind the head, is sclerotized and contains the legs (usually six) and wings on adult insects and it is responsible for the locomotion. In the wings dark thickened lines are present: they are called wing veins and are very important characters for identification in some groups. Adult flies have a single pair of wings. In beetles the wings are covered and protected by hard, shell-like structures called elytra, whose colour, shape and texture can be very useful in species identification.

The abdomen follows the thorax and contains genitalia and other specialized external structures; internally it contains many of the essential body systems (respiratory, reproductive, digestive and circulatory organs). In particular small oval spots, called spiracles, may be present along each side of the abdomen; maggots also have a thoracic spiracle in each side of the body and a pair of posterior spiracles at the tip of the abdomen. Their coloration and shape are important in determining the species.

Insect development pass through a series of stage, from egg to adult. The appearance and the length of these stages varies according to species and environmental conditions. In figure 1 life cycle of forensically important insects (Diptera and Coleoptera) is shown. Flies begins life as eggs, usually laid in large numbers on carrion or decaying material. The eggs hatch after roughly 24 hours at room temperature, producing first instar maggots. They moult again about a day later to give rise to second instars, which live for a further day or two. The second instars then moult into third instars, which live for five or six days after which they stop feeding. They then leave the corpse and wander about for two or three days. The maggots' skin darkens, contracts and hardens to form the puparium, within which the maggot pupates. After a week or so, the flies emerge by breaking the front end of the puparium. Puparia are durable structures and may last unchanged for hundreds of years. Morphological features of larvae are retained on the outer surface of the puparium and could be distinctive enough to allow a species identification.

The periods of time given above are approximate and vary considerably between species and at different environmental temperatures. It can take a maggot two or three months to complete its development at relatively low temperatures.

## INSECTS AND CORPSES

Insect are the first organisms to arrive on a body after death; they are attracted to a body immediately after death, often within minutes and colonize it in a predictable sequence. (Erzinclioglu 1983, Smith 1986, Anderson and VanLaerhoven 1996, Haskell 1997, Anderson 2001). The corpse progresses through a well known sequence of decompositional stages, from fresh to skeletal; each of these stages is attractive to a different group of insects. Some are attracted by the corpse, that is used as food or to lay eggs, others are attracted by insects they use as food.

According to Smith (1986), four ecological categories can be identified in a carrion community:

1. Necrophagous species, feeding on the corpse tissues.
2. Predators and parasites of necrophagous species, feeding only on carrion entomofauna.
3. Omnivorous species feeding both on the corpse and its colonizers (wasps, ants and some beetles).
4. Adventives or incidental species, such as springtails and spiders, which use the corpse as an extension of their normal habitat.

For the purposes of forensic entomology, the first two groups are the most important. They include mainly species from the orders Diptera (flies) and Coleoptera (beetles) (Table 1).

**Table 1. Some forensic important insects. The five families of insects most commonly associated with corpses are underlined**

| Order/family | General |
|---|---|
| DIPTERA/FLIES | |
| *Calliphoridae* | Calliphora, Chrysomya, Cochliomyia, Lucilia, Phormia |
| Drosophilidae | Drosophila |
| Ephydridae | Discomyza |
| Fanniidae | Fannia |
| Heleomyzidae | Heleomyza, Neoleria |
| *Muscidae* | Hydrotaea, Musca, Muscina, Ophyra |
| Phoridae | Conicera, Megaselia |
| Piophilidae | Piophila, Stearibia |
| *Sarcophagidae* | Liopygia, Sarcophaga |
| Sepsidae | Nemopoda, Themira |
| Sphaeroceridae | Leptocera |
| Stratiomyidae | Hermetia, Sargus |
| Trichoceridae | Trichocera |
| COLEOPTERA/BEETLES | |
| Cleridae | Necrobia |
| *Dermestidae* | Attagenus, Dermestes |
| Geotrupidae | Geotrupes |
| Histeridae | Hister, Saprinus |
| *Silphidae* | Necrodes, Nicrophorus, Silpha |
| Staphylinidae | Aleochara, Creophilus |

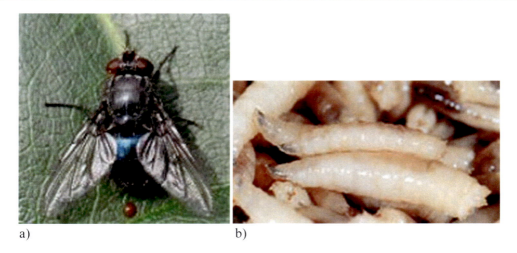

Figure 2. a) Calliphora vomitoria, a blue bottle fly. b) blow flies maggots.

Majority of forensically important fly species belong to the families Calliphoridae (blow flies), Sarcophagidae (flesh flies), and Muscidae (house flies) and are considered to be the most important decomposers of carrion (Payne 1965). Among Coleoptera, the Silphid beetles and the Dermestid beetles are the most forensic important families.. The succession on corpses can be divided into different waves over the various stages of decay, although this has been debated (Schoenly and Reid 1987).

During the initial decay the corpse appears normal outside, but it begins to decay inside due to cellular death and microbial activity. The first insects to arrive on the scene are the Diptera, specifically Calliphorids (blow flies), attracted by odor produced during decomposition (Wall and Warnes 1994, Fisher 1998, Anderson 2001), even over large distances (Braack 1981, Erzinclioglu 1996). The blow fly family includes the familiar green bottle flies (genus Phaenicia) and blue bottle flies (genus Calliphora) (figure 2a). There are more than 1000 known species of blow flies, comprising one of the largest groups of flies in the world. They can be found on almost every continent. Depending on weather conditions, these flies can lay eggs within minutes of death. The presence of ammonia-rich compounds and hydrogen sulphide are important stimulants for oviposition, as well as moisture, some pheromones, and tactile stimulants (Ashworth and Wall 1994, Fisher 1998, Anderson 2001). Diptera do not oviposit in dehydrated or mummified tissue, as eggs and larvae need moisture for successful development (Introna and Campobasso 2000). Oviposition first occurs at the orifices or wounds of the corpse. Their activity is generally limited to daylight hours. Adult calliphorids usually are 6-14 mm in length, have bright metallic coloration, with colors ranging from green, blue, bronze or black. They have three segmented antennae with a plumose or hairy arista on the final portion. The mature larvae of blow flies (figure 2b) are 8-23 mm in length, they are white or cream colored. The terminal segment of the maggot body usually has six or more conic tubercles, which constitute the breathing apparatus. The slits within each spiracle is inclined towards the centre of the larva.

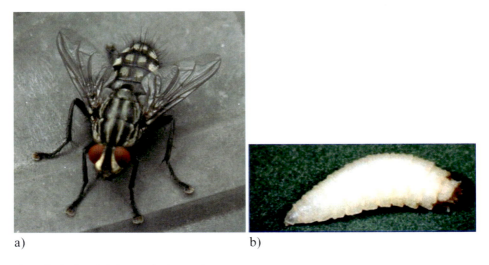

Figure 3. a) flesh fly adult insect. b) Sarcophaga maggot.

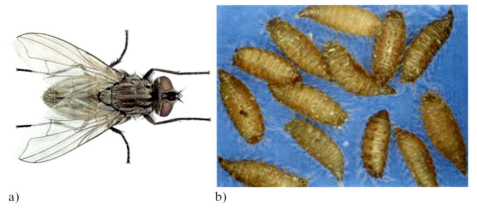

Figure 4. a) adult muscid fly. b) Fannia maggots.

The next insects to colonize the corpse are Diptera, specifically Sarcophagids (flesh flies) (though blow flies are still attracted) followed closely by Coleoptera (Staphylinids and Silphids). Flesh flies also use the body as a breeding ground, but they are larviparous, meaning they lay larvae, not eggs. The big difference in this stage is the feeding material. All of these insects (flesh fly larvae and adult beetles) are predaceous and feed on the eggs and larvae of other insects. There are more than 2000 known species of flesh flies, widespread all around the world. Flesh flies are 2-14 mm in length and have gray and black longitudinal stripes on the torax and a checkerboard pattern on the abdomen (figure 3a). They have not a metallic coloration and the arista is plumose only at the base. Their body is bristly and the eyes are separated. In the maggots the posterior spiracles are located in a depression at the tip of the abdomen, which is edged with fleshy tubercles. Sarcophagid species are very similar in both the adult and larval stages and are very difficult to identify. Maggots (figura 3b) should always be reared to the adult stage to facilitate species identification.

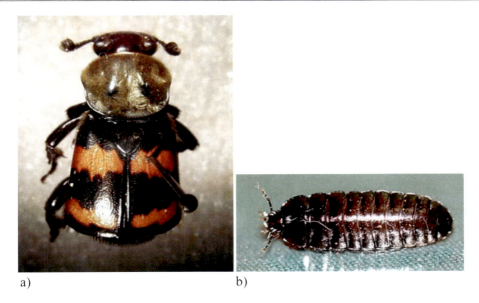

Figure 5. a) Silphid beetle. b) larva.

House flies (family Muscidae) belong to a family with over than 700 species and are of great forensic importance because of their wide distribution, ubiquitous nature and synanthropy (close association with man). They arrive at the corpse after the blow flies and flesh flies and lay eggs in natural body openings, at wound sites or in fluid-soaked clothing. Maggots feed on carrion, but in some species show predacious behaviour as they mature. Muscid flies are 3-10 mm in length and are dull gray to dark in colour (figure 4a). Most muscid larvae have the typical cylindrical shape, tapering from the tail end towards the head. Mature larvae are 5-12 mm in length and are white, yellow or cream colored. The maggot surface is generally smooth, although members of genus Fannia are flattened and have ornate projections (Figure 5b).

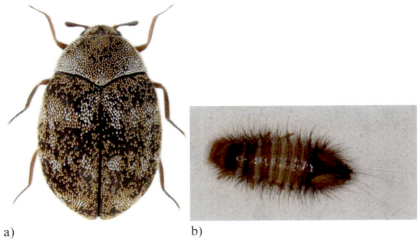

Figure 6. a) Dermistid beetle. b) dermestid maggot.

Shortly after the arrival and colonization of a corpse by dipteran flies, the "second wave" of carrion-frequenting insects (*i.e.*, beetles) quickly become associated with decaying remains (Greenberg 1991). A significant portion of the beetles inhabiting a corpse are predators (*i.e.* Histeridae, Silphidae, and Staphylinidae) of fly larvae and/or other visiting arthropods. However, the scavenging families Dermestidae, Scarabaeidae, and Cleridae are also abundant and represent the second most important carrion decomposers (DeSouza and Linhares 1997). The Coleoptera are characterized by having hard wings covers (elytra) that protect their wings. The larvae are called grubs. The carrion beetles (Silphidae) have a worldwilde distribution and are 10-35 mm in length. Adults vary greatly in size and shape and certain physical features can be useful in their identification. The body is usually broader towards the posterior end and it is black, with yellow, orange or red patches (figure 5a). Antennae are clubbed and either knob-like or broaden gradually. Elytra are often short and leave some abdominal segments exposed. The terminal portion of each leg has five segments. Larvae are generally 15-30 mm long and flattened (figure 5b). Dermistid beetles have a worldwide distribution. They are generally small beetles, 2-12 mm in length, rounded to oval in shape and covered with scales that may form colourful and distinctive patterns (figure 6a). Larvae are 5-15 mm in length and they are generally covered with tufts of long, dense hair (figure 6b). Larvae are found on corpses during the dry and skeletal stages of decomposition; the presence of dermestid beetles is often an indication that considerable time has elapsed since death.

## PMI ESTIMATION

Determining the time of death of a body is one of the most difficult aspects of forensic science, yet it is so often one of the most important problems that has to be resolved in a criminal investigation.

If a post-mortem is held within two or three days after death, in many cases the pathologist's expertise is sufficient to determine the time of death by means of the classical pathological indicators: onset and passing away of rigor mortis, the drop of body temperature to the ambient temperature and the order in which the various organs decompose. When human remains are found days, weeks, or even longer after death, body temperature, and conditions such as rigor mortis or livor mortis are no longer appropriate for estimating time since death. Entomology can often be of use in time of death estimation in such cases. In fact the ages of insect immature stages found on a dead body can provide evidence for the estimation of a minimum PMI ranging from 1 day up to more than 1 month, depending on the insect species involved and the climatic conditions at the death scene. However, this period will not always match the exact PMI, since the age of the maggot can not indicate when the flies arrived at the body after the victim's death but when insect colonisation of the corpse took place. Exact species identification of insect samples is the first essential and crucial step in estimating the age of the larvae found, since insect larvae differ in growth rates and biology. The misidentification of a specimen could produce a PMI estimate that, depending on the species and temperature, could be off by more than a week.

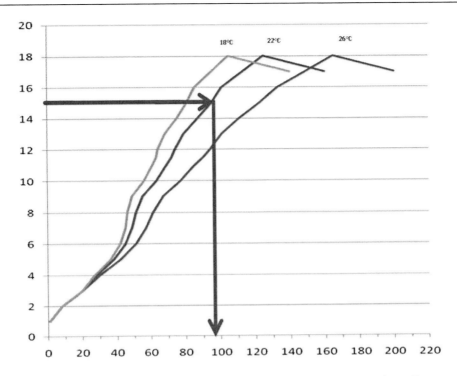

Figure 7. Growth-curve at different temperature (18, 22 and 26°C) for the estimation of larva age. On the Y-axes is reported the maggot size (mm) while X-axes represents time (hours).

For estimating the minimum PMI, the age of the immature larval stages must be determined. Various procedures for estimating their age exist, but they are all based on the fact that the rate of development depends on the ambient temperature (Amendt 2004). In fact the age of a maggot and its stage of development are very different things. A maggot developing at a high temperature may be at a more advanced stage of development than another maggot developing at a low temperature. The latter may be chronologically older, yet still be at an earlier stage of development. Therefore, the age of a maggot is based on a consideration of two aspects: its stage of development, which is discovered by dissection of the maggot, and the temperature at which it was developing. Larval growth rates are the central variable of most estimates of the post-mortem interval.

There are two approaches to estimate the PMI: the calculation ca be based on succession models, or by using maggot age and development. Calculating the PMI from insect succession is the least accurate of the two models, usually limited to a month or season, but in cases where the body is more than two months and several years old, this may be the only method available. The succession method is based on well-documented patterns that insects follow when colonizing remains. According to the evidence of which groups of insects have colonized the body (determined by the presence of larvae/adults and empty or occupied pupal cases of many species), an approximate indication of the post-mortem interval can be ascertained. Calculations based on maggot development are a more precise mean of determining the date of death, usually to a day or less, or at the most a range of days. The development of insects is temperature dependent and can easily be visualised in growth-curves for various constant temperatures, for example in the so called isomorphen diagram, that illustrates the points of morphological changes during the development of the fly depending on temperature. If the reference model for species development is a growth-curve the best estimate of larva age is the value corresponding to its size on the curve, i.e. horizontal line from the value of length or weight of the larva intersects the growth-curve directly above its age (red line) (figure 7). For more details on PMI estimation see the book Forensic Entomology, The utility of Arthropods in Legal Investigation, by Byrd and Castner.

## MOLECULAR IDENTIFICATION OF FORENSICALLY IMPORTANT INSECTS: COMMON USED MARKERS

As previously said, accurate identification of an insect specimen is the crucial first step in a forensic entomological analysis since insects differ in growth rates and biology. Morphological methods are usually used (Smith 1986; Povolny and Verves 1997). However, these techniques require specialized taxonomic knowledge. Although identification keys are available, only a few experts are able to identify the larvae of forensically relevant insects to species level. Furthermore, for some groups of insects (i.e. Sarcophagidae) differentiation at the larval stages using morphological criteria is still not possible. Time consuming rearing of the larvae to adults for identification may delay the criminal investigation or cause significant problems when rearing fails.

At a time when several aspects of forensic science are dominated by recent advances in the field of molecular biology, it is no surprise that DNA technology should also became a tool of the forensic entomologist.

DNA-based identification of organisms has some advantages over classical methods: it is possible at any life stage and can greatly reduce the time need to identify an insect; DNA sequence-reading facilities are common, while fly experts are rare; DNA can be recovered even from dead maggots, or parts of them, while in order to raise a maggot to adulthood it needs to be alive and healthy. Moreover courts are more incline to accept evidence based on numbers and probabilities as opposed to an expert's personal opinion. Using DNA to determine larva species results in a probability that can be presented in court ("The maggot has a 99.3% probability to belong to the species Calliphora vicina according to its DNA sequence"), while using the morphological keys does not provide any probability estimate.

Mitochondrial DNA (mtDNA) is particularly well suiteable as a marker for species identification, since it is a small molecule relative resistant to degradation; hundreds of copies are generally present in each cell and it has a mutation rate high enough to provide sequence differences between closely related species (Avise 1991). Moreover the availability of conserved mtDNA primers (Simon 1994) made it easy to obtain mtDNA sequence data from many insect species. The result was an explosive growth in mtDNA sequence data (Caterino 2000).

The mtDNA of a calliphorid fly closely resembles that of Drosophila yakuba, the first fly species for which the entire mtDNA sequence was described (Clary and Wolstenholme 1985). Insect mtDNA is a small circular molecule with very little non coding portion; the major non coding region is called A+T rich because of the high proportion of adenine and thymine bases. MtDNA contains the genes for some of the protein and ribonucleic acid (RNA) molecules needed for mitochondrial functions (figure 8). Mitochondrial DNA is haploid and it passed down through the generations by maternal inheritance. Because there is no genetic recombination an organism has the same mtDNA haplotype as other members of its maternal line. Investigators do not typically sequence the whole mtDNA molecule, but they examine a region that shows variation that is appropriate for their purposes. Protein-coding genes in the mtDNA are most often used to recognize species; although there is little evidence that one of the protein-coding genes is a more effective marker than the others, the need to compare results has lead to concentrate study on just few regions. For insects some or all of the cytocrome oxidase subunits one and two (COI+COII) are usually analyze, because the majority of published insect mtDNA sequences cover some portion of these genes (Caterino 2000). Coincidentally, the 5 end of COI is also the site of the proposed universal animal DNA barcode (Herbert PD 2003).

In addition to COI and COII genes, frequently investigated mtDNA genes are also NADH dehydrogenase subunit 5 (ND5), NADH dehydrogenase subunit 1 (ND1), 12S and 16S ribosomal RNA genes as well as nuclear gene for 28S ribosomal RNA (Stevens J 2001) and the ribosomal internal transcribed spacer regions (ITSI and II) (Ratcliffe 2003).

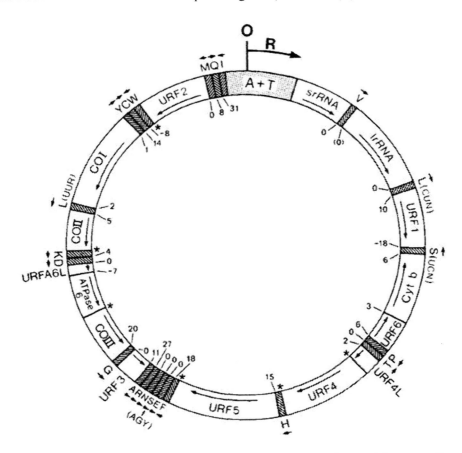

Figure 8. Insect mtDNA molecule structure illustrating the coding portions and the non-coding A+T rich reagion.

Sperling (1996) was the first to demonstrate that mtDNA sequence data from easy-to-identify adult specimens of forensically important flies could be used to identify immature forms of the same species. He analyzed a 2.3kb region of mtDNA comprising the COI and COII genes and the tRNA leucine (UUR) gene and found levels of DNA sequence divergence consistent with the established phylogenetic relationship between examined insects. Moreover nucleotide variations among the blow flies mtDNA were not uniformly distributed, but some regions showed a higher degree of sequence divergence than others. Many substitutions were present throughout the COI and COII genes and in the short sequence between tRNA leucine and COII genes, while the tRNA leucine gene and the beginning of COII gene showed no differences. Using the same techniques Wells and Sperling (1999) found that calliphorid species taxonomically difficult to separate even in the adult stage have distinctly different mtDNA. During their studies, Wells and Sperling have collected COI+COII sequence data on several carrion flies species found in North America, making them publicly available. Two years after, they proposed a method for identifying all forensically important species in the blow fly subfamily Chrysomyinae (Diptera: Calliphoridae) likely to be found in a human corpse in Canada or the USA (Wells and Sperling 2001). This test relies on a short region (~300bp) of the COI sequence from an evidence specimen and maximum parsimony phylogenetic analysis (Swofford 1996) to potentially associate a sequence from an unidentified specimen with a sequence from an identified specimen. In almost all cases, closely related species can be separated using this short region, but for some insects this is not true. In fact a locus that works well for diagnosing species of one taxonomic group may not be so effective for a different group. For this reason some authors suggest to include more than one locus in the analysis (Stevens JR 2002, Stevens JR 2003, Wallman 2005).

## MOLECULAR IDENTIFICATION OF FORENSICALLY IMPORTANT INSECTS: TECHNIQUES

Nowadays genetic examination of DNA markers is based on the popular process invented in 1983 by Kary Mullis, the Polymerase Chain Reaction (PCR). Even for genetic species identification of forensically important flies PCR amplification of suitable regions of the genome, is the usual and recommended method. Prior to be submitted to PCR reaction, DNA has to be isolated from the specimen. This can be done by various well established methods including phenol/chloroform extraction (Sambrook and Russel 2001), CTAB extraction (Stevens and Wall 1996), Chelex extraction (Junqueira 2002), or using commercial extraction kits. DNA can be recovered from insect collected at any stage of development, even from eggs, empty puparia or from dead organism. After DNA extraction, PCR and subsequent analysis of the amplicons obtained can be performed.

Two types of analysis are routinely performed to identify species of forensically important flies: restriction fragment lenght polymorphism (PCR-RFLP) analysis or sequence analysis.

**Sequences producing significant alignments:**
(Click headers to sort columns)

| Accession | Description | Max score | Max ident |
|---|---|---|---|
| AY097333.1 | Calliphora vomitoria isolate NTU-kh cytochrome oxidase subunit | 920 | 100% |
| AJ417702.1 | Calliphora vicina mitochondrial COI gene for cytochrome oxidase | 909 | 97% |
| AF259505.1 | Cynomyopsis cadaverina cytochrome c oxidase subunit 1 (COI) | 848 | 96% |
| AF295557.1 | Eucalliphora latifrons cytochrome oxidase subunit 1 (COI) gene, | 837 | 96% |
| AF295553.1 | Protophormia terraenovae cytochrome oxidase subunit 1 (COI) c | 821 | 95% |
| L14946.1 | Protophormia terraenovae cytochrome oxidase I gene, partial cd | 821 | 95% |

Figure 9. Result of a BLAST search showing sequences producing significant alignments. As showed by the value in the "max ident" column the query sequence matches entirely the Calliphora vomitoria sequence allowing species identification of the unknown insect. The others species can be excluded because of >3% variation.

By applying PCR-RFLP, where specific restriction patterns are produced according to different restriction sites in the sequences, only limited information about a small region within the sequence (i.e. the restriction site) is achieved. In cases of intraspecific variation occurring at a certain restriction site, this may lead to false exclusions because a new restriction pattern may occur, although the other parts of the sequence are identical. Although this technique offers fast and cheap results, it cannot be used for direct and unambiguous species determination.

The technique of sequence analysis has become very popular in recent years. Sequence analysis is relatively easy thanks to analysis kits, computer-based sequencers and software analysis of the sequences generated. Moreover, many companies offer sequence analysis for a relatively small price. Sequence analysis is the recommended method for species determination. Once sequence data are obtained from an unknown specimen, it can be compared to a large number of identified sequences by performing a BLAST search of the GenBank/EMBL/DDBJ database. When a sequence of an unknown insect matches a reference sequence (figure 9) it can be concluded that these two insects belong to the same species. If not, different species can be assumed because, in most cases, considerable differences between species can be observed. However, where differences occur, information about the intraspecific vs the interspecific variation is necessary in order to evaluate these differences. According to some reports (Wells and Sperling 1999, 2001, Wells 2001, Vincent 2000) insects belonging to the same species exhibit less than 1% intraspecific differences in COI and COII sequences; on the contrary insects beloging to different species exhibit about 3% intraspecific differences. Since intraspecific variation will mostly be smaller than interspecific variation, unambiguous identification at the species level may be possible. However, these data have to be seen as preliminary because an overlap of intraspecific and interspecific sequence variation cannot be excluded, so careful interpretation should be employed until more data are available. Furthermore geographic variation among insects from the same species is also possible (Stevens 2002). If the unknown evidence is a species not found in the reference sequence database, phylogenetic analysis can provide useful information for an investigator. The most reliable DNA-based identification of evidence samples employs phylogenetic analysis (Wells 2007). Sequence data from the unknown insect is compared to reference sequences from identified adult specimens, analyzing them by any of the commonly used phylogenetic software packages such as PAUP (Swofford 1998). The goal of such an analysis is to identify the reference sequence that is the closest relative of the unknown sample. If the unknown specimen is one of the species represented in the reference database then the closest relative will be the same species as the unknown specimen. Using common software to apply statistical methods (e.g., the bootstrap) allows to objectively express how much the DNA evidence supports a "sister group" relationship between known and unknown sequences. If the support is too weak, then additional data are needed.

## COMMON ERRORS IN DNA-BASED SPECIES IDENTIFICATION

There are numerous potential pitfalls in attempting DNA forensic insect species identification. The most common beginner mistake is species identification by an uncritical BLAST search. In fact a BLAST search returns the sequences with the highest percent of similarity to the questioned sequence and it is a fast and valid way to get an idea of what the sample may be, but to date it is still an unreliable method because of errors and gaps present in the database. In fact sequences contained in the database are not representative of all known insect species, so the analyst should have enough familiarity with the taxonomy and biology of the relevant insect to notice that a candidate species (i.e. one that the evidence sample might be given the genetic results and the circumstances of its collection) is not present in the database. Until the database is not complete, one can not be sure that all close relatives can be identified by a genetic test.

Moreover when investigators submit their results to GenBank only gross errors are automatically detected and the sequence rejected; submitters have the charge to avoid other sequence errors and to properly identify the organism. Therefore the source of a reference sequence must be known before it can be trusted and this requires scrutiny of the publication from which it was drawn and checking if species was identified by a taxonomic expert, if the work was replicated, if voucher material have been submitted to further analysis and if there is agreement between independent submissions attributed to the same species.

The use of phylogenetic analysis of mtDNA sequence data for species determination requires an assumption of reciprocal mtDNA monophyly among species included in the data set (Moritz 1996, Palumbi 2001). In other words, unless each analyzed species corresponds to a single mtDNA lineage, it will not be possible to assign at least some sample haplotypes to a single species. A study by Stevens and Wall (1996) shows well this problem. They examined the calliphorids Lucilia (=Phaenicia) cuprina and L. sericata using randomly amplified nuclear DNA and 12s rRNA. A study by Wells (2007) performed an analysis of COI+II reference data for Lucilia specimens: the results of this work was a pairing of a Hawaiian L. cuprina haplotype with that of a L. sericata from Canada rather than with another L. cuprina from Australia. He further explored this using a worldwide sample of both species and by also sequencing the nuclear locus 28s ribosomal RNA and he found a clear conflict between the phylogenetic tree based on nuclear DNA and that based on mitochondrial DNA. This data suggested that a lack of COI+COII reciprocal monophyly is common within the genus Lucilia making species diagnosis based on the commonly used cytochrome oxidase I gene (COI) less straightforward than initially thought. This example make clear that regional sampling, particularly of isolated populations, is a necessary step for evaluating these methods.

## CONCLUSION

More research is required before forensic entomologists can use DNA to identify maggots instead of the traditional method of raising them to adult flies to evaluate their morphological features. For instance, investigators are trying to find which genes are best to identify fly species. A locus that is more polymorphic than COI+II might still be useful. The perfect genes are those that differ among individuals of different fly species, but are the same for individuals of the same species.

Many authors have proposed DNA-based methods for identifying an insect specimen associated with human remains, however, almost no attempt has been made to validate these methods using additional observations (Wells 2007). Validation is the process used by the scientific community to acquire the necessary information to assess the ability of a procedure to reliably obtain a desired result, determine the conditions under which such results can be obtained, and determine the limits of the procedure (Technical Working Group on DNA Analysis Methods, 1995).

Although a strong measure of support, such as a bootstrap value, , may seem to indicate a reliable test to link the evidence specimen to a known reference specimen, this result does not say anything about how well the same analysis is likely to work with a future specimen. Therefore, validation of any molecular genetic species test for insects requires a population and geographic survey of the target locus. A strong effort should be made to obtain specimens and genetic data covering a geographic range as wide as possible to determine if this species-diagnostic procedure could be widely applied. These data will be used to complete the database; until then one can not be sure that all close relatives can be identified by a genetic test.

For all these reasons the genetic identification of forensically important insects still need to be supported and confirmed by traditional identification performed by an expert entomologist, until a complete and error-free reference sequence database will be available and/or more robust DNA markers are found.

## COMPETING INTERESTS

The authors declare that they have no competing interests. The authors alone are responsible for the content and writing of the paper.

## REFERENCES

Amendt, J; Krettek, R; Zehner, R. Forensic entomology. *Naturwissenschaften*, 2004, 91, 51-65.

Anderson, GS. The use of insects in death investigations: An analysis of cases in British Columbia over a five year period. *Can Soc Forensic J*, 1995, 28, 277-292.

Anderson, GS; VanLaerhoven, SL. Initial studies on insect succession on carrion in southwestern British Columbia. *J Forensic Sci*, 1996, 41, 617–625.

Anderson; GS. Succession on carrion and its relationship to determining time of death. In: Byrd JH, Castner JL (eds). *Forensic entomology: the utility of arthropods in legal investigations*. CRC, Boca Raton, Fla, 2001, 143–175.

Ashworth, JR; Wall, R; Responses of the sheep blowflies Lucilia sericata and L. cuprina to odour and the development of semiochemical baits. *Med Vet Entomol*, 1994,8, 303–309.

Avise, JC. Ten unorthodox perspectives on evolution prompted by comparative population genetic findings on mithocondrial DNA. *Annual review of genetics*, 1991, 25, 45-69.

Braack, LEO. Visitation patterns of principal species of the insect complex at carcasses in the Kruger National Park. *Koedoe*, 1981, 24, 33–49.

Byrd J.H., & Castner J.L. (1996) *Forensic Entomology The utility of Arthropods in Legal Investigation*. CRC Press. Boca Raton. Fla.

Caterino MS, Cho S, Sperling FAH. 2000. The current state of insect molecular systematics: a thriving tower of Babel. *Annu. Rev. Entomol.* 45:1–54.

Catts EP, Haskell NH. (1990) *Entomology and Death: A Procedural Guide* (1st ed). South Carolina Joyce's Print Shop.

Clary, DO; Wolstenholme, DR. The mitochondrial DNA molecule of Drosophila yakuba: nucleotide sequence, gene organization and genetic code. *J Mol Evol*, 1985,22, 252-271.

De Souza, AM; Linhares AX. Diptera and Coleoptera of potential forensic importance in southeastern Brazil: relative abundance and seasonality. *Med. Vet. Entomol*, 1997,11, 8-12.

Erzinclioglu, YZ. The application of entomology to forensic medicine. *Med Sci Law*, 1983, 23, 57–63.

Erzinclioglu, YZ. *Blowflies*. Richmond Publishing, Slough, UK, 1996.

Erzinçlioglu, YZ. Forensic entomology. *Clinical Medicine*, 2003, 3.

Fisher, P; Wall, R; Ashworth, JR. Attraction of the sheep blowfly, Lucilia sericata (Diptera: Calliphoridae) to carrion bait in the field. *Bull Entomol Res*, 1998, 88, 611–616.

Greenberg, B. Flies as forensic indicators. *J. Med. Entomol*, 1991,28, 565-577.

Goff, ML. Comparison of insect species associated with decomposing remains recovered inside dwellings and outdoors on the island of Oahu, Hawaii. *J. Forensic Sci*, 1991, 3, 748-753.

Hall, RD; Doisy, KE. Length of Time after Death: Effect on Attraction and Oviposition or Larviposition of Midsummer Blowflies (Diptera: Calliphoridae) and Flesh Flies (Diptera: Sarcophagidae) of Medicolegal Importance in Missouri. *Annals of the Entomological Society of America*, 1993, 86, 589-593.

Haskell, NH; Hall, RD; Cervenka, VJ; Clark, MA. () *On the body: insect's life stage presence, their postmortem artifacts*. In: Haglund WD, Sorg MH (eds) *Forensic taphonomy: the postmortem fate of human remains*. CRC, Boca Raton, Fla; 1997; 415–448.

Herbert, PD; Cywinska, A; Ball, SL; De Waard, JR. Biological identifications through DNA barcode *Proc R Soc London Sci B*, 2003, 270, 313-321.

Introna, F; Campobasso, CP; Difazio, A. Three case studies in forensic entomology from Southern Italy. *J Forensic Sci*, 1998, 43, 210-214.

Introna, F; Campobasso, CP. Forensic dipterology. In: Papp L, Darvas B (eds) *Contributions to a manual of palaearctic diptera 1: General and applied dipterology*. Science Herald, Budapest; 2000; 793–846.

Junqueira, ACM; Lessinger, AC; Azeredo-Espin, AML. Methods for the recovery of mitochondrial DNA sequenze from museum specimens of myiasis-causing flies. *Med Vet Entomol,* 2002,16, 39–45.

Lord, W.D., & Stevenson, J.R. (1986) *Directory of forensic entomologists, 2nd ed.* Defense Pest Management Information Analysis Center, Walter Reed Army Medical Center, Washington, D.C.

Moritz, C. The uses of molecular phylogenies for conservation. In: Harvey PH, Leigh Brown AJ, Maynard Smith J, Nee S (eds) *New uses for new phylogenies.* Oxford University Press,; Oxford; 1996; 203–214.

Palumbi, SR; Cipriano, F; Hare, MP. Predicting nuclear gene coalescence from mitochondrial data: the three-times rule. *Evolution,* 2001, 55, 859–868.

Payne, JA. A summer carrion study of the baby pig Sus scrofa Linnaeus. *Ecology,* 1965, 46, 592-602.

Povolny, D; Verves, Y. The flesh-flies of central Europe. *Spixiana Suppl,* 1997, 24, 1–260.

Ratcliffe, ST; Webb, DW; Weinzievr RA, Robertson HM PCR-RFLP identification of Diptera (Calliphoridae, Muscidae and Sarcophagidae)-a generally applicable method. *J Forensic Sci,* 2003, 48, 783-785.

Sambrook, J., Russel, D.W. (2001) *Molecular cloning: a laboratori manual.* Cold Spring Harbor Laboratory Press, Cold Spring Harbor, N.Y.

Schoenly, K; Reid, W. Dynamics of heterotrophic succession in carrion arthropod assemblages: discrete series or a continuum of change? *Oecologia,* 1987, 73, 192–202.

Simon, C; Frati, F; Beckenbach, A; Crespi, B; Liu, H; Flook, P. Evolution, weighting and phylogenetic utility of mitochondrial gene sequences and a compilation of conserved polymerase chain reaction primers. *Ann. Entomol. Soc. Am.* 1994, 87, 651–70.

Smith KGV (1986) *A manual of forensic entomology.* British Museum, London

Sperling, FAH; Anderson, GS; Hickey, DA;. A DNA-based approach to the identification of insect species used for postmortem interval estimation. *J. Forensic Sci.* 1994, 39:418–27. Erratum. 2000. *J. Forensic Sci.* 45:1358–59

Stevens, JR; Wall, R. Species, sub-species and hybrid populations of the blowflies Lucilia cuprina and Lucilia sericata (Diptera: Calliphoridae). *Proc R Soc Lond B,* 1996, 263, 1335–1341.

Stevens, J; Wall, R. Genetic relationships between blowflies (Calliphoridae) of forensic importance. *Forensic Sci Int,* 2001, 120, 116-123.

Stevens, JR; Wall, R; Wells, JD. Paraphyly in Hawaiian hybrid blowfly populations and the evolutionary history of anthropophilic species *Insect Mol Biol,* 2002, 11, 141-148.

Stevens, JR The evolution of myiasis in blowflies (Calliphoridae) *Int J Parasitol,* 2003, 33, 1105-1113.

Swofford, DL; Olsen, GJ; Waddell, PJ; Hillis, DM. (1996) *Phylogenetic inference.* In: Hillis DM, Moritz C, Mable BK (eds, 407–514) *Molecular systematics.* Sinauer, Sunderland.

Swofford, DL. (1998). P-AUP, phylogenetic analysis using parsimony (and other methods). Version 4. Sinauer, Sunderland, MA.

Technical Working Group on DNA Analysis Methods. Guidelines for a quality assurance program for DNA analysis. *Crime Lab. Digest,* 1995, 22:21–43.

Vincent, S; Vian, JM; Carlotti, MP. Partial sequencing of the cytochrome oxydase b subunit gene I: a tool for the identification of European species of blow flies for postmortem interval estimation. *J Forensic Sci,* 2000, 45, 820–823.

Wall, R; Warnes, ML. Responses of the sheep blowfly Lucilia sericata to carrion odour and carbon dioxide. *Entomol Exp Appl,* 1994,73, 239–246.

Wallman, JF; Leys, R; Hogendoorn, K. Molecular systematics of Australian carrion-breeding blowflies (Diptera: Calliphoridae) based on mitochondrial DNA. *Invertebrate Systematics,* 2005,19, 1-15.

Wells, JD; Sperling, FAH. Molecular phylogeny of Chrysomya albiceps and C rufifacies. *J Med Entomol,* 1999,36, 222-226.

Wells, JD; Pape, T; Sperling, FAH. DNA based identification and molecular systematics of forensically important Sarcophagidae (Diptera). *J Forensic Sci,* 2001, 46, 87–91.

Wells, JD; Sperling, FAH. DNA-based identification of forensically important Chrysomyinae (Diptera: Calliphoridae). *Forensic Sci Int,* 2001, 120, 109–114.

Wells, JD; Wall, R; Stevens, JR. Phylogenetic analysis of forensically important Lucilia flies based on cytochrome oxidase I sequence: a cautionary tale for forensic species determination. *Int J Legal Med,* 2007, 121, 229233.

In: Forensic Genetics Research Progress
Editor: F. Gonzalez-Andrade

ISBN: 978-1-60876-198-2
© 2010 Nova Science Publishers, Inc.

*Chapter 13*

# MOLECULAR TECHNIQUES FOR THE IDENTIFICATION OF NON-HUMAN SPECIES IN FORENSIC BIOLOGY

## *Antonio Alonso*[*]

Instituto Nacional de Toxicología y Ciencias Forenses, Departamento de Madrid, Servicio de Biología, C/ Jose Echegaray 4 – 28232 - Las Rozas - Madrid, Spain

## ABSTRACT

It seems clear that the biological remains from animals, plants, algae, fungi and microorganisms are becoming, increasingly relevant in the field of forensic biology and alternative disciplines such as other forensic sciences (forensic toxicology, forensic botany, forensic microbiology, ... ) and study at the molecular level could help with a broad variety of forensic studies of legal interest. There is currently a substantial number of technical protocols and genetic markers (nuclear DNA, mitochondrial DNA and chloroplast DNA) and various DNA databases that makes extremely reliable the genetic identification (at species, lineage, or individual levels) of non human species. This could overcome many of the limitation of classical non human species analysis based on morphological, biochemical or inmunological techniques. This issue outlines the different technologies and DNA markers currently used in the genetic identification of non-human species and its usefulness in a great variety of forensic cases.

## 1. INTRODUCTION

Biological human remains are not the sole kind of evidence faced by forensic laboratories. The analysis of biological remains from animals, plants, algae, fungi and

---

[*] E-mail: a.alonso@mju.es

microorganisms can provide knowledge of considerable interest for solving many different forensic cases. Unfortunately, conventional techniques routinely used for identifying the species that provides the biological traces of forensic interest are based on immunological procedures for the identification of individual protein species (in the investigation of animal remains) morphological (for insects, fungi and higher plants) or viability assays in culture and biochemical and serological tests (in the occurrence of microorganisms) and have severe limitations: These techniques can be nonspecific and rarely reach the stage of identification of the species. In various cases, they cannot be applied to the forensic specimen under study nor can they acquire details on the individual origin of biological traces. However, the most current practice of DNA technology developed in humans and especially the newest techniques of DNA extraction, PCR amplification and high-resolution electrophoretic analysis of fragments and sequencing, has overcome the limitations of standard techniques for the genetic identification of non-human species. There is currently a substantial number of technical protocols and genetic markers (nuclear DNA, mitochondrial DNA and chloroplast DNA) and various DNA databases that makes extremely reliable the genetic identification (at species, lineage, or individual levels) of non human species. The biological remains from animals, plants, algae, fungi and microorganisms are becoming, increasingly relevants in the field of forensic biology and alternative disciplines such as other forensic sciences (forensic toxicology, forensic botany, forensic microbiology, ... ) and study at the molecular level could help with a broad variety of forensic studies of legal interest, among which are:

*Animals*
- Relate the suspect with the crime scene and / or victim
- The identification of the attacker in attacks by animals on humans
- The identification of cadaveric remains of animal origin
- The investigation of poaching and illicit trade in protected species
- Investigation of food fraud and/or health in the composition of food
- The determination of the postmortem interval in forensic entomology
- Studies of ancient DNA
- Studies of pedigrees and paternity

*Plants*
- Criminal investigation to link suspects and victims in a specific area where a felony was committed
- Identification of illicit trafficking of plants that contain psycho-tropic substances
- Investigation of food fraud and / or health in the composition of food
- Identification of poisonous plants
- Studies of ancient DNA

*Algae*
- Identification of plankton in cases of death by drowning

*Higher Fungi*
- Identification of toxic mushrooms
- Identification of hallucinogenic mushrooms

*Microorganisms*
- Research and recognition of microorganisms causing deaths of possible infectious etiology

- Identification of microorganisms used in the manufacture of biological weapons.
- Studies of ancient DNA

This issue outlines the different technologies and DNA markers used currently in the genetic identification of non-human species and its usefulness in a great variety of forensic cases.

## 2. ANIMALS

### 2.1. Species Identification

The genetic identification of animal species is based on analysis of the sequence of DNA markers moderately preserved (with a high degree of inter-species genetic polymorphism and a moderate degree of intra-species variability) so that comparative analysis of the sequence obtained from biological traces with a collection of reference sequences from different species, allowed identification of the species based on the value of the observed sequence homology.

The genetic marker most widely used in forensic identification of animal species, which meets the characteristics of genetic polymorphism mentioned above, is the cytochrome b gene (Cyt b) of the mitochondrial DNA, of approximately 1140 bp in size, which is part of the set of genes involved in the process of oxidative phosphorylation. Moreover, the Cyt b, which is a mitochondrial marker, has a high number of copies per cell, which is of special interest in the forensic analysis of individual samples with small DNA content (such as samples of hair, bones, ... ). The analysis is based on PCR amplification of the most informative region of the gene (between 300–500 bp, depending on the different primers used) using universal primers (which amplify all species) and dye-terminator sequencing of PCR products and subsequent analysis by capillary electrophoresis and laser-induced detection using automated sequencers [Parson et al., 2000]. The comparison of the sequence obtained in each individual case with the collection of sequences of animal species placed in the public database GenBank (http://www.ncbi.nlm.nih.gov/) using the BLAST (Basic Local Alignment and Search Tool), allows to achieve reliable results for identification. A validation study conducted with 44 different species of animals including the five main groups of vertebrates (mammals, birds, reptiles, amphibians and fish) permitted the determination of all the species that were represented in the database with a sequence similarity higher than 99% [Parson et al., 2000]. Analysis of the sequence of the gene Cyt b is often applied for the identification of the species in the analysis of pet hair samples obtained from the crime scene, the victim or suspect. This analysis is also used for the genetic identification of unknown cadaveric remains from animals. The Cyt b has also been applied in the genetic identification of samples of skin, pulverized debris, bones, horns ... for the investigation of illegal trafficking of products derived from protected species (many of them for therapeutic and ornamental uses) [Hsieh et al. 2003; Wong et al., 2004; Wetton et al., 2004]. Trade with products derived from protected species is a worldwide problem, and the Convention on International Trade in Wild Species of Wild Flora and Fauna in Danger of Extinction (CITES: The Convention on International

Trade in Endangered Species of Wild Fauna and Flora) (www.cites.org) provides a listing of species whose trade is prohibited or subject to stringent regulations.

The sequence analysis of two other mitochondrial genes, such as genes for subunits I and II of cytochrome c oxidase (COI and COII) has been applied to the identification of the species from the larvae of insects that colonize the corpse after death. This diagnosis is extremely difficult using morphological techniques and is essential to define the post-mortem (or date of death) since the periods of growth of the larvae are highly variable even between closely related species [Wells et al. 2001; Harvey et al., 2003].

It has recently been described other methods for mammalian species identification from highly degraded forensic samples, as well as ancient DNA samples based on the analysis by PCR amplification of short regions (120 bp) of mitochondrial DNA of different genes such as: Cyt b, the genes of ribosomal RNA (RNAr 12S and RNAr 16S) and genes of the different subunits of NADH dehydrogenase (ND1, ND2 and ND5) [Pereira et al. 2006; Alonso et al. 2006].

## 2.2. Genetic Profiling of Domestic Animals in the Criminal Investigation

Domestic animals like cats and dogs living in a human habitat, detach and deposit in the environment hair samples which can be effortlessly, transferred between suspect, victim and scene. Therefore, genetic analysis of these hairs can provide data to place a suspect at the crime scene, to link the suspect with the victim or to associate the victim with a primary scene of the crime.

In the case of *Canis Familiaris* (dog) study of sequence polymorphisms of the hypervariable regions (HV1 and HV2) of mitochondrial DNA control region allows to retrieve genetic identification data in samples of hair when it is not possible to perform analysis of nuclear DNA [Savolainen et al. 1997; Wetton et al. 2003; Pereira et al. 2004; Eichmann et al., 2007]. This method has a mean power of exclusion exceeding 90% and it is possible to estimate the likelihood ratio of matched haplotypes by counting the occurrence of matching haplotypes in databases of the variants of the mitochondrial DNA control region of the dog. It has been recently proposed specific recommendations to standardize the nomenclature of the haplotypes in the forensic field [Pereira et al. 2004]. In addition, the Spanish and Portuguese Group of the International Society of Forensic Genetics (GEP-ISFG) has coordinated various proficiency exercises for the standardization of the method for analyzing the sequence polymorphisms of the mitochondrial DNA control region from dog forensic samples between forensic genetics laboratories of Spain, Portugal and Latin America.

In the case of samples where it is feasible to obtain nuclear DNA (e.g., remnants of saliva in bites from dog attacks on people), the application of STR polymorphisms provides a greater discrimination power than mitochondrial DNA analysis. 15 STR markers for forensic genetic identification have been sequenced in samples from Canis Familiaris [Eichmann et al, 2004]. STR polymorphisms are equally used in studies of paternity.

In the case of *Felis catus* (cat) it has been developed a multiplex-PCR system (called "MeowPlex") that allows the concurrent analysis of a panel of 11 STR markers and a sex marker (SRY) which provides a power of discrimination in the range of $10^{-7}$ - $10^{-13}$ [Butler et al. 2002]. On the other hand, it has been proposed a real-time PCR system for quantification of specific nuclear DNA samples obtained from cats [Menotti-Raymond et al., 2003]. The STR profile obtained from a cat hair sample found at the crime scene, and its coincidence with the STR profile obtained from a sample of hair from a cat that lived with the suspect was instrumental in solving the murder of a woman in Canada [Menotti-Raymond et al., 1997].

Analysis of the sequence of the mitochondrial DNA control region is more complex in the case of the cat, due to the existence of a long repetitive sequence (long tandem repeat) polymorphism of 80 bp in length, which makes it awkward to achieve reliable sequence results in forensic samples (e.g., hair). If it is not viable to analyze the polymorphism of the repetitive sequence, the power of discrimination is not very high (in a sample of 167 specimens, 70% of cats are represented by only 3 major haplotypes) [Halverson et al. 2005].

Sequence analysis of mitochondrial DNA control region is a technique used for the identification of genetic lineages of additional species of domesticated animals such as *Equs caballus* (horse). However, a key problem for the application to the forensic field of polymorphism of the hypervariable regions of mitochondrial DNA in other species of domestic animals is the lack of representative DNA databases that allow a reliable biostatistical assessment. In the case of the horse, different STRs panels have also been developed (such as the Horse 17-Plex Genotyping Kit, Applied Biosystems), which are used commonly on studies of paternity and pedigree [Dimsoski, 2003]. Various STR markers in goat, sheep and pigs have also been developed following the standards of the International Society for Animal Genetics (www.isag.org.uk).

## 3. PLANTS

The genetic analysis of plants has potentially very different forensic applications:

1. Allows you to link suspects and victims in a certain area (and even a brief period), where a crime was committed.
2. It is a method of identifying the illegal plants that contain psycho-tropic substances.
3. Is used in the investigation of food fraud and / or health in the structure of food.
4. Studies of Ancient DNA

Specific methods have been developed for extracting DNA from plant material, as well as different genetic testing for detection of species and for the diagnosis of individualization. However, its use is less widespread in forensic biology laboratories and a lesser degree of standardization and validation of the methods is applied.

### 3.1. Species Identification

Although there is no a degree of standardization in forensic botany as this achieved in the determination of animal species with respect to Cyt b, there are two types of molecular targets that exhibit the characteristics suitable for application to the forensic diagnosis of species from plant remains: certain genes of chloroplasts and some regions of nuclear ribosomal RNA.

Chloroplast genes, such as the rbcL gene (ribulose bis-phosphate carboxylase 1.5), the atpB gene (ATP synthase B) or the nadhF gene (subunit 5 of NADH dehydrogenase) are located in the genome of the chloroplast and therefore, are in a high number of copies in each cell, and also show intra-species conserved sequences with inter-species genetic polymorphism. rbcL (approximately 1400 bp) is one of the best characterized genes. There is an extensive collection of thousands of sequences obtained from different species in Genebank (http://www.ncbi.nlm.nih.gov/) that allow an identification of genus or species depending on the circumstances. The analysis is by PCR amplification of the most informative gene fragment, and subsequent characterization by automated sequencing techniques followed by comparison of the sequence with reference sequences in the Genebank using BLAST program [Bever et al. 2001]. Analysis of the sequence of the rbcL gene has been successfully applied to forensic samples such as samples of dried leaves and ancient pollen samples [Bever et al. 2005]. The analysis of short sequence fragments (80-157 bp) of the rcbL gene has further been applied to the study of intestinal contents of the Neolithic mummy (Ötzi) of the Alps [Rollo et al. 2002] and the analysis of 11,000 - 28,500 years old coprolites [Hofreiter et al. 2000].

The genes of the nuclear ribosomal RNA, such as rRNA 18S (18S subunit gene for ribosomal RNA) or regions ITS1 and ITS2 (Internal transcribed spacer) that flank the coding region of rRNA 5.8S, are also used in taxonomic studies and evolution of plants and have been applied to species recognition in the forensic field. In the latest analysis is by PCR amplification and following characterization of PCR products by automated sequencing techniques and comparing the sequence with reference sequences in the Genebank using BLAST program.

## 3.2. Genetic Individualization of Plants

There are essentially three methods for analyzing DNA polymorphisms used to distinguish different plants in the field of forensics:

a) Analysis of Randomly Amplified Polymorphic DNA (RAPDs)
b) Analysis of Amplified fragment length polymorphisms (AFLPs)
c) Analysis of Short Tandem repeats (STRs)

The principal advantages of the top two methods (RAPD and AFLP) are:

1. These are universal methods (applicable to any kind of species)
2. You do not demand prior knowledge of information from the DNA sequence.

### 3.2.1. RAPDs

The generation of multi-loci profiles using the RAPDs technique is performed through a standard PCR reaction in which primers are used with random sequences of tiny size (8-15 nucleotides) that aneal in several regions of the genome to generate a substantial number of PCR products of different sizes that are analyzed by different electrophoretic methods. The RAPD method produces complex multi-loci patterns that offer exceptional power of discrimination, but are hard to interpret (visually and statistically). An additional problem of this method for forensic applications is the low inter-laboratory reproducibility offered because small variations in PCR conditions produce changes in electrophoretic patterns. Nor are they applicable to mixtures. The RAPDs method has nevertheless been used in some forensic cases, both criminal and civil. One of the earliest cases documented in the literature is the case of Palo Verde in which the RAPD patterns of seeds found in the trunk of the suspect vehicle matched the RAPD patterns of seeds found in the body of the victim, allowing to relate the suspect with the crime scene [Yoon, 1993]. This method was further used in the investigation of the illegal marketing of a protected species of strawberries [Congiu et al. 2000].

### 3.2.2. AFLPs

The technique of AFLPs has been used for the individualization of plants, insects, birds and bacteria. The AFLPs were generated by cutting the genomic DNA with one or more restriction enzymes and subsequently joining sequences (adapters) at the sites of cutting restriction enzymes. The use of PCR primers (tagged with fluorescent dyes) that specifically anneal with the sequence of adapters allows to obtain DNA fragments of varying sizes (in the range of 50-400 bp). The PCR products were separated by capillary electrophoresis and detected by laser-induced fluorescence using automatic sequencers. The method of AFLPs has been validated for the individualization of *Cannabis sativa* (marijuana) plants. AFLPs patterns databases have also been built that have confirmed the constancy of the genetic profiles retrieved from clonally propagated plants as well as the variability of the AFLP patterns obtained from unrelated *Cannabis* plants (Miller Coyle et al. 2003]. The technique has been applied in the genetic identification of marijuana caches [Miller Coyle et al. 2005]. The major disadvantage of this method for implementation in the forensic field is that they involve substantial amounts of DNA (10-20 ng) that is not degraded.

### 3.2.3. STRs

The recent discovery in plants of short tandem repeat sequences (STRs) that show variability in the amount of repetitions (such as those used in the genetic identification of forensic human genetics), opens the doorway to an increasing use of such markers in the individualization of plants in the forensic field. Several STR markers have been described in Cannabis Sativa [Hsieh et al. 2003, Gilmore et al. 2003; Alghanim and Almirall 2003] including an hexa-nucleotide STR with high degree of variability (between 3 and 40 repeat units) and a high power of discrimination (index of heterozygosity: 87%) [Hsieh et al. 2003]. The use of STR markers has been recently described in the investigation of a double murder (of a pregnant woman) that provided input to exclude the possibility that the plant remains found in the vehicle of the suspect (*Quercus Geminata*) come from the place where the victim was found based on the different STR profiles obtained from each sample. [Craft et al. 2007]. It is anticipated that the use of STR markers will increase in the nearby future in forensic laboratories as a test for the individualization of plant samples due to:

a) The high power of discrimination in PCR-multiplex systems,
b) Their applicability to degraded samples
c) The proper statistical assessment (independence of loci and the product rule for evaluating the probability of match)

d) Compatibility with the technology used in forensic analysis of human samples.
e) Possible application in mixtures

It will be necessary, however, carry out appropriate validation studies (population studies, database development, independence between loci, sensitivity, specificity, ...) before its implementation in routine forensic biology laboratories. The main disadvantage of STRs for use in genetic identification of plants is that the development of these systems require prior knowledge of the sequence of the flanking regions to design specific primers to each particular species, and subsequently the development of population databases for each marker which, because of the wide variety of existing plant, would be a human effort and financial investment that is difficult to address. It is expected therefore the development of STRs only for those plant species that have more significance in the forensic field.

## 4. ALGAE

The genetic identification of diatoms and other phytoplankton algae in cases of death by drowning (both freshwater and salt water) recovered from certain tissues and organs of the victim of drowning is another example of the potential usefulness of molecular techniques for the identification of non human species in the forensic field. It had been proposed the following markers and methods:

a) PCR amplification of the gene of the 16S subunit ribosomal RNA (16S ARNr) using universal phytoplankton primers and subsequent analysis by sequencing [Kane et al. 1996].
b) Amplification by PCR with primers specific for diatoms (eg gene for APO protein of chlorophyll) and electrophoretic detection of PCR products. [Abe et al. 2003]
c) PCR amplification of the 16S gene from plankton followed by DGGE analysis (Denaturing Gradient Gel Electrophoresis) [He et al. 2007]

## 5. FUNGI

The genetic identification of poisoning mushroom by analysis of ITS regions-1 and ITS-2 (Internal Transcriber Spacer) ribosomal RNA gene [Iturralde et al., 2003] is another example of application of forensic DNA analysis of non-human species. The method involves PCR amplification of each of the ITS region with universal primers (specific for higher fungi) followed by cycle sequencing of PCR products with dye-terminators, and subsequent detection of the sequencing reactions by using automated sequencers. The identification of magic mushrooms, specifically the identification of species of the genus *Psilocybe*, which synthesizes hallucinogens (psilocin and psilocybin, which are illegal substances in various laws around the world) is another example of the application of DNA technology to the identification of fungi with forensic purposes. Other molecular methods for the genetic identification of higher fungi are:

a) RAPDs & ALFPs techniques, as well as PCR techniques with specific dye-labeled primers for the ITS regions and subsequent analysis by capillary electrophoresis and laser induced detection [Linacre et al. 2002]
b) PCR amplification and subsequent sequencing of the ITS-1 region and the 5′region of the large subunit of nuclear ribosomal RNA (nLSU rRNA or 28s) [Nugent et al. 2003]
c) Testing of real-time PCR with Taqman probes for detection of the nLSU rRNA region [Maruyama et al. 2006]

## 5. MICROORGANISMS

Molecular techniques for identification of species have become a triple interest in forensic microbiology laboratories. On one side they have developed DNA tests that are used in the investigation of possible infectious etiology of unexplained and sudden deaths (adult and infant).

On the other hand, it have developed various molecular tools for detection and identification of microorganisms to deal with bio terrorism and the use of biological weapons. In 2001, at least five people died in the United States by inhaling anthrax spores that were inoculated by alleged Islamist terrorist groups, in anonymous letters that were addressed to each of the victims. The U.S. government then launched a specific program of microbiology and forensic genetics in order to respond to bio-terrorist attacks. At the present time have developed different genetic testing for the genetic identification of Bacillus anthraces, *Yersinia pestis*, *Francisella tularensis*, *Brucella spp.* and *Burkholderia spp.* [Jones et al., 2005].

Finally, analysis of DNA from ancient organisms (mainly bacteria) isolated from human paleontological and archaeological remains is a tool that can help to clarify questions about a wide variety of infectious diseases suffered by various human populations throughout history. In fact there are several scientific papers describing the isolation of bacterial DNA from archaeological human remains, such as the molecular identification of *Mycobacterium Tuberculosis* in mummified human remains [Spigelman et al. 1993, Salo et al. 1994; Faerman et al. 1997], the identification of *Mycobacterium leprae* DNA from bone remains [Rafi et al. 1994] or, more recently, the identification of *Yersinia pestis* from human dental remains of the fourteenth century as a causative agent of plague medieval pandemic known as "black death" [Raoult et al. 2000]. One of the fundamental limitations of such studies is the difficulty to differentiate between the DNA of ancient microorganisms and opportunistic pathogen DNA from soil microorganisms that can colonize the bones in later times [Rollo et al. 1999]. The most used molecular techniques currently in forensic microbiology can be classified into three groups:

1. Real-time PCR Techniques for detection of single genes, using primers and probes specific to the species. This is a method of high sensitivity and specificity, which provides fast and easily automate.
2. Sequencing of the bacterial rRNA 16S with universal primers.
3. AFLPs techniques

## 6. FUTURE PROSPECTS OF MOLECULAR ANALYSIS OF NON-HUMAN SPECIES IN FORENSICS

It seems clear that the genetic identification of non-human species is an emerging tool in forensic biology laboratories and the number of applications that can be addressed is growing. It is predictable for the various disciplines involved (veterinary forensics, forensic botany, forensic microbiology ,...) to develop (according to standards developed in forensic human genetics) measures for the validation and standardization of the genetic markers and analytical techniques applied, and the standardization of the nomenclature used to describe the genetic profiles and the statistical criteria in the assessment of them and for presentation of proof in court. In the near future, it is also vital for the development of a DNA Database Reference to perform a reliable statistical assessment of the similarities observed between the genetic profile of the remnant under study and a reference sample. The application of genetic typing platforms of high performance (both STR markers and SNPs) as well as automation and miniaturization of analytical systems (which are two current trends of development and advancement of forensic human genetics) is likely to also have an impact on some applications of molecular analysis of non-human species for the area coroner.

## COMPETING INTERESTS

The author declares that he has no competing interests. The author alone is responsible for the content and writing of the paper.

## REFERENCES

Abe et al. *Med Sci Law*. 43, 23-3 (2003).
Alghanim y Almirall. *Analytical and bioanalytical Chemistry*. 376, 1225-1233 (2003).
Alonso et al. *Electrophoresis*.27(24):5101-9 (2006).
Bever et al. *Proceedings from the 12$^{th}$ International Symposium on Human Identification. Promega* (2001).
Bever et al. In: *Forensic Botany: Principles and Applications to criminal casework*. Ed: Heather Miller Coyle. CRC Press (2005).
Butler et al. *Profiles in DNA*. 5, 7-10 (2002).
Craft et al. *Forensic Science International*. 165, 64-70 (2007).
Congiu et al. *Mol. Ecol.* 9, 229–232 (2000).
Dimsosky et al. *Croatian Medical Journal*. 44, 332-335 (2003).
Eichmann et al. *International Journal of Legal Medicine*. 118, 249-266 (2004).
Eichmann et al. *Int J Legal Med.* 121:411-6 (2007).
Faerman et al. *Ancient Biomolecules* 1: 205-214 (1997).
Gilmore et al. *Forensic Science international*. 131, 65-74 (2003).
Halverson et al. *Croatian Medical Journal*. 46, 598-605 (2005).
Harvey et al. *Forensic Sci. Int*. 131, 134–139 (2003).
He et al. *Forensic Sci. Int*. [Epub ahead of print] (2007).

Hofreiter et al. *Mol. Ecol.* 9, 1975-1984 (2000).
Hsieh et al. *Forensic Science international*. 131, 53-58 (2003).
Iturralde et al. *Bol. Soc. Micol. Madrid*, 27, 189-198 (2003).
Jones et al. *Croatian Medical Journal* 46, 522-529 (2005).
Kane et al. *Int J legal Med.* 108:323-326 (1996).
Linacre et al. *Science & Justice* 42, 50-54 (2002).
Maruyama et al. *Forensic Science international*. 163, 51-58 (2006).
Menotti-Raymond et al.. *Nature* 386, 774 (1997).
Menotti-Raymond et al. *Croatian Medical Journal*. 44, 327-331 (2003).
Miller Coyle et al. *Croatian Medical Journal* 44, 315-312 (2003).
Miller Coyle et al. In: *Forensic Botany: Principles and Applications to criminal casework.* Ed: Heather Miller Coyle. CRC Press (2005).
Nugent et al. *Forensic Science International* 140, 147–157 (2004).
Parson et al.. *Int. J. Legal Med.* 114, 23–28 (2000).
Pereira et al. *International Congress Series* 1288, 103-105 (2006).
Pereira et al. *Forensic Sci Int.* 141, 99-108 (2004).
Rafi et al. *Lancet* 343, 1360-1361 (1994).
Raoult et al. *Proc Natl Acad Sci.* 97, 12800-12803 (2000).
Rollo et al. *Phil Trans R Soc Lond* B 354, 111-119 (1999).
Rollo et al. *Proc. Nat. Acad. Sci.* 99, 12594-12599 (2002).
Savolainen et al. *Journal of Forensic Sci.* 42, 593-600 (1997).
Spigelman et al. *Int J Osteoarcheology* 3, 137-143 (1993).
Salo et al. *Proc Natl Acad Sci* USA 91: 2091-2094 (1994).
Wells et al. *Forensic Sci. Int.* 120, 110–115 (2001).
Wetton et al.. *Forensic Sci. Int.* 140, 139–145 (2004).
Wong et al. *Forensic Sci. Int.* 139, 49–55 (2004).
Yoon. *Science.* 260, 894-895 (1993).

In: Forensic Genetics Research Progress
Editor: F. Gonzalez-Andrade

ISBN: 978-1-60876-198-2
© 2010 Nova Science Publishers, Inc.

Chapter 14

# LOCAL DNA DATABASES IN FORENSIC CASEWORK

*José Luis Ramírez*[1,2,*], *Miguel Angel Chiurillo*[3], *Noelia Lander*[2], *Maria Gabriela Rojas*[2] *and Marjorie Sayegh*[2]

[1]United Nations University Program Biotechnology for Latin America and the Caribbean, UNU/BIOLAC, Venezuela
[2]Laboratorio de Polimorfismos Genéticos, Instituto de Estudios Avanzados, MppCT, Carretera Nacional Hoyo de la Puerta, Caracas 1080ª, Venezuela
[3]Decanato de Ciencias de la Salud, Universidad Centro-occidental Lisandro Alvarado, Barquisimeto 3001, Estado Lara, Venezuela

## ABSTRACT

Like many applications of molecular diagnostics, the field of forensic DNA typing is undergoing a period of growth and diversification. In contrast to strictly technological advances there have been a number of forensic-specific applications of existing techniques that have been raised in response to a particular research need, and that have had considerable impact on the field. The range of molecular markers and the analytical methods used in forensic genetics is continuously increasing. In Venezuela rising crime rates are outweighing state security systems, moreover, many mass disasters have recently occurred highlighting the necessity of implementing techniques for DNA analysis for the resolution of criminal cases, as well as the determination of genealogy and disaster victim identification. However, in this country despite having the human resources and training institutes and centers to conduct these tests, there has been a significant delay in the implementation of genetic technology in forensic science.

In response to these needs, in the last six years we have generated mitochondrial DNA (mtDNA) control regions, and autosomal and Y-chromosome Short Tandem Repeats (STR) databases from the admixed population of Caracas (capital city of Venezuela), and its use has allowed a better statistical analysis of forensic casework. Like many other countries, legislation is being adapted to technological innovations, and the creation of a Venezuelan forensic DNA national database is under discussion. In this work we highlight some of the most important cases analyzed, including disaster victim identification, criminal investigation, missing person cases and ancient DNA.

Firstly, we compare markers unbalance between mitochondrial DNA and chromosome Y in the Venezuelan population, confirming the colonization patterns reported for other Latin American countries; also we report in our population unique mtDNA haplotypes of phylogenetic significance. Second we describe the use of forensic genetic techniques and the databases in the identification of victims of an air disaster. Finally, we describe and discuss the experience of our attempts to recover the hypervariable sequences HVRI, HVRII, and HVRIII of the mtDNA control region from ancient hair samples of more than 140 years using technologies such as Phi29 DNA polymerase amplification protocols, and PCR analysis of reduced size fragments.

Although in our laboratory the number of forensic cases that has been processed has increased during the last five years, there is not yet a high output identification technology in place, and to this aim we are starting with the specific database for personal under high risk jobs, namely the Caracas Firefighters Squad. Finally, we are frequently testing standard methods used in forensic genetics, and each new case represents a new challenge for us and a contribution to the accumulated experience that is passed into other parts of the Venezuelan society. In this regard we acknowledge the outstanding contribution of the the Spanish and Portuguese Working Group of the International Society for Forensic Genetics (GEP-ISFG) without which these advances could not be possible.

## INTRODUCION

DNA typing technologies are rapidly evolving but still in human identification the most frequently used markers are autosomal Short Tandem Repeats (STR) PCR assays coupled to the automated capillary DNA sequencer. Among reasons for this preference there are: robustness, reproducibility, and existence of large number of databases.

In Latin America forensic genetics researchers have embraced this technology in full, and in a very short period most laboratories of the region switched from traditional polyacrylamide gel electrophoresis, to automated sequencers. In this technological evolution the activities of the GEP have been a decisive factor. In an approach of convincing rather than demanding, GEP has contributed to the implementation of better forensic genetics practice in the region.

In the particular case of Venezuela, forensic genetics was carried out with home made assays and markers derived from medical genetics studies. Starting in the year 2000 some laboratories began using commercial kits for autosomal markers in polyacrylamide gels, and by 2004, five laboratories were using automated capillary electrophoresis and commercial kits. However, the application of this technology was not accompanied by the development of local population databases with the frequencies of STR markers. Convinced that this type of databases could be useful for local forensic studies, we started the construction of the first database of autosomal markers for the two largest Venezuela cities, namely Caracas [1] and Maracaibo [2], then together with the Unit of Medical Genetics from the School of Medicine

---

[*] E-mail: ramjoseluis@gmail.com

of the University of Zulia, we completed the first chromosome Y database [3], and finally more recently we published the first Venezuelan population mitochondrial DNA database [4].

## VENEZUELAN DATABASES

### STR Database

In 2003 we published the first autosomal-STR Venezuelan database by genotyping 255 unrelated subjects. We used the AmpFlSTR® Identifiler® PCR Amplification Kit that includes the core Genetic Loci of the Combined DNA Index System (CODIS) of the United States Federal Bureau of Investigation (FBI) [1]. In this database we registered the allele frequencies for STRs D2S1338 y D19S433 not previously reported in any Latin American population. Also, we found and characterized a new allele for STR locus D21S11 [5]. However we scored, without further characterization, many other atypical markers. Another interesting observation was that the Caracas city database when compared with a similar database from Maracaibo city (Northwest of Venezuela), with a stronger Amerindian presence [2]; did not show statistically significant differences.

### Chromosome Y Database

For the construction of chromosome Y database we selected 62 individuals living in Caracas city, and used the PowerPlex® Y System (Promega) consisting of 12 Y-STR markers [3]. We found 58 haplotypes with frequencies of 0.0161 for those found once, and of 0.0322 for those found twice. Haplotype diversity (HD) indicated that these markers were highly discriminative for Caracas population (0.9979) i.e. by using these markers there is a probability higher than 99.6% for discriminating between two unrelated males.

When allele and haplotype frequencies from Caracas city were compared with those from Maracaibo city, except for DYS19 and DYS385a/b markers, the allele frequencies for these two populations had similar distributions [6]. The genetic distance between both populations was not significant. Our data is available at the Y Chromosome Haplotype Reference Database site (www.yhrd.org).

### Mitochondrial DNA Database

The most recent database released by our laboratory corresponds to the mitochondrial DNA profiles of individuals living in the North Central region of Venezuela [4]. To this end, we collected a total of 100 blood samples from unrelated individuals. Mitochondrial DNA fragments for hypervariable regions (HVR) I (520pb), II (401pb) and III (478pb) were obtained and sequenced. The sequence analysis for assignment of haplogroups was performed following the guidelines for mtDNA typing [7, 8, 9]. Finally, the haplotypes were deposited to the EMPOP project (www.empop.org).

Although the analysis of region HVRIII was useful for assignation of some haplogroups, HVIII mutations added little to the capacity to differentiate among haplotypes and to the discrimination power of the database (Table 1).

**Table 1. Comparative statistical parameters of Venezuelan mtDNA database ($N= 100$) when hipervariable region III is included**

|  | HVR I + II | HVR I + II + III |
|---|---|---|
| Number of unique haplotypes | 65 (86.7%) | 66 (86.4%) |
| Number of different haplotypes | 75 | 76 |
| Discrimination power | 0.9744 | 0.9764 |
| Random match probability (%) | 2.56 | 2.36 |

As for the data itself, the most frequent kind of mutation was the transition 263 (100%) followed by an insertion, 315.1C (98%), we also reported a new mutation that according to Anderson's reference sequence [10] corresponds to 115d. This mutation was scored in three individuals of the database and in one case we could track that it was present in the female ancestors two generations ago. The individuals harboring the 115d mutation came from the Andean region of Venezuela and belong to Native American haplogroup C1c. Further characterization of this lineage is underway at our laboratory.

The information gained from the mitochondrial studies not only proved to be useful in determining and resolving cases where autosomal STR analysis is insufficient, but also has allowed us to have a better insight of the genetic backgrounds of our population and its relationship to other populations in the continent.

## Admixture and Asymmetry in Maternal and Paternal Human Lineages in Venezuela

The high phylogeographic information content of both Y-chromosome and mtDNA markers has been investigated in depth, allowing the reconstruction of past demographic and evolutionary events, such as human migrations and admixture processes [11, 12, 13]. In admixed populations, mtDNA sequences and Y-chromosome haplotypes can be assigned to a continent of origin [14].

The present-day population of Venezuela is the result of interbreeding between Amerindians, Europeans (mostly Spaniards) and Africans, whom came in contact for five centuries, interacting and mingling. The Spaniards have been coming to Venezuela ever since the conquest, and during the last century, other Europeans, mostly Italians and Portuguese, have also contributed to the gene pool of Venezuela. The African migration, mostly from sub-Saharan region, was restricted to 16th, 17th and 18th centuries, when slave trade was active.

In particular the city of Caracas, founded in 1567, has been an important economic attraction pole for people coming from the country side and abroad, both European and Latin American. The city, located in the north-central region of Venezuela and with an estimated population of four million people, was selected for a preliminary characterization of the parental genetic contributions of chromosome Y and mitDNA markers. Haplogroups of mtDNA and Y chromosome were assigned by direct comparison with the literature, and confirmed with the programs mtDNAmanager (http://mtmanager.yonsei.ac.kr) [15] and Haplogroup Predictor (http://www.hprg.com/hapest5/hapest5a/hapest5.htm), respectively.

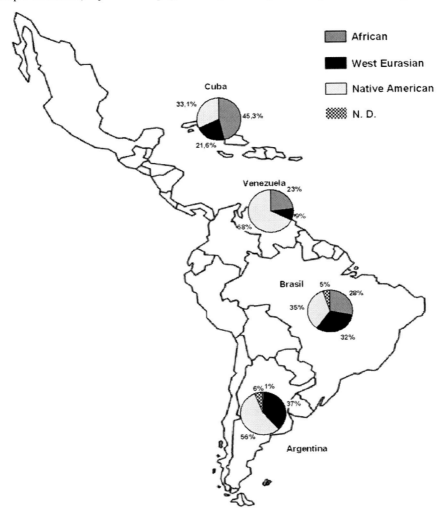

Figure 1. Frequency of mitochondrial lineages in Latin American countries: African (dark gray), West Eurasian (black), Native American (gray) and not determined (black and white squares).

The structure of the Y-chromosome lineages in Caracas shows that 66.8% of the haplotypes analyzed can be traced back to the West Eurasian gene pool, whereas the African fraction accounts for 25.4% of lineages [3]. Among the West Eurasian fraction, the vast majority of individuals belong to West European haplogroup R1, whereas the Native Americans barely represent 7.9% of lineages (Q haplogroup). For mtDNA, the most common haplogroups were assigned to Amerindians (34% A, 5% B, 20% C, 8% D) and Africans (20% L, 3% U6), while the haplogroups corresponding to Europeans maternal line ancestors represented 9% (H, U, J, K, R and T) [4]. Although mtDNA and Y-chromosome analysis show evidence of Amerindian genetic contribution to the population of the city of Caracas, the paternal contribution of Native Americans was substantially lower (7.9%) than the maternal one (67%). Thus there has been a biased gene flow in Caracas that matches the historical reports indicating that during the Spanish colony men came alone, and practiced polygamous unions with Native American women.

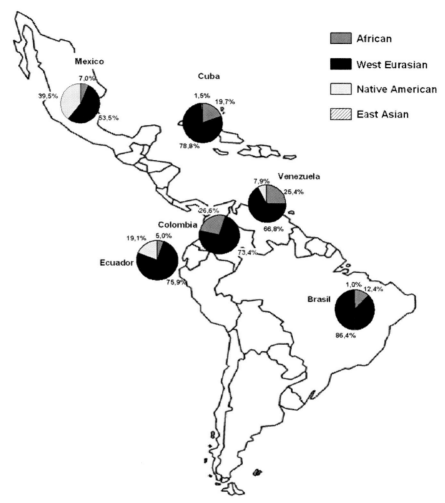

Figure 2. Y-chromosome lineages found in Latin American countries: African (dark gray), West Eurasian (black), Native American (gray) and East Asian (diagonal lines).

The mtDNA haplogroups distribution for other Latin American populations showed a similar trend. In the city of La Plata (Argentina) Amerindian haplogroups contributions was of 56%, but those of African origin accounted for less than 1% [16]. In the case of the Brazilian study there is a distribution of 35% for Amerindian haplogroups, 28% for African origin, and up to 32% for Europeans [17]. However, the authors discuss a possible bias because the sample consisted of individuals coming from the upper-middle class. In the case of Cuba, 45% of mtDNA sequences are of African origin, 33% of Native Americans, and 22% from West Eurasian origin [18] (Figure 1).

In all populations considered, West Eurasian chromosome Y haplogroups were predominant, corresponding to 53.5%, 76.7%, 78.8%, 79.8%, and 86.4% for the male populations of Mexico, Colombia, Ecuador, Cuba and Brazil, respectively [18, 19, 20, 21, 22]. The Amerindian component was important in Mexico City with 39.5% and Quito (Ecuador) 19.2% (Figure 2). The most important African haplotypes contribution was registered in the very racially mixed populations of Colombia (21.6%), Cuba (19.7%) and Brazil (12.4%).

In conclusion, most Latin American populations showed similar trends in chromosome Y and mtDNA haplogroups distributions, and the deviations to this pattern obey not only the process of conquest, but of the Europeans migrations occurring in the last two centuries.

## SPECIAL FORENSIC CASES

### Identification of Airplane Crash Victims

With the availability of local databases and all forensic tests dully certified, our laboratory started to receive special forensic cases from the National Attorney Major Office, such as the identification of human body remains from a plane crash that occurred at the beginning of 2008. Santa Barbara Airlines Flight 518 ATR YV-1449 with 46 people aboard collided against a mountain in Venezuela's Andean region, with no survivors. The passengers' resulting remains were heavily fragmented and scattered in a wide zone of difficult access, therefore the collection of the evidence was done by well trained mountaineers, but with no experience in forensic evidence collection. An additional complication was that many Venezuelan air-carriers including the one in this investigation, failed to comply with seat assignment demanded by the National Aviation Regulatory Agency. Despite these limitations forensic anthropologists and dentists managed to establish the identity of 43 passengers, demanding DNA typing for just three victims.

From 13 non-matched body remains, identified as M1 to M13, bone samples were dissected and sent to our laboratory (Figure 3) together with two *pre-mortem* evidences and nine blood samples collected in FTA cards from the unidentified victims' relatives (FTA 14 to FTA 22). As a double check procedure, duplicated samples were sent to CeSAAN (Centro de Secuenciación y Análisis de Ácidos Nucleicos, Instituto Venezolano de Investigaciones Científicas). Isolation of DNA from the skeletal remains was carried out by crushing the bones in liquid nitrogen, followed by extraction by phenol-chloroform method, and purification by Microcon YM-100 (Millipore). Additionally, for three samples DNA was isolated from partially decomposed bone marrow swabs spread onto FTA cards (Figure 4) and processed with FTA Purification Reagent (Whatman). All remains samples and peripheral blood in FTA cards were tested for 15 autosomal STRs markers using AmpFlSTR® Identifiler™ kit (Applied Biosystems). Since there was a possibility that the *pre-morten* samples could be contaminated with DNA from other individuals, we opted to process the samples from living relatives first.

When the genetic profiles of the bone samples were compared with the relatives' samples (Figure 5), two out of the 13 had a match. Despite not having samples from one parent in the three victims, the high discrimination power achieved by using a 15 STR markers system, combined with the use of a Venezuelan database allowed us to obtain high likelihood ratio scores to confirm the matching profiles, so it was not necessary to use the *pre-mortem* samples. Moreover, the quality of the DNA profiles obtained from bone marrow swabs was identical to the corresponding bone samples, confirming the utility of this faster technique whenever medullar tissue is available. The independent results obtained for both participant laboratories had a perfect match, confirming the truthfulness of the study. This experience has been the first mass disaster investigation where DNA analysis has been entirely made by local experts.

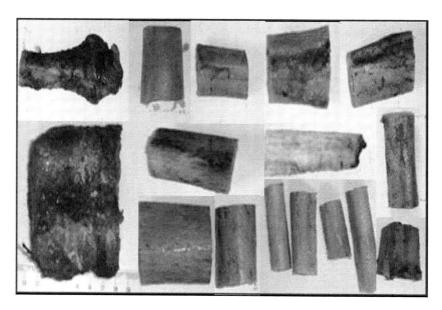

Figure 3. Skeletal remains samples from airplane crash sent to our laboratory.

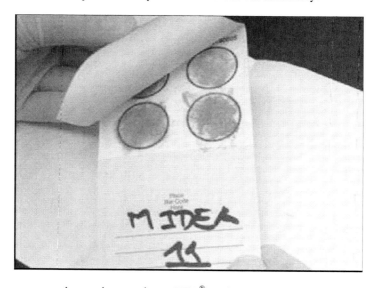

Figure 4. Bone marrow swab sample spread onto FTA® card used in the study of identification of human remains from a plane crash.

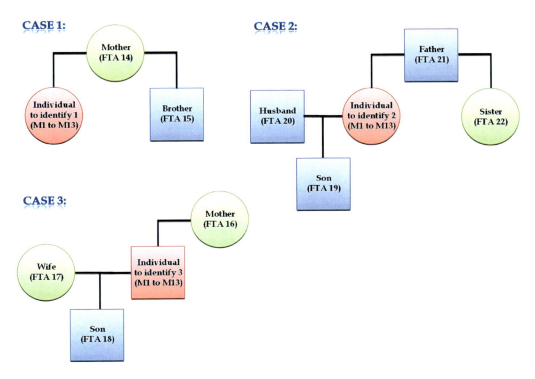

Figure 5. Family diagram of relatives and victims of the airplane crash.

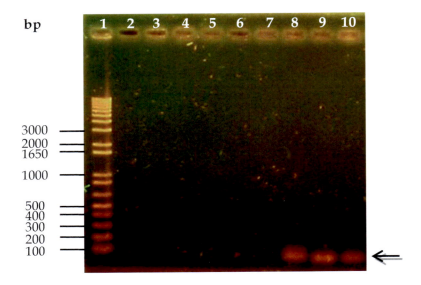

Figure 6. PCR products from HVR I, II and III of mtDNA from ancient hairs and blank controls. Lanes are: 1, Ladder 1 Kb Plus (Invitrogen); 2-4, HVRI-III from ancient hair shaft 1; 5-7, HVRI-III from ancient hair shaft 2; 8-10, HVRI-III blank controls. Arrow points out primer dimmers present in negative controls.

## DNA Analysis from Ancient Hair Samples

Mitochondrial DNA (mtDNA) has been widely used in phylogenetic and population-genetic studies of ancient samples [23, 24, 25]. These studies have been focused either on the control hipervariable regions (HVRI, HVRII), or whole-genome mtDNA. The term "ancient DNA" (aDNA) has been applied to DNA samples from evidences of 60 or more years, coming from different animal origins, including hominids [24, 26]. Hair shafts are an excellent source of aDNA because the low quantities of free water associated with the keratin-packaged hair cells reduce hydrolytic damage of DNA [26]. On the other hand, hair samples have been preserved for long periods in a variety of natural environments and many of them are available in taxonomic collections and museums [24, 26].

After finishing the mitochondrial database of the Caracas population, a challenging forensic case was presented to our laboratory. In this experience, we had the opportunity of analyzing the genetic material from a hair sample of approximately 140 years old. The sample consisted of three human hair shafts from the same origin, which had been conserved at a local museum and had reliable chain of custody. Despite the age of the three hair shafts (without roots) they looked like a modern hair, dark brown, straight, brilliant and flexible, between 4-6 cm long. The sample was handled under strict laboratory conditions, in an isolated environment, following recommendations of Cooper and Poinar (2000) [27] for ancient DNA samples manipulation. To this end, a brand new laboratory located at an isolated building was equipped for aDNA extraction. Macroscopic analysis and hair handling before proteolytic digestion was performed in a security DNA-free hood and operator staff wore security clothes (disposable coat, muffler and cap) during the complete aDNA isolation protocol.

Hairs were individually processed and washed in deionized sterile water to remove any kind of biological material that could be adhered to the sample. Proteolytic digestion was performed by incubating hair over night at 56°C in lysis buffer (10 mM Tris HCl, 10 mM EDTA, 50 Mm NaCl, 2 % SDS) containing Dithiothreitol (DTT) and Proteinase K. Thereafter, DNA extraction was performed by phenol/chloroform/isoamyl alcohol (25:24:1) protocol and a Microcon YM-100 (Millipore) unit was used for washing and concentrate DNA.

Amplification of the three hypervariable regions (HVRI, HVRII and HVRIII) from human mitochondrial DNA was performed as described before [4] using aDNA extracted from a single hair shaft. For PCR optimization, $MgCl_2$ concentration was adjusted to 3 mM. In a first attempt, it was not possible to amplify any hypervariable region of mtDNA. Interestingly, we noted here the absence of primer dimmers in the lanes corresponding to the PCR products from the ancient sample, despite that these dimmers were present in the negative controls (Figure 6). This fact suggested the presence of an inhibitory agent in the ancient hair sample. The inhibitory effect was confirmed by performing additional assays, where addition of control modern DNA to the PCR reaction mix containing the aDNA did not amplify either.

A second amplification attempt was performed by purifying aDNA present in the complete failed PCR reaction using ionic interchange columns from kit Concert™ Rapid PCR Purification System (GIBCO BRL). Purified DNA was used as template for PCR reamplification of HVR I, II and III, and the corresponding PCR product was obtained just for the shortest 401 bp region HVRII (Figure 7, lane 6). We also tested without success two additional purification protocols namely DNeasy® Blood & Tissue kit (Qiagen) and DNA IQ™ System (Promega).

The HVRII fragment was purified and sequenced by dye chemistry and capillary electrophoresis using an automatic genetic analyzer. Thereafter, *in silico* sequence edition and analysis was performed and mutations presented at the hypervariable region II of mtDNA from the ancient hair were successful established following guidelines of the ISFG [7, 8], as 73G 150T 152C 263G 295T 309.1C 315.1C. Then using program mtDNAmanager [15] we determined the haplotype affiliation corresponding to haplogroup J2, which is mainly found in Eurasian lineages localized around the Mediterranean, Greece, Italy/Sardinia and Spain [28, 29]. Despite that all individual mutations have been reported in the mtDNA database from Caracas population [4], this haplotype J2 was missing in this database

In view of the amplification failures for HVRI and HVRIII regions from aDNA and assuming that the sample was in good shape but in low concentration, we used the kit REPLI-g (QIAGEN), which works with the very processive enzyme phi29 DNA polymerase, for amplifying the complete mitochondrial genome. REPLI-g reaction product was then used as template for amplifying HVR I, II and III fragments, but again, it was not possible to amplify any of them (Figure 8). These result led us to conclude that the aDNA present in these hair shafts was degraded, and as recommended by manufacturers the phi29 DNA polymerase protocol is not useful in this type of material. In this sense, shotgun sequencing has been demonstrated to be a better strategy for obtaining the whole-mitochondrial genome sequence from ancient samples [24].

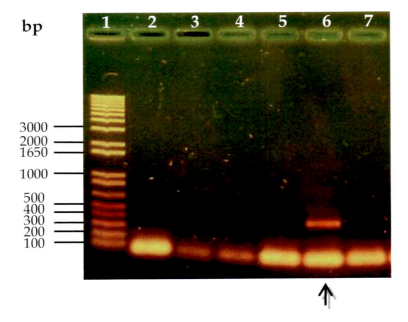

Figure 7. PCR products from HVR I, II and III of mtDNA from blank controls and ancient hairs. Lanes are: 1, Ladder 1 Kb Plus (Invitrogen); 2-4, HVRI-III blank controls; 5-7 HVRI-III from ancient hair shaft 1. Arrow points to the lane where HVRII amplified fragment from aDNA was observed.

Finally, we carried out a third attempt for amplifying mtDNA from the ancient hair sample. The last methodology we tested consisted in amplification of seven small DNA fragments (137 – 173 bp) overlapping to the hypervariable regions I and II of the human mitochondrial control region. Mini-primer set used for these PCR amplifications was reported by Lee et al. (2008) [30]. These primers were tested with DNA control samples and PCR resulted in amplification of expected bands for six out of the seven fragments (Figure 9). However, when PCRs were performed using aDNA from hair shafts we observed several diffuse bands instead of discrete expected PCR products (Figure 10). The electropherograms obtained for sequencing reactions of these amplicons were of a very low quality and it was not possible to type the mitochondrial DNA control region using mini-primer set methodology, thus supporting the idea that the DNA in this sample was damaged. The specific ancient hair sample used in this study could have received a *post-mortem* treatment to preserve the macroscopic appearance of the specimen, and this treatment may have caused the inhibitory effect on aDNA amplification. This inhibitory effect was only eliminated when interchange ionic columns from kit Concert™ Rapid PCR Purification System were used.

Finally, it is important to warn about the high level of mtDNA contamination generated by the use of phi29 DNA polymerase. The levels of contamination generated are so severe that its use in laboratories for routine forensic evidence processing should be avoided.

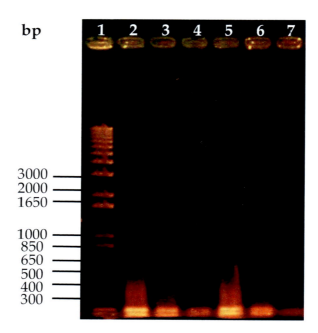

Figure 8. PCR products from HVR I, II and III of mtDNA using REPLI-g reaction products as template. Lanes: 1, Ladder 1 Kb Plus (Invitrogen); 2-4, HVRI-III from ancient hair shaft 1; 5-7 HVRI-III from ancient hair shaft 2.

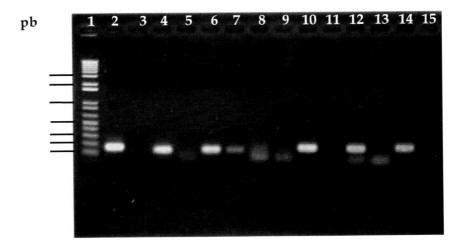

Figure 9. PCR products from seven small fragments of mtDNA amplified using mini-primers set in a sample of modern DNA used as positive control.
Each assay is shown with its negative on the right side. 1, Ladder 1 Kb Plus (Invitrogen); 2-3, M11; 4-5, M12; 6-7, M13; 8-9, M14 (no amplification); 10-11, M21; 12-13, M22; 14-15, M23. Characteristics of the fragments are described in Lee et al. (2008).

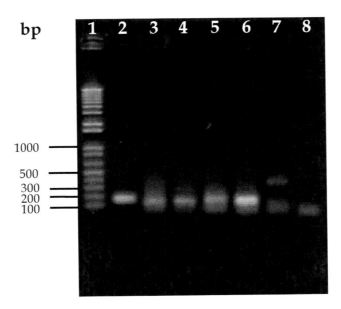

Figure 10. PCR products from seven small fragments of mtDNA amplified using mini-primer set and ancient DNA as template.
1. Ladder 1 Kb Plus (Invitrogen); 2-8, M11, M12, M13, M14, M21, M22 and M23. Except lane 8 (M23) were not PCR product was observed, diffused bands were obtained in all lanes. The characteristics of the fragments are described in Lee et al. (2008).

## DNA and the Venezuelan Legal System

In general Venezuelan public perception is very favorable to DNA tests, and we could even say that due in part to American TV series on crime labs, common people to wrongly believe that other forensic tests are not as reliable as DNA, thus causing potentially serious work loads on public and private laboratories. At the same time public interest has been ahead of the legal system demanding more and better forensic laboratories, and pressing legislators to incorporate modern forensic techniques into the new laws (*Código Civil de Protección a la Familia* http://biogafias.bcn.cl/alegislativo/pdf/cat/lext/5816-07/664.pdf.). However, the creation of a national criminal DNA database has been a contentious issue not yet resolved, and the appropriate legislation is still missing. Despite these restrictions, the construction of databases for personal in high risk jobs have been welcomed by the affected community, and we are currently working in the Caracas firefighters DNA database.

## COMPETING INTERESTS

The authors declare that they have no competing interests. The authors alone are responsible for the content and writing of the paper.

This work was sponsored by Grants FONACIT-Venezuela G-99000035 and IDEA-MPPCT Plan Operativo 0012.

## REFERENCES

[1] Chiurillo MA, Morales A, Mendes AM, Lander N, Tovar F, Fuentes A, Ramírez JL. Genetic profiling of a Central Venezuelan Population using 15 STR markers that may be of forensic importance. 2003. *Forensic Sci Int.* 136 (1-3): 99-101.

[2] Bernal LP, Borjas L, Zabala W, Portillo MG, Fernandez E, Delgado W, Tovar F, Lander N, Chiurillo MA, Ramirez JL, Garcia O. Genetic variation of 15 STR autosomal loci in the Maracaibo population from Venezuela. 2006. *Forensic Sci Int.* 161(1): 60-3.

[3] Tovar F, Chiurillo MA, Borjas L, Lander N, Ramírez JL. Chromosome Y haplotypes database in a Venezuelan population. 2005. International Congress Series. *Progress in Forensic Genetics* 11. 1288: 246-248.

[4] Lander N, Rojas MG, Chiurillo MA, Ramírez JL. Haplotype diversity in human mitochondrial DNA hypervariable regions I–III in the city of Caracas (Venezuela). *Forensic Sci Int Genet.* 2008. 2(4):61-64.

[5] Lander N, Tovar F, Chiurillo MA, Ramirez JL. A new allele of the short tandem repeat locus D21S11 in a Venezuelan population. 2006. *J Forensic Sci.* 51(3): 695.

[6] Borjas L, Bernal LP, Chiurillo MA, Tovar F, Zabala W, Lander N, Ramírez JL. Usefulness of 12 Y-STRs for forensic genetics evaluation in two populations from Venezuela. *Leg Med* (Tokyo). 2008; 10(2):107-12.

[7] Carracedo A, Bar W, Lincoln P, Mayr W, Morling N, Olaisen B, Schneider P, Budowle B, Brinkmann B, Gill P, Holland M, Tully G, Wilson M. DNA commission

of the international society for forensic genetics: guidelines for mitochondrial DNA typing. 2000. *Forens. Sci. Int.* 110 (2): 79–85.

[8] Parson W, Bandelt HJ. Extended guidelines for mtDNA typing of population data in forensic science. 2007. *Forensic Sci Int Genet.* 1(1): 13-9.

[9] Bandelt H-J, Parson W. Consistent treatment of length variants in the human mtDNA control region: a reappraisal. *Int. J. Legal Med.* 2008; 122: 11–21.

[10] Andrews RM, Kubacka I, Chinnery PF, Lightowlers RN, Turnbull DM, Howell N. Reanalysis and revision of the Cambridge reference sequence for human mitochondrial DNA, *Nat. Genet.* 1999; 23: 147.

[11] Behar DM, Garrigan D, Kaplan ME, Mobasher Z, Rosengarten D, Karafet TM, Quintana-Murci L, Ostrer H, Skorecki K, Hammer MF. Contrasting patterns of Y chromosome variation in Ashkenazi Jewish and host non-Jewish European populations. *Hum Genet.* 2004; 114(4):354-65.

[12] Pakendorf B and Stoneking M. Mitochondrial DNA and human evolution. *Annu Rev Genomics Hum Genet.* 2005; 6:165–183.

[13] Walsh B. Estimating the time to the most recent common ancestor for the Y chromosome or mitochondrial DNA for a pair of individuals. *Genetics.* 2001; 158:897–912.

[14] Berniell-Lee G, Plaza S, Bosch E, Calafell F, Jourdan E, Cesari M, Lefranc G, Comas D: Admixture and sexual bias in the population settlement of La Reunion Island (Indian Ocean). *Am J Phys Anthropol.* 2008; 136(1):100-107.

[15] Lee HY, Song I, Ha E, Cho SB, Yang WI, Shin KJ. mtDNAmanager: a Web-based tool for the management and quality analysis of mitochondrial DNA control-region sequences. 2008. *BMC Bioinformatics.* 9:483.

[16] Martínez-Marignac VL, Bertoni B, Parra EJ, Bianchi NO. Characterization of admixture in an urban sample from Buenos Aires, Argentina, using uniparentally and biparentally inherited genetic markers. *Hum Biol.* 2004;76(4):543-57

[17] Alves-Silva J, da Silva Santos M, Guimarães PE, Ferreira AC, Bandelt HJ, Pena SD, Prado VF. The ancestry of Brazilian mtDNA lineages. *Am J Hum Genet.* 2000; 67(2):444-61.

[18] Mendizabal I, Sandoval K, Berniell-Lee G, Calafell F, Salas A, Martínez-Fuentes A, Comas D. Genetic origin, admixture, and asymmetry in maternal and paternal human lineages in Cuba. *BMC Evol Biol.* 2008 ;8:213.

[19] Luna-Vázquez A, Vilchis-Dorantes G, Aguilar-Ruiz MO, Bautista-Rivas A, Pérez-García A, Orea-Ochoa R, Villanueva-Hernández D, Muñoz-Valle JF, Rangel-Villalobos H. Haplotype frequencies of the PowerPlex Y system in a Mexican-Mestizo population sample from Mexico City. *Forensic Sci Int Genet.* 2008, 2(1):e11-3.

[20] Brión M, Sanchez JJ, Balogh K, Thacker C, Blanco-Verea A, Børsting C, Stradmann-Bellinghausen B, Bogus M, Syndercombe-Court D, Schneider PM, Carracedo A, Morling N. Introduction of an single nucleodite polymorphism-based "Major Y-chromosome haplogroup typing kit" suitable for predicting the geographical origin of male lineages. *Electrophoresis.* 2005; 26(23):4411-20.

[21] Pereira RW, Monteiro EH, Hirschfeld GC, Wang AY, Grattapaglia D. Haplotype diversity of 17 Y-chromosome STRs in Brazilians. *Forensic Sci Int.* 2007;171(2-3):226-36.

[22] Baeza C, Guzmán R, Tirado M, López-Parra AM, Rodríguez T, Mesa MS, Fernández E, Arroyo-Pardo E. Population data for 15 Y-chromosome STRs in a population sample from Quito (Ecuador). *Forensic Sci Int.* 2007; 173(2-3):214-9.

[23] Ricaut FX, Bellatti M, Lahr MM. Ancient mitochondrial DNA from Malaysian hair samples: some indications of Southeast Asian population movements. 2006. *Am J Hum Biol.* 18(5):654-67.

[24] Gilbert MT, Tomsho LP, Rendulic S, Packard M, Drautz DI, Sher A, Tikhonov A, Dalén L, Kuznetsova T, Kosintsev P, Campos PF, Higham T, Collins MJ, Wilson AS, Shidlovskiy F, Buigues B, Ericson PG, Germonpré M, Götherström A, Iacumin P, Nikolaev V, Nowak-Kemp M, Willerslev E, Knight JR, Irzyk GP, Perbost CS, Fredrikson KM, Harkins TT, Sheridan S, Miller W, Schuster SC. Whole-genome shotgun sequencing of mitochondria from ancient hair shafts. 2007. *Science.* 317(5846):1927-30.

[25] Gilbert MT, Kivisild T, Grønnow B, Andersen PK, Metspalu E, Reidla M, Tamm E, Axelsson E, Götherström A, Campos PF, Rasmussen M, Metspalu M, Higham TF, Schwenninger JL, Nathan R, De Hoog CJ, Koch A, Møller LN, Andreasen C, Meldgaard M, Villems R, Bendixen C, Willerslev E. Paleo-Eskimo mtDNA genome reveals matrilineal discontinuity in Greenland. 2008. *Science.* 320(5884):1787-9.

[26] Gilbert MT, Wilson AS, Bunce M, Hansen AJ, Willerslev E, Shapiro B, Higham TF, Richards MP, O'Connell TC, Tobin DJ, Janaway RC, Cooper A. Ancient mitochondrial DNA from hair. 2004. *Curr Biol.* 14(12):R463-4.

[27] Cooper A, Poinar HN. Ancient DNA: do it right or not at all. 2000. *Science.* 289(5482):1139.

[28] Logan I. Mitochondrial DNA (mtDNA). 2007. website at http://www.ianlogan.co.uk/mtDNA.htm.

[29] Logan J. The subclades of mtDNA Haplogroup J and proposed motifs for assigning control-region sequences into these clades. 2008. *J Genet Geneol.* 4:12-26.

[30] Lee HY, Kim NY, Park MJ, Yang WI, Shin KJ. A modified mini-primer set for analyzing mitochondrial DNA control region sequences from highly degraded forensic samples. 2008. *Biotechniques.* 44(4): 555-6, 558.

In: Forensic Genetics Research Progress
Editor: F. Gonzalez-Andrade

ISBN: 978-1-60876-198-2
© 2010 Nova Science Publishers, Inc.

Chapter 15

# *IN VITRO* STUDIES OF DNA RECOVERED FROM INCINERATED TEETH

*Paola León-Sanz[1,*], Carolina Bonett[2], Raúl Suárez[3], Yolanda González[3], James Valencia[3], Ignacio Zarante[4]*

[1] Dentistry Faculty, Pontificia Universidad Javeriana, Bogotá Colombia
2. Forensic Medicine Department, Administrative Department of Security (DAS), Bogotá, Colombia
3. Fiscalía General de La Nación, Bogotá, Colombia
4. Institute of Genetics, Hospital San Ignacio, Bogotá, Colombia

## ABSTRACT

### Aim

To compare the quality of DNA extracted of molars and premolars teeth burned to temperatures between 300°C to 700°C, and provide the initial and detailed knowledge to handle the identification of incinerated bodies by dental DNA. This knowledge is advantageous to avoid delays in the scientific investigation of criminal caseworks.

### Material and Methods

It included sixty-six teeth, upper and lower premolars and molars, of patients under extraction therapeutic, orthodontic treatment or periodontal disease. The samples were divided into six groups randomly, as follows: no burn teeth (control group); teeth incinerated at 300° C, at 400° C, at 500° C, at 600° C and at 700° C. The first group, control, was washed according the described protocol and using Alconox[©] at 1%. Samples were pulverized individually into a cryogenic impact grinder with self-contained liquid nitrogen. DNA was extracted by the organic of method phenol-chloroform-

---
[*] E-mail: paolaleon3@hotmail.com

isoamilic alcohol. PCR was carried out using Amelogenin 10X first pair (2µM) fluorescein. Statistical analysis was tested three different models of logistic regression, which allow us predict about the appearance or absence of DNA on the variables sex, temperature, washing and tooth type.

## Conclusion

It can isolate DNA of good quality in burned teeth, only when the heat reached 300° C or below, if the sample has not been handled or washed beforehand. The quality of the DNA will not vary with the gender, type of tooth or previous washes in the extraction process. It would recommend: do not wash to the teeth that have a high degree of destruction or where it suspects by their morphological features they have been exposed to heat above 300° C.

**Keywords:** DNA, burned teeth, PCR, temperature, human identification, forensic genetics, human remains, DNA extraction

## INTRODUCTION

For numerous decades, the investigators used the teeth for the identification of corpses. Postmortem teeth are the most solid structures, and can be used to achieve different information like age, identity, sex and genetic data [1]. DNA testing is essential to link the ante-mortem records, dental charts, radiographs, study models and the evolution of dental treatment to burned bodies [2]. Victims of incineration challenge forensic scientists when coronal restorations are no longer seem to compile postmortem data. At this point, the standard method of identification such as fingerprinting is not convenient and it is necessary to rely on forensic science specialist [3]. The meaning of DNA testing increased with the time, and currently is the basis for the identification of bodies incinerated [4]. Several reasons exist for identify human remains and have been described widely [5].

Mineralized tooth structures resist degradation postmortem as incineration [6], deterioration, decay [7], disfigurement or the intentional maiming [8]. This ability to survive these changes deliberate, accidental or naturally led to forensic scientists to concentrate on the teeth as a leading source of DNA [9]. The burned DNA can be extracted from different sources, including soft tissues [10], stains, bones [11] and tooth structure [12]. The stability of the purified DNA is very reliable but environmental and biological factors that occur after death can be degraded [13] and fragmented [14]. DNA can persist for prolonged periods of time if it is not damaged [15]. The teeth meet the burden of encapsulating the DNA in it and isolate it from the environment. Therefore, they are the most valuable source of DNA postmortem and in particular cases, the single available for analysis. The boundaries of the preservation and retrieval of DNA from degraded samples have not already been completely determined.

The fire is one of the most devastating forces, but we do not understand much about nature and its effects on DNA extracted from dental structures [16]. Researchers have greatly augmented knowledge regarding the effects of extreme heat on skeletal remains and teeth. As a result, of this effort, enhanced interpretation on such issues as the degree of recovery, reconstruction, trauma, individual identification, size reduction, thermal effect on histological structures, color variation, the determination if remains were burned with or without soft tissue, DNA recovery and remaining weight is now possible [17]. Cremated teeth exhibit a range of colors ranging from white through gray to reach the black target [18]. This coloration can be definitively attributed to the temperatures at which each set of teeth was exposed, since they were not surrounded by any fabric protector, which would isolate them from the heat [19]. The same can be said about the patterns of fracture-induced warming, ranging from the integrity of fracture lines through the enamel, loosening of the coronal segment of the enamel or of the entire crown to the explosion and the wreckage they leave dental DNA exposed at the surface so that it will degrade by the influence of heat [20].

Determining the gender of the source of forensic DNA evidence is based on the Amelogenin test [21]. It is a STR marker commonly used with forensic purposes and is a protein produced by ameloblast, which are founded in tooth enamel. It is the most plentiful protein of enamel matrix [22]. It is relatively modest size marker that can be amplified by PCR techniques, even in highly degraded material [23]. For this reason, is used to explore alternative methods and techniques, in DNA of a satisfactory quality.

The aim of this paper is to compare the quality of DNA extracted of molar and premolar teeth burned to temperatures between 300°C to 700°C, and provide the starting and detailed knowledge to handle the identification of incinerated bodies by dental DNA. This knowledge is advantageous to avoid delays in the scientific investigation of criminal caseworks. .

## MATERIAL AND METHODS

*Sample size:* It included sixty-six teeth, upper and lower premolars and molars, of patients under extraction therapeutic, orthodontic treatment or periodontal disease. All patients signed the Informed Consent. The samples were divided into six groups randomly, as follows: no burn teeth (control group); teeth incinerated at 300° C, at 400° C, at 500° C, at 600° C and at 700° C.

*Incineration:* the teeth were subjected to incineration in a preheated programmable oven (model 120-096, Dentaurum™, Ispringen, Germany).

*Washes:* The first group, control, was washed according the next protocol: a) Each sample was submerged in a 15 ml Falcon™ tube, with 3 ml of Alconox© at 1% (Alconox, Inc., White Plains, NY. Alconox© is a biodegradable detergent powder used like a precision cleaner). b) It was brushed to remove remain impurities and washed with distilled water for one minute, by three times to remove the remaining residues. c) It submerges in Sodium Hypochlorite at 5% for 30 seconds and it washes again in distilled water by three times for one minute. d) It was submerged in 80% ethanol (fixative) by two times. e) It was left to dry in the cabin of extraction for four hours. The remains burned teeth were distributed into two new groups: A, washed and B, without wash [11].

*Spraying*: samples were pulverized individually into a cryogenic impact grinder with self-contained liquid nitrogen (SPEX SamplePrep Freezer/Mill 6750) with a pre-cool cycle of 15 minutes until to reach the temperature of liquid nitrogen, in which they were embedded raise -170° C. Then samples were crushed every three cycles of two minutes, with an interval of two minutes of pause [24].

*DNA Extraction:* the DNA was extracted by the organic of method phenol-chloroform-isoamilic alcohol, followed by filtration in Microcon® centrifugal filtration devices of 100 kDa NMWL, (Millipore Inc., Beverly, MA, USA), after this DNA were re-suspended in a final volume of 60 µL [25].

*PCR:* It was carried out using Amelogenin 10X first pair (2µM) fluorescein (Promega, Wisconisn USA) according to manufacturer's instructions. The amplification conditions were: 96° C for 1 minute, 94° C for 30 seconds; 68 seconds to raise 60° C maintained for 30 seconds, 50 seconds to climb to 70° C maintained for 45 seconds for 10 cycles. Then at 90° C for 30 seconds, 60 seconds to climb 60° C maintained for 30 seconds, 50 seconds to climb 70° C maintained for 45 seconds for 20 cycles. Then at 4° C rinse [26].

*Electrophoresis:* It was carried in a polyacrylamide gel at 6%, for one hour to 50° C, to 2000 volt, 40 amp and 80 watts for 50 min. After the electrophoresis, the gels were scanned on a **FMBIO II Multi-View** fluorescent image analyzer **(Hitachi** Software Engineering) to visualize the PCR products, at 505 nm of fluorescence.

*Statistical analysis*: It was tested three different models of logistic regression, which allow us predict about the appearance or absence of DNA on the variables sex, temperature, washing and tooth type. The first one is a model with all the variables, it has an effectiveness of 81.8%; the second model handles varying temperature, washing and tooth type, which also has an effectiveness of 81.8%; and finally a third model manages the temperature and wash the tooth as independent variables able to predict the presence of DNA or not, with a 86.4% effectiveness. Finally, the used model was as follow:

$D = 0.909 + 2.41L - 0013T$

Where if D is greater than 1 is expected the presence of DNA; where L is a dichotomous variable that takes values of 0 when the tooth is not washed and 1 when it is washed; and T a variable that measures the temperature in degrees Celsius. For any combination of these two will result in a forecast 86.4% of the actual presence of DNA in the tooth. The most important level of significance is given to 8% for the variables temperature and washing, which are the variables that were finally left for the model.

*Test of Hypothesis:* 1) Null hypothesis, the percentage of DNA obtained of the teeth from the control group is the same that the DNA obtained from the other groups, at different temperatures. H1: The percentages differ significantly, $z = 4.57825726$. As z is greater than 1.96, the null hypothesis is rejected. This means that there are significant differences in the percentage of teeth which DNA is obtained from the control group and the studied groups at different temperatures. 2) Null hypothesis, the percentage of DNA derived from teeth of men is the same as that obtained in women. H1: The percentages differ significantly, $z = -0.07659459$. As z is less de1.96, not reject the null hypothesis. There is no significant difference in the percentage of DNA obtained from the teeth in men and women. 3) Null hypothesis, the percentage of DNA obtained in the teeth cleaned by washes (group control) is the same as that obtained with no washing. H1: The percentages differ significantly, $z = -0.82458781$. As z is less de1.96, not reject the null hypothesis. Therefore there is no significant difference in the percentage of DNA obtained of the teeth cleaned by washes with respect to that obtained with no washing. 4) Null hypothesis, the percentage of DNA obtained of premolar teeth is the same as that obtained from molar teeth. H1: The percentages differ significantly, $z = 1.93520818$. As z is less de1.96, not reject the null hypothesis. Therefore there is no significant difference in the percentage of DNA obtained of premolar teeth with respect to that obtained for molar teeth. z is obtained from the following formula: P1 - P2. Total P x Q x total (1/n1 + 1/n2). [P1 = percentage of temperature control, P2 = percentage of the groups temperature of 300 ° to 700 °, P = percentage of total teeth where DNA was obtained, Q total = 1-P total, n1 = sample size in the control group, n2 = sample size of other groups].The confidence level for all tests is 95%.

## RESULTS AND DISCUSSION

### Morphological Changes

About the color it can remark that cremated teeth exhibit a range of colors ranging from white through gray to reach the black. This tooth coloration can be definitively attributed to the temperatures at which each group was exposed, since they were not surrounded by any fabric protector, which would isolate them from the heat. In this vein, describing the scope of colors is an acceptable predictor for estimating the temperature at which the teeth were exposed (See figure 1). Teeth subjected to direct effect of heat at temperatures above 500° C suffer disturbances in the crown-root integrity, ranging from the release until the explosion of the whole structure. There were significant differences ($p < 0.05$) with temperatures above 300° C; the samples amplified for amelogenin marker until 300°C. Table 1 shows the macroscopic changes of the teeth observed at the set temperatures. It shows the variations in the crown, root and integrity.

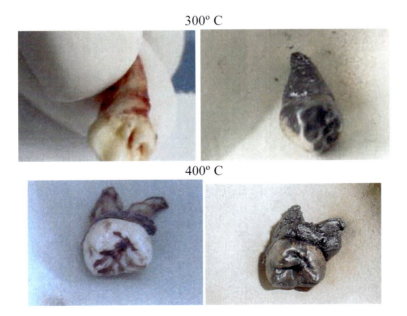

Figure 1. (Continued)

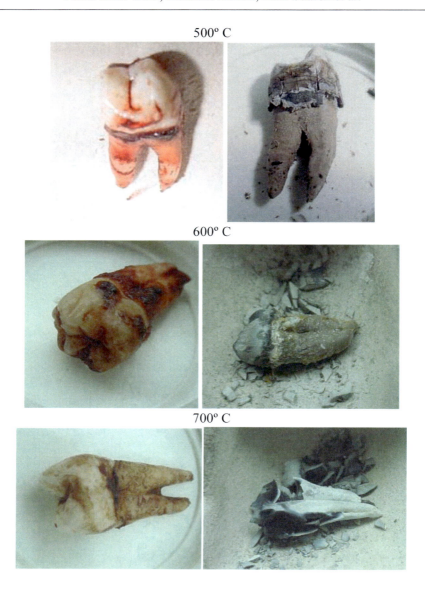

Figure 1. Pictures before and after of the incineration at different temperatures.

Figure 2 shows the assessment of Amelogenin marker. Control group displays the positive control, the allelic ladder, the samples 1-1 to 1-6 bands (XY) males, samples 1-7, 1-8 and 1-10 not amplified, samples 1 -9 to 1-11 show only 1 band (XX) females, the control of isolation and the negative control are appropriate. The 300° C group displays the positive control, the allelic ladder, the samples 2-1, 2-2, 2-4, 2-5, 2-7, 2-8 and 2-10 not amplified, the samples 2-3 2-6 and two bands (XY) males, and 2-9 and 2-11 show only 1 band (XX) female. The negative control is adequate. The 400° C group displays the allelic ladder, the samples 3-2 and 3-11 show two bands (XY) males. The remains do not amplified them.

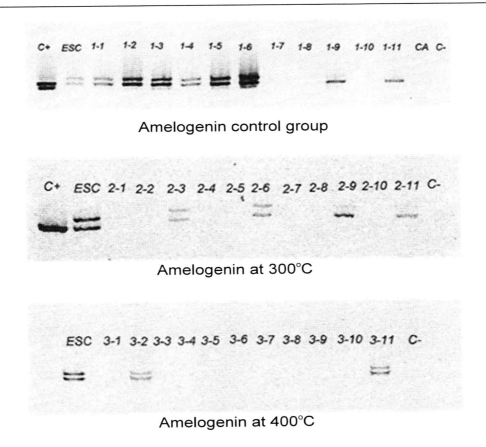

Figure 2. Amelogenin marker amplification by temperature.

## Patterns of Fracture

They are warm-induced, range from the integrity through to destruction. They went by different stages: a) integrity, b) enamel fractures, c) loosen of the coronal segment of the enamel, d) loosen of the crown, e) fragmentary explosion, and f) destruction. They leave dental DNA exposed at the surface so that it will degrade by the influence of heat. Table 3 explains the variables analyzed in each tooth incinerated.

## Quality of DNA

Table 2 shows the quality in the percentage of the DNA purified from incinerated teeth. It obtained DNA of suitable quality for the group was not subjected to incineration. It obtained DNA in 72.7% of the samples. In 36.4% of the samples at 300°C DNA as available, 18.2% of the group of 400°C and 0% for groups of 500, 600 and 700°C.

## Table 1. Morphological changes observed by group and temperature

| Variable | Control | 300° C | 400° C | 500° C | 600° C | 700° C |
|---|---|---|---|---|---|---|
| Crown | Without burning | turning brown in the vestibular area and black in the occlusal pits and grooves rather than on the slopes | Brownish pigmentation | Grey and brown pigmentation, multiple longitudinal fracture lines extended to the cement | Crown explosion of the enamel with the remaining dentinal gray ash | Crown explosion, gray-white pigmentation |
| Root | | Generalized black pigmentation | Generalized black pigmentation, bubblish shape | Grey pigmentation, with homogeneous surface (lack of emanel) | Brown pigmentation, surface with lumps and cracks | Root explosion, grey-white pigmentation on surface and deeper black color with root fragments |
| Integrity | | Preserved | Preserved | Rupture of the enamel from the corona | Is denoted by the line amelo - cementaria the difference in color with respect to dentinal cementum | Tooth explosion |

## Table 2. Quality of the DNA obtained

| Temperature | Positive | Negative | % DNA purified |
|---|---|---|---|
| Control | 8 | 3 | 72.7 |
| 300°C | 4 | 7 | 36.4 |
| 400°C | 2 | 9 | 18.2 |
| 500°C | 0 | 11 | 0 |
| 600°C | 0 | 11 | 0 |
| 700°C | 0 | 11 | 0 |
| Total | 14 | 52 | |

## Gender, Washes and Type of Tooth

There was no significant difference in gender variable ($p > 0.05$) as it was not a relevant factor to adjust the amplification of DNA in either group. There was no statistical difference in tooth type of the variable ($p > 0.05$) as it was not a relevant factor to convert the amplification of DNA in either group. There was no statistical difference in the variable washing ($p > 0.05$), although it was noted that the samples in which DNA was obtained after

300° C had not been subjected to the task of washing, where it can be concluded that washing influences negatively.

### Table 3. Samples by variables analyzed

| No. | °C | Sex | Washes | Type | DNA |
|---|---|---|---|---|---|
| 1-1 | 37 | M | 1 | 1 | 1 |
| 1-2 | 37 | M | 1 | 1 | 1 |
| 1-3 | 37 | M | 1 | 1 | 1 |
| 1-4 | 37 | M | 1 | 2 | 1 |
| 1-5 | 37 | M | 1 | 1 | 1 |
| 1-6 | 37 | M | 1 | 1 | 1 |
| 1-7 | 37 | M | 1 | 2 | 0 |
| 1-8 | 37 | M | 1 | 2 | 0 |
| 1-9 | 37 | F | 1 | 1 | 0 |
| 1-10 | 37 | F | 1 | 2 | 1 |
| 1-11 | 37 | F | 1 | 1 | 1 |
| 2-1 | 300 | F | 0 | 1 | 0 |
| 2-2 | 300 | F | 1 | 1 | 0 |
| 2-3 | 300 | M | 0 | 2 | 1 |
| 2-4 | 300 | M | 1 | 2 | 0 |
| 2-5 | 300 | M | 0 | 2 | 0 |
| 2-6 | 300 | M | 1 | 1 | 1 |
| 2-7 | 300 | M | 0 | 1 | 0 |
| 2-8 | 300 | F | 1 | 2 | 0 |
| 2-9 | 300 | F | 0 | 2 | 1 |
| 2-10 | 300 | F | 1 | 2 | 0 |
| 2-11 | 300 | F | 0 | 1 | 1 |
| 3-1 | 400 | F | 1 | 2 | 0 |
| 3-2 | 400 | M | 0 | 1 | 1 |
| 3-3 | 400 | F | 0 | 2 | 0 |
| 3-4 | 400 | F | 1 | 2 | 0 |
| 3-5 | 400 | M | 0 | 1 | 0 |
| 3-6 | 400 | M | 1 | 1 | 0 |
| 3-7 | 400 | M | 0 | 2 | 0 |
| 3-8 | 400 | M | 1 | 2 | 0 |
| 3-9 | 400 | M | 0 | 2 | 0 |
| 3-10 | 400 | M | 1 | 1 | 0 |
| 3-11 | 400 | F | 0 | 1 | 1 |
| 4-1 | 500 | M | 0 | 1 | 0 |
| 4-2 | 500 | M | 0 | 1 | 0 |
| 4-3 | 500 | M | 1 | 2 | 0 |
| 4-4 | 500 | M | 1 | 2 | 0 |
| 4-5 | 500 | F | 0 | 2 | 0 |

**Table 3. Continued**

| No. | °C | Sex | Washes | Type | DNA |
|---|---|---|---|---|---|
| 4-6 | 500 | F | 1 | 1 | 0 |
| 4-7 | 500 | F | 1 | 1 | 0 |
| 4-8 | 500 | M | 0 | 2 | 0 |
| 4-9 | 500 | M | 0 | 2 | 0 |
| 4-10 | 500 | F | 0 | 2 | 0 |
| 4-11 | 500 | F | 1 | 1 | 0 |
| 5-1 | 600 | M | 1 | 1 | 0 |
| 5-2 | 600 | M | 1 | 1 | 0 |
| 5-3 | 600 | M | 1 | 1 | 0 |
| 5-4 | 600 | M | 0 | 2 | 0 |
| 5-5 | 600 | M | 0 | 2 | 0 |
| 5-6 | 600 | M | 1 | 2 | 0 |
| 5-7 | 600 | F | 1 | 2 | 0 |
| 5-8 | 600 | M | 0 | 1 | 0 |
| 5-9 | 600 | M | 0 | 1 | 0 |
| 5-10 | 600 | M | 0 | 2 | 0 |
| 5-11 | 600 | M | 0 | 2 | 0 |
| 6-1 | 700 | M | 1 | 1 | 0 |
| 6-2 | 700 | M | 0 | 2 | 0 |
| 6-3 | 700 | M | 0 | 2 | 0 |
| 6-4 | 700 | M | 0 | 2 | 0 |
| 6-5 | 700 | F | 1 | 1 | 0 |
| 6-6 | 700 | F | 1 | 1 | 0 |
| 6-7 | 700 | F | 0 | 2 | 0 |
| 6-8 | 700 | F | 0 | 2 | 0 |
| 6-9 | 700 | F | 1 | 2 | 0 |
| 6-10 | 700 | M | 0 | 1 | 0 |
| 6-11 | 700 | M | 1 | 1 | 0 |

M= male, F= female;
Washed: 0= no-wash, 1= with wash;
DNA: 0 =absent; 1= present;
Type of tooth: 1= premolar, 2= molar.

It would recommend, when it try to retrieve DNA from burning teeth, the following:

a) Do not wash to the teeth that have a high level of impairment or where it suspects by their morphological features they have been exposed to heat above 300° C.
b) The logistic regression have to stay used to handling the temperature and washes as independent variables, capable of predicting the appearance of nuclear DNA or not, with a 86.4% effectiveness.
c) Soft tissues protect the teeth in the vocal cavity; in order to implement these results in the future, it will be necessary advanced studies with teeth covered by soft tissues, in a kind of preliminary taphonomic analysis.

d) Mitochondrial DNA can be extracted in greater quantity in the teeth that in cells, for that, it will be necessary extend this analysis to mitochondrial DNA.

## CONCLUSION

It can isolate DNA of good quality in burned teeth, only when the heat reached 300° C or below, if the sample has not been handled or washed beforehand. The quality of the DNA will not differ with the gender, type of tooth or previous washes in the extraction process.

## AKNOWLEDGMENTS

The authors would like to thank technical and scientific staff of the Forensic Genetics Laboratory of the *Fiscalia General de la Nación* and Human Genetics Institute from the *Pontificia Universidad Javeriana de Colombia*, for his continuous and committed support of research and progress in molecular forensic science.

## COMPETING INTERESTS

This research was funding and supported by the Forensic Genetics Laboratory of the *Fiscalía General de la Nación,* Bogotá, Colombia.

## REFERENCES

[1] Dobberstein RC, Huppertz J, von Wurmb-Schwark N, Ritz-Timme S. Degradation of biomolecules in artificially and naturally aged teeth: implications for age estimation based on aspartic acid racemization and DNA analysis. *Forensic Sci Int.* 2008 Aug 6;179(2-3):181-91.

[2] Sweet D, Sweet C: DNA analysis of dental pulp to link incinerated remains of homicide victim to crime scene. *J Forensic Sci.* 1995; 40(2): 310-14.

[3] Pretty IA, Sweet D: The role of teeth in the determination of human identity. *Brit Dent J* 2001; 190(7):359-66.

[4] González-Andrade F, Sánchez D. DNA typing from skeletal remains following an explosion in a military fort – first experience in Ecuador (South- America), *Legal Med* (Tokyo) Oct 2005; 7 (5): 314-318.

[5] Pavel I, Maya I: *Identification of human decomposed remains using the STR systems: effect of typing results.* Institute of molecular biology, Russian Academy of sciences, Mooscow, Russia. P: 18-21.

[6] Mayers Sl, Williams Jm And Jodgers JS: Effects of extreme heat on teeth with implications for histologic processing. *J Forensic SCI* 1999, 44(4): 805-809.

[7] Graham EA, Turk EE, Rutty GN.Room temperature DNA preservation of soft tissue for rapid DNA extraction: an addition to the disaster victim identification investigators toolkit? *Forensic Sci Int Genet.* 2008 Jan;2(1):29-34.

[8] Loreille OM, Diegoli TM, Irwin JA, Coble MD, Parsons TJ. High efficiency DNA extraction from bone by total demineralization. *Forensic Sci Int Genet.* 2007 Jun;1(2):191-5.

[9] Sweet D, Hildebrand D, Phillips D. Identification of skeleton using DNA from teeth and a PAP smear. *J Forensic Sci* 1999; 44(3):630-633.

[10] Tsuchimochi T, Iwasa M, Maeno Y, Koyama H, Inoue H, Isobe I, Matoba R, Yokoi M, Nagao M. Chelating resin-based extraction of DNA from dental pulp and sex determination from incinerated teeth with Y-chromosomal alphoid repeat and short tandem repeats. *Am J Forensic Med Pathol.* 2002 Sep;23(3):268-71.

[11] Dragan P, Simun A, Marija D.G. Identification of War victims from mass graves in Croatia, Bosnia and Herzegovina by the use of standard forensic methods and DNA typing. *J Forensic Sci.* 1996:41 (5): 891-4.

[12] Schwartz Tr, Schwartz E, Mieszerski L: Characterization of Deoxyribonucleic Acid (DNA) obtained from teeth subjected to various environmental conditions. *J Forensic Sci* 1991, 36(4): 979-990.

[13] Westen AA, Gerretsen RR, Maat GJ. Femur, rib, and tooth sample collection for DNA analysis in disaster victim identification (DVI): a method to minimize contamination risk. *Forensic Sci Med Pathol.* 2008; 4(1):15-21.

[14] Delattre V. Burned beyond recognition: systematic approach to the dental identification of charred human remains. *J Forensic Sc.* 2000; 45 (3): 589-596.

[15] Colotte M, Couallier V, Tuffet S, Bonnet J. Simultaneous assessment of average fragment size and amount in minute samples of degraded DNA. *Anal Biochem.* May 2009. 388 (2): 345-7.

[16] Pretty IA. Forensic dentistry: 1. Identification of human remains.*Dent Update.* 2007 Dec; 34(10):621-2, 624-6, 629-30 passim. Review.

[17] Ubelaker DH. The forensic evaluation of burned skeletal remains: a synthesis. *Forensic Sci Int.* 2009 Jan 10; 183(1-3):1-5.

[18] Gaytmenn R, Sweet D. Quantification of forensic DNA from various regions of human teeth. *J Forensic Sc.* 2003; 48 (3): 1-4.

[19] Butler JM, Shen Y, McCord B. The development of reduced size STR amplicons as tools for analysis of degraded DNA. *J Forensic Sc.* 2003, 48(5): 1-11.

[20] Roffey P, Eckhoff C, Kuhl J. A rare mutation in the amelogenin gene and its potential investigative ramification. *J Forensic Sc.* 2000; 45 (5): 1016-9.

[21] Young D, Tun Z, Honda K. Identifying Sex chromosome abnormalities in forensic DNA testing using amelogenin and sex chromosome short tandem repeats. *J Forensic Sc.* 2001; 46(2): 346-8.

[22] La Fountain M, Schwartz M, Cornier J, Buel E. Validation of capillary electrophoresis for analysis of the X-Y homologous amelogenin gene. *J Forensic Sc.* 1998; 43(6): 1188-1194.

[23] Hanaoka Y, Minagushi K. Sex determination from blood and teeth by PCR amplification of the aplhoid satellite family. *J Forensic Sc.* 1996; 41(5): 855-858.

[24] Sweet D, Hildebrand D: Recovery of DNA from Human teeth by criogenic grinding. *J Forensic Sci* 1998;43(6): 1199-1202.

[25] Hochmeister M, Budowle B, Borrer U, Rudin O, Bohnert M, Dirnhofer R. Confirmation of the identity of human skeleton remains using multiplex PCR amplification and typing kits. *J Forensic Sci* 1995;40(4): 701-705.

[26] Soares J, Correia A, Miazato E. Postmortem Forensic identity testing: application of PCR to the identification of FIRE victim. *Sao Paulo Med J/Rev Paul Med* 2000; 118 (3):75-7.

In: Forensic Genetics Research Progress
Editor: F. Gonzalez-Andrade

ISBN: 978-1-60876-198-2
© 2010 Nova Science Publishers, Inc.

*Chapter 16*

# PROMISING PROSPECTS OF CHINESE MEDICAL SEMIOLOGY ON FORENSIC GENETICS

## *Ahmed Youssif El Tassa*[*]

The Chinese Academy of Social Sciences (CASS), 5, Jianguomennei Dajie, Beijing, 100732, China

## ABSTRACT

The present chapter starts by citing ancient semiologies, particularly by providing background knowledge on Chinese medical semiology. The intention is to stress their importance and value as assets to any Forensic Genetics researches performed today around the world. As an outcome, this chapter draws attention to the practical usefulness of Chinese Medical Semiology on Forensics and on Forensic Genetics.

It begins by presenting a discussion about the philosophical principles of typology in general and human typology in particular, and by portraying some analogies between nature and the human being. After a short introduction on the basic logics behind those universal principles, called *yin* and *yang*, literally *shadow* and *light*, which also could be resembled to *time* and *space*, each principle is compared to elements or phenomena from nature and human being, stressing the importance of this background towards Genetics and Forensic Genetics.

Inferred from the two fundamental principles (*yin/yang*) a categorization system is dialectically developed, transforming those two into five archetypes. Next, a peculiar typological system based on these five archetypes is then proposed to classify the five basic human races, classifying them according to the relative quantities of *yin* and *yang* they impart and to which they are connatural.

It is remembered that this approach of depicting nature is not exclusive to the East, given that in ancient Greece, a similar categorization method based in five elements was also traditionally used. The East called the five archetypes being: wood, fire, earth, metal and water, and the West labeled them as being: fire, air, earth, water and ether.

---

[*] E-mail: ayelt@yahoo.com

By contrasting an assertive, or direct approach on human typology performed throughout Western history to the moral, or indirect treatment of the same subject in ancient China, this article demonstrates the bio-ethical convenience of the later. When human types are primarily portrayed from a moral point of view, instead of an assertive, legal or a "normal" one, as the genome-wide association (GWA) studies tends to set down, *free will* embodied by each individual is appropriately emphasized as pre-requisite for a *free society*.

## INTRODUCTION

One of the most amazing breakthroughs in modern science is, with no doubt, that, once unsolvable crimes or historical enigmas of the past are today being fairly elucidated, thanks to genetic analysis and to the increasing sophistication in Forensic Genetics. Nevertheless, the challenge persists. Increasingly "perfect crimes", or so-called *cold cases* have been continuously obliging forensic technologies to utilize ever more tiny DNA samples necessary to obtain reliable profiles with trustworthy analysis sensibility. This fact, as we might expect, sooner or later will set us before a kind of material limitation, e.g., a cytological dilemma, when epithelium, sperm, blood, bone or hair traces are so insignificant and almost impossible to be purged from cross contamination between victims, suspects and/or bystanders that will make any visual, chemical or cytological forensic technique, microscopically speaking, not viable to be properly performed or trusted. *PROMISING PROSPECTS OF CHINESE MEDICAL SEMIOLOGY ON FORENSIC GENETICS* intends to add on top of *trace DNA, mRNA, STRs, SNPs, miniSTRs* and many other cutting edge forensic methods and analyses, some philosophical, anthropological, medical, psychological, legal and ethical approaches to the matter, addressing it in a new, fresh and multidisciplinary look to the human element.

To shed light to the potential of ancient medical semiologies, in general, in helping modern scientific and bio-ethical issues, and to the prospects of Chinese medical semiology, in particular, to assist Forensic Genetics professionals, background knowledge on both is needed.

Along the history of mankind innumerous typological systems were constructed to sort out different groups of humans, classifying them by two, three, four, five or by their multiples according to the criteria and the categorization system chosen to depict human nature.

Thousands of years ago, since Socrates, Plato, Aristotle and Hippocrates up to these 21st century days, where partial findings of the Genome Project guarantee to be unarguably a *turning point* to some and a *cornerstone* to many just born scientific fields, the desire to directly define normality of human behavior, including his overall physiology, psychological profiles and moral trends included, indeed, never ceased to flourish among us in the Western world.

The same desire to grasp what's normal in human being thrived throughout history in a quite opposite way in the East. Instead presenting, analyzing and discussing the matter vis-à-vis, Eastern scholars from ancient times seemingly preferred to treat this controversial subject in a "negative" fashion, e.g., by showing what's immoral let people indirectly envisage normalcy.

Works and lessons from Pythagoras[1] (580-572 BC), Empedocles[2] (c.490-430 BC), Hippocrates[3] (c.460-c.377 BC), Plato[4] (428-347 BC) and Aristotle[5] (384-322 BC) have paved the way for Galen[6] (129-c.216), Geber[7] (c.721-c.815), Al-Farabi (c.873-950), Avicenna[8] (980-1037), and Ibn Arabi[9] (1165-1240), and later on inspired Gall[10] (1758–1828), Heymans[11] (1857-1930), Wiersma[12] (1858-1940), Jung[13] (1875-1961), Le Senne[14] (1882-1954), Kretschmer[15] (1888-1964), Szondi[16] (1893-1986), Mario Ferreira dos Santos[17] (1907-1968), Eysenck[18] (1916-1997), Olavo de Carvalho[19,20] (1947- ) and others, to base their characterological sciences and practices on essentially the same fundamental semiological principles, besides their different living times and places.

Traditionally, Western as well as Eastern semiologies like the Greco-Roman, Perso-Arabic and Indo-Chinese were all founded on five natural archetypes, which some call: *fire, air, earth, water* and *ether*, and others: *wood, fire, earth, metal* and *water*.

The relationship drawn between nature and the human being among early traditions was based in analogies between inherent properties of primeval archetypes and the properties of individuals themselves, being them corporal or psychological, e.g., the constitutions and temperaments. The classical doctrine of the five primal elements, responsible for human body constitutions and psychological temperaments, used to be taught as the basic semiology in the medical schools for at least more than two thousand years (from Antiquity up to end of the Renaissance, XVI century).

At the same time, a similar semiological system was developed in the East, which also was footed into five primordial elements as well: wood, fire, earth, metal and water[21].

The crucial point to be stressed here is that the fundamental difference between these two similar typological systems is that the psychological features of the Chinese five types were depicted "negatively" in the Chinese Medicine Canon called *Huangdi Neijing*, or *Yellow Emperor's Internal Classic[22]*. This fact itself makes this *classical* work an exceptional primary source for Forensics. The philosophical and semiological principles laid down by the *Yellow Emperor's Internal Classic* are universal.

Humans from this XXI century and people who lived during the Spring/Autumn and Warring States Eras[23], more than 2500 years ago, enjoyed and continue to enjoy the same biological genetic substrate; at least, up to now, neither anthropologists nor paleontologists seemed to disagree on that, nor anyone discovered any exclusively "prehistoric amino-acid", nor any previously unknown nitrogenated base or nucleotide that could refute such sameness.

As matter of fact, since antiquity that same biological or genetic matter had never died away to be the pre-requisite for individuals' psycho-somatic features to be expressed, being them anatomical, physiological or psychological, and for all its derived behavior patterns, being them instinctive or chosen.

According to early known and today's newest studies in Genetics, it is difficult to argue that genetic expressions (anatomical and physiological) and genetic structures (base pairing) are not "two faces of the same coin", or in other words, the genetic code itself.

Despite what sociologists, anthropologists or historians dispute among each other about the diverse origins, development, history and fall of cultures; it certainly is the genetic substrate that's the precondition for their history, including their development, climax and extinction, including their crimes and all other forensic issues. For that reason, it is difficult to argue that molecular biology does not precede ideological, sociological and economical arguments, or any further historical phenomena.

Being the utmost foundation of our material life, the genetic code, as we understand it today, is materially the same for everyone on Earth, regardless of the phenotypic differences between whites, blacks, yellows, mulattos, griffes or any other race blend resulting from combinations between these five basic phenotypes scattered around the world throughout centuries of human history since immemorial times. Singular skin colors, cultural peculiarities, different religions and diverse likes and dislikes are not result of any essentially different genetic substance. The differences rely solely on combinatorial sequences of amino acids (tri-nucleotides) located in various loci (codons), and not on any odd genotype for each phenotype at all.

From thinking about the genetic code, the first thing that comes to mind is that this "code" is, basically, a biological matter. Being a biological matter, the "code" pertains to and it is restricted by the same space-time category, laws and circumstances which governs any existent matter in universe. Its spatial and temporal features are remarkably expressed within its double facet: the genetic code is a chemical mixture of different amounts of sugar, protein and minerals extant in space, and yet, at the same time, it is a specific informational sequence orderly tailored throughout time.

Therefore, it is easy to understand that DNA, being a biological matter, is subjected not only to space and time restraints, but by being their related product, it is also a space-temporal restrictor factor itself, e.g., where and when the DNA express or not a particular trait is by rule a matter of space and time conjunction.

Consequently, it can be inferred that different individuals at different times, or even same individuals at different periods of development could experience time and space through different psychological perceptions, trends and insights. That's especially true when we talk about males and females, youngsters and elders, whites and griffes, blacks and mulattos, Westerners and Easterners, etc.

This inextricable duality between time and space, or the interconnection among positive and negative forces is the most basic physiological tenet in Chinese Medicine that has been taught for centuries by the world's oldest and still accessible medical textbook called *Yellow Emperor's Internal Classic*. The idea of balance amid opposite but complementary forces (*yin-yang*) and its relationship to the body and mind health of an individual is embedded through all its 162 chapters.

These opposites, yet inter-reliant forces, called *yin-yang*, literally *shadow-light*, a concept explicited by the *Yellow Emperor's Internal Classic*, can represent not only a wide range of paradoxical pairs or matching concepts theoretically constructed by human science, such as the opposition between negatively and positively electrically charged ions, anions and cations; electrons and protons; photons and bosons; strong and weak nuclear forces, etc; but also can represent macroscopic physical phenomena, normally occurring in nature, such as the antagonism involving acid and alkali; water and fire; ice and mist; winter and summer or day and night.

There are innumerable ways to understand what could be the *yin-yang* of an object or phenomenon in Genetics, and by extension in Forensic Genetics, depending on the point of view from which we depart to analyze a specific concept. Therefore, a precise context is always a must. For instance, if we re-take the aforementioned spatial and temporal categories intermingled and inherent to the genetic code, on one hand, we may represent its "space" by its body of nucleotides (which really and substantially exists in and occupies a space), and on the other hand, we may represent its "time" part by the function of its respective codons (which is just a virtual concept, realized or not from time to time by the actual sequences of nucleotides). In this sense, we may say, using the words of Chinese Medicine, that the nucleotides are the *yang* portion while its codons are the *yin* portion of the DNA. But in another sense, we can also represent the amino acid itself as being the *yang* and the respective tri-nucleotide sequence (code) as being the *yin* portion. Meaning the *yang* of a phenomena or object is, by rule, objectively measurable and quantifiable, whilst the *yin* is subjected to convey a kind of order, concept or information which is not always necessarily realized or enacted. In other words, *yang* is an act inhabiting space or frame, and *yin* is its potency dwelling in time, or the virtual path of a process.

Hence, it is fairly simple to understand that, hypothetically, the real differences among people, such as the differences between the five basic human phenotypes or "races" (whites, blacks, yellows, mulattos and griffes) could eventually be reduced to different combinatorial amounts of *yin* and *yang* embodied by the amino acids and polypeptides which constitute each to these groups and/or by the respective information actualized or not in the final expression of their genetic code.

As we have indicated before, populations, cultures and civilizations presuppose necessarily the existence of actors for these facts to happen, and the individuals, in turn, presuppose the inevitable presence of their own genetic codes. And, as we have also pointed out, any natural object or phenomena in existence is subjected to *time* and *space* constraints, or in Chinese terms, subjected to nature's law of *yin-yang*.

The very first pair of opposites or the two groups of humans that can roughly exemplify such difference in the relative amounts of expressed *yin-yang* is the men and the women populations. Nevertheless, this natural fact can also be observed in many other opposite groups or pairs that usually exerts a morally accepted, legally permitted and culturally expected relationship in human life: a group who, by being "more" *yang*, naturally tends in their world-view to prioritize the category of *space*, while the other, by being "more" *yin*, is instinctively inclined to give primacy to *time*. For example: men and women; husbands and wives; parents and children; brothers and sisters; youngsters and elders; young women matching old men; old women matching young men; etc. However, what's important here is to know that complementarity and opposition between the priorities of each human group are sources for peace and prosperity, but they also can be reason for war and crime, or in other terms, they are and should be seen as the first and the fundamental rationale or the *a priori* background in Forensic issues.

These examples are just few forms to express the universal dialectic principle that permeates every object and phenomenon in the universe. This principle was called above as being the inextricable duality between the categories of time and space, i.e., existent objects in space and their function along their time of existence. In fact, despite of opposite and complementary differences among the populations of men and women, or youngsters and elders along with the whole myriad of different social roles in which they interact with each other, there are other anthropological and genetic instances where *yin* and *yang* (or time and space) are expressed in distinct combinations.

The *Yellow Emperor's Internal Classic* classifies not only the human population, but innumerable facts and phenomena concerning nature and human body according to a dialectic, qualitative and quantitative distribution of *yin-yang*.

See figure 1.

| | NATURE |
|---|---|---|---|---|
| colspan="3" | YIN - | | YANG + |
| YIN > YANG | ONLY YANG | YIN = YANG | YANG > YIN | ONLY YIN |
| | THE FIVE METAPHYSICAL DIMENSIONS |
| WOOD | FIRE | EARTH | METAL | WATER |
| | THE FIVE FORCES IN THE UNIVERSE |
| WEAK | STRONG | UNNAMED | ELECTRO MAGNETIC | GRAVITY |
| | THE FIVE SUBATOMIC PARTICLES |
| BOSONS | PHOTONS | NEUTRONS | ELECTRONS | PROTONS |
| | THE FIVE ATMOSPHERIC FORCES |
| WIND | HEAT | MOIST | DROUGHT | FROST |
| | THE FIVE SEASONS |
| SPRING | SUMMER | MUGGY SUMMER | FALL | WINTER |
| | THE FIVE CARDINAL POINTS |
| EAST | SOUTH | CENTRE | WEST | NORTH |
| | THE FIVE COLORS |
| GREEN | RED | YELLOW | WHITE | BLACK |
| | THE FIVE FLAVORS |
| SOUR | BITTER | SWEET | PUNGENT | SALTY |
| | THE FIVE MUTATIONS |
| BIRTH | GROWTH | TRANSFORMATION | DECAY | DEATH |
| | HUMAN BEING |
| colspan="3" | YIN ℵ | | YANG ⌐ |
| YIN > YANG | ONLY YANG | YIN = YANG | YANG > YIN | ONLY YIN |
| | THE FIVE HUMAN RACES |
| WOOD | FIRE | EARTH | METAL | WATER |
| | THE FIVE RELATIONSHIPS |
| DAUGHTER | FATHER | IN-LAW | SON | MOTHER |
| | THE FIVE ORGANS |
| LIVER | HEART | SPLEEN | LUNGS | KIDNEYS |
| | THE FIVE ENTRAILS |
| GALL BLADDER | SMALL INTESTINE | STOMACH | LARGE INTESTINE | BLADDER |
| | THE FIVE HUMOURS |
| BILE | BLOOD | DIGESTIVE ENZYMES | LYMPH | URINE/FAECES |
| | THE FIVE TISSUES |
| TENDONS | VESSELS | MUSCLES | SKINS | BONES |
| | THE FIVE METABOLISMS |
| HEPATOBILIAR | CARDIO VASCULAR | GASTRO INTESTINAL | BRONCHO PULMONARY | GENITO URINARY |
| | THE FIVE SENSES |
| VISION | GUSTATION | PROPRIO CEPTION | OLFACTION | AUDITION |
| | THE FIVE EMOTIONS |
| ANGER | EXCITEMENT | ANXIETY | SADNESS | FEAR |
| | THE FIVE TEMPERAMENTS |
| CHOLERIC | SANGUINEOUS | APATHETIC | PHLEGMATIC | MELANCHOLIC |

Figure 1. The five categories' taxonomy in Nature and Humans.

For instance, chapter 64 in book II of the *Yellow Emperor's* treatise depicts the whole human population into five human races[24]: wood; fire; earth; metal and water. Each of them is described according to an anatomical, psychological, and behavioral approach, as follows[25]:

> "Humans made of wood... like the green emperor...lazy...liars... Humans made of fire... like the red emperor...untrustful...loathers... Humans made of earth... like the yellow emperor...unconcerned...profit seekers... Humans made of metal...like the white emperor...cruel...dictators... Humans made of water... like the black emperor...irreverent...tricksters... ." [26]

The syllogistic development of the *yin-yang* concept into five variations exemplified by this chapter confirms the inherence of both categories and their anthropological expressions in the study of the human being, including all complex semiological or psychological nuances of different people. Nevertheless, what makes this passage most remarkable and highly laudable is that it gives room to the liberty of the individual by tacitly acknowledging his *free will* independently of any compulsory phenotypic consideration, since the passage does not affirm in absolute terms that each type "is" or "has" the respective attribute, instead it just indicates by analogy that each of the five races share analogous *likenesses* with its respective and possible vice expression.

On the other hand, on the basis of phenotypic differences among individuals in the human population, studies of genetic variation across the entire human genome has been designed to identify genetic complex association with several semiological and psychological traits and other nuances. According to Pearson & Manolio[27], in the past years, there has been a dramatic increase in genomic complex association discoveries robustly identified and replicated in many genome-wide-association (GWA) studies. The GWA approach, increasingly fashionable today, particularly helped by the ever-growing genome-wide database of patterns of common human genetic sequence variation among the population (the International HapMap Project)[28,29], has a high risk to conduct future Genomics at large, and by extension Forensic Genetics, to the perverse dead-end of *eugenics*, where genetic "gold standards" could with no doubt dictate racial discrimination as a rule, supposedly based in scientific findings.

Through this possibility, the traditional rule-of-law and principle of justice that grants individual innocence *a priori* despite of any forensic charge could be easily jeopardized, and finally inverted upside down, by the likelihood of, for example, criminalizing individuals according to the presence in their DNA of a specific Single-Nucleotide-Polymorphisms (SNPs) linked to some immoral tendencies of a particular ethnic group.

Such sort of logical non-sense can occur by the simple inversion of an *object* or *phenomenon* and its *attributes*, provided that it is logically impossible to have vices before having the virtues to what they negatively relate to. This, added to the fact that in Genetics, molecular biology works with both: actual (*yang*) and virtual (*yin*) findings (i.e.: nucleotides and codons), and not in the midst of unforeseen abstract possibilities, the genome-wide-association (GWA) studies, broadly performed today, would be ethically misleading if they set *a priori* standards for normalcy only according to genetic findings, overlooking the truth that at the end tendency does not mean actuality nor certainty.

## CONCLUSION

After thousands of years of wisdom, humans are living today on the verge of a complete perversion of *yin-yang* relationships, such as nature and human being; time and space; biology and logics and many others. The traditional understanding of precedence of the human element towards nature is being derelict.

The reason for this situation is the inconstancy of criteria that devastates whichever field in science and society. Only through invariable criteria one would be able to analyze dialectical and variable factors, like *yin-yang*, time-space, codons and nucleotides, etc, with the required scientific neutrality.

Scientific neutrality defines science, and science means freedom to pursue further understanding about its subject of study. Therefore, if some scientific findings of a particular scientific field threat the scientific freedom as a whole, the entire matter should be readdressed multidisciplinarily. For example, recent advances in molecular sequencing technology, gene polymorphisms, such as single-nucleotide polymorphisms (SNPs), and especially SNPs that occur in gene regulatory or coding regions (cSNPs) added by biochemical and semiological studies to assess whether these genomic polymorphisms have phenotypic consequences[30], may spell a kind of "racist typology" that gives no room for individual liberty.

By bluntly laying down the immoral affinities of each human "race", the 64th chapter in Book II of the *Yellow Emperor's Internal Classic*, at its time in history, seems to having been trying to buster away from society for more than two millennia the danger of *yin-yang* perversion and the lost of freedom. This old Chinese medical textbook rooted out any possibility of cataloging people by bias or bigotry based on an ideal "physiological" or "normal" standards, and by doing this, it prevented people from popular discussions about supposedly "better" or "not-so-good" temperaments and constitutions, once that all five human predispositions described by the treatise are equally immoral, but not compulsory.

However, the ever-recurring temptation of preemptively labeling people according to their inheritance haunts today's Genomics. This is a fact that could grow and become dangerously serious, especially if we loose from our sight angular definitions of what are intrinsically immoral and legally illogical by being, day after day, increasingly more convinced that what is eugenically desirable or ideal can be genetically measured, manipulated and achieved.

The Chinese medical semiology approaches this prickly issue in a much more modest and pedagogical way. It does not try to square normal or ethical standards to human types or human behaviors; instead, it just indicates by means of reasoning *ad absurdum* their pathological tendencies.

The truth of the matter is, some genetic polymorphisms could indeed be found in the neuro psychochemistry of human brain's metabolism, linking them to some moral dispositions discovered on the basis of phenotypic differences among races. So, the question to be raised by the present chapter on Forensic Genetics is: Would some mRNA, SNPs or cSNPs be valuable enough compared to the precedence of the individual freedom?

Failing to rightfully answering this, sooner or later, will bring the specter of racism and mutating it into a scientific credo to the last human society.

## COMPETING INTERESTS

The author declares that he has no competing interests. The author alone is responsible for the content and writing of the paper.

## REFERENCES

[1] Pythagoras. D' Olivet F. *The Golden Verses of Pythagoras*. Transl. from French, 2$^{nd}$ ed, Putnam, 1925.
[2] Empedocles. Wright. M.R. *Empedocles: The Extant Fragments*. Bristol, London, 1995.
[3] Hippocrate. Jouanna, J. *Oeuvres completes*. 2$^{ème}$ Ed. Belles Lettres, Paris, 1990.
[4] Plato. Cooper, J.M. Hutchinson, D.S. *Plato Complete Works*. Hackett Publishing Company, 1997.
[5] Aristotle. Barnes, J. *Complete Works of Aristotle*, Vols.1, 2, Princeton University Press, 1971, 1984.
[6] Galen. Walzer R. Frede, M. *Three Treatises on the Nature of Science*. Hackett Publishing Company, 1985.
[7] Jabir Ibn Hayyan. Russell, R.*The Alchemical Works of Geber*. Weiser Books, 1994
[8] Ibn Sina. *Canon of Medicine*. Kazi Publications, 1999.
[9] Ibn Arabi, M. Hirtenstein, S. *The Four Pillars of Spiritual Transformation*. Anqa Publishing, 2009.
[10] Gall, F.J. *On The Functions Of The Cerebellum*. Alofsin Press, 2009.
[11] Heymans, G. Gerritsen, T.J.C. *La philosophie de Heymans*, Alcan, Paris, 1938.
[12] Wiersma, E.D. *Lectures on Psychiatry*. 1$^{st}$ ed., Lewis, 1932.
[13] Jung, C.G. *Psychological Types*. 9$^{th}$ ed., Princeton University Press, 1990.
[14] Le Senne, R. *Traité De Caractérologie*. 7$^{ème}$ Ed., Presses Universitaires De France, 1963.
[15] Kretschmer, E. *Physique And Character*. Dick Press, 2007.
[16] Szondi, L. *Diagnostic expérimental des pulsions*. Presses Universitaires de France, Paris, 1952.
[17] Santos, M.F. Curso de Integração Pessoal. Editora Logos, São Paulo, 1963.
[18] Eysenck, H. *Dimensions of Personality*. Transaction Publishers, 1997.
[19] Carvalho, O. *O Caráter como Forma Pura da Personalidade*. Astroscientia Ed., Rio de Janeiro, 1993.
[20] Carvalho, O. *Curso de Astrocaracterologia*. São Paulo, Rio de Janeiro, 1989, 1991.
[21] El Tassa, A.Y. *Philosophical Foundations of Huangdi Neijing's Typology*. Chinese Academy of Social Sciences, Beijing, 2006.
[22] Huang Di Nei Jing, Su Wen,Wang Bing.*People's Health Publishing House copy*, Beijing, 1956.
[23] This is the estimated age in which the world's oldest medical textbook called *Yellow Emperor's Internal Classic* was written in ancient China.
[24] El Tassa, A.Y., Yellow Emperor's "Manner" life model and its clinical significance, Master's Degree Thesis, Chinese Academy of Social Sciences, Beijing, 2008.

[25] More *yin* than *yang* = wood; only *yang* = fire; *yin* and *yang* = earth; more *yang* than *yin* = metal; only *yin* = water.
[26] Huang Di Nei Jing Su Wen, Wang Bing.People's Health Press, photocopying, Beijing, 1956.
[27] Pearson TA, Manolio TA. *How to interpret a genome-wide association study*. JAMA. 2008; 299 (11):1335-1344.
[28] International HapMap Consortium. *A haplotype map of the human genome*. Nature. 2005; 437(7063):1299-1320. PUBMED..
[29] Frazer KA, Ballinger DG, Cox DR; et al, International HapMap Consortium. *A second generation human haplotype map of over 3.1 million SNPs*. Nature. 2007; 449(7164):851-861. PUBMED.
[30] http://www.sciencemag.org/feature/data/1044449.shl

# INDEX

## A

abortion, 241
absorption, 2, 198
abstinence, 121, 125
acceptor, 111
accidental, 294
accreditation, ix, 74, 89
accuracy, viii, 36, 40, 44, 205, 222, 232
acetate, 8
acid, x, 7, 15, 26, 75, 78, 91, 92, 93, 98, 108, 109, 110, 112, 113, 114, 119, 120, 134, 156, 164, 165, 168, 169, 171, 194, 198, 225, 226, 232, 256, 303, 309, 310, 311
acidic, 92
ACM, 263
acquisitions, 9
activation, 83, 210
active site, 110, 115
addiction, xiii, 245
adducts, 206
adenine, 16, 256
adenosine, 208
adipose, 7, 16, 18, 26, 29
administration, 55
administrative, 58
administrators, 58, 69
adsorption, 157
adult, xiv, 71, 226, 228, 245, 247, 249, 252, 258, 259, 261, 273
adulthood, 256
adults, xiii, 245, 255, 256
Africa, 175
African American, 213, 214, 218
African Americans, 218
age, xiii, 4, 26, 32, 121, 153, 157, 158, 165, 180, 245, 254, 255, 286, 294, 303, 315
agent, 81, 273, 286

agents, 25, 159, 246
aggregates, 157, 170
aggression, 79, 119, 130
aging, 11, 165
aid, vii, 39, 42, 44, 46, 48, 126, 136, 147, 214, 246
aiding, 129, 214
air, xv, xvi, 8, 16, 17, 119, 201, 278, 283, 307, 309
albumin, 155, 170
alcohol, xv, 7, 8, 15, 81, 286, 294, 296
algae, xiv, 265, 272
algorithm, 95, 219
aliphatic compounds, 93
alkali, 310
alkaline, 39, 81, 200
allele, vii, viii, 35, 40, 41, 42, 43, 44, 50, 84, 85, 87, 88, 124, 125, 134, 138, 139, 140, 141, 145, 146, 148, 149, 191, 194, 195, 196, 198, 199, 200, 202, 203, 204, 206, 207, 209, 210, 213, 216, 217, 218, 219, 221, 222, 226, 227, 233, 235, 238, 240, 279, 290
alleles, 38, 40, 41, 42, 43, 44, 45, 87, 124, 137, 140, 141, 144, 147, 194, 195, 198, 199, 200, 201, 203, 205, 206, 209, 212, 215, 221, 224, 235, 237, 238, 239, 242
alpha, 26, 33, 170
Alps, 270
alternative, vii, xi, xiv, 1, 79, 122, 133, 135, 139, 143, 207, 209, 213, 265, 266, 295
alternatives, 41
Alzheimer's disease, 198
amendments, 147
amino, 81, 86, 93, 156, 159, 167, 194, 198, 309, 310, 311
amino acid, 81, 86, 93, 156, 167, 194, 198, 310, 311
amino acids, 81, 86, 93, 167, 310, 311
amino-groups, 159
AML, 263

ammonia, 251
amphibians, 267
Amsterdam, 70, 225, 228
AMT, 48
amylase, 3, 7, 26
analysts, 31
analytical techniques, 274
anatomy, 85
animals, xiv, 152, 246, 265, 266, 267, 268, 269
annealing, 139, 140, 182, 200
antagonism, 310
antenna, 248
anthrax, 273
anthropological, 135, 148, 153, 183, 191, 308, 311, 313
anthropology, 153, 219, 220, 226
antibody, 3
antigen, x, 3, 15, 117, 120
ants, 250
APO, 272
apoptotic cells, 37
appropriate technology, 222
aqueous solution, 156
archeology, x, 91
Argentina, 282, 291
arginine, 110
Aristotle, 308, 309, 315
aromatic rings, 93
arrest, 56, 57
arson, 185
arthropod, 246, 263
arthropods, xiii, 245, 246, 247, 254, 262
ash, 300
Asia, 175
Asian, 54, 174, 180, 191, 197, 282, 292
Asian countries, 54
assault, x, 2, 27, 28, 31, 74, 77, 81, 117, 118, 119, 120, 121, 122, 123, 124, 125, 127, 129, 132, 211
assessment, 53, 60, 63, 64, 164, 170, 219, 220, 229, 269, 271, 274, 298, 304
assets, xv, 307
assignment, 235, 279, 283
asthma, 197
asymmetry, 124, 291
ATP, 86, 175, 208, 270
attacker, 266
attacks, 136, 148, 212, 266, 268, 273
attempted murder, 71
aura, 69
Australia, 9, 47, 51, 54, 57, 58, 60, 62, 63, 260
Austria, 53, 54, 217
authentication, 153, 155, 162
authenticity, xi, 151, 152, 154, 162, 163, 164

auto theft, 36
automation, xii, 3, 48, 135, 193, 205, 209, 216, 221, 222, 274
autopsy, 246
autosomes, 194, 212, 218
availability, xiv, 119, 163, 246, 256, 283
awareness, viii, 35, 54, 58, 63, 65, 66, 67, 68, 70
azo dye, 7

# B

back, 2, 3, 46, 65, 71, 105, 106, 152, 176, 184, 185, 212, 247, 281
backscattered, 164
bacteria, x, 76, 91, 113, 195, 246, 271, 273
bacterial, 113, 114, 154, 160, 273
bacterial contamination, 154
banks, xi, 133, 141
barriers, 62, 63, 69
base pair, 85, 86, 98, 195, 309
beetles, 248, 249, 250, 251, 252, 254
behavior, 168, 309
behaviours, 60
Beijing, 307, 315
Belarus, 231, 234
Belgium, 53, 54
benefits, ix, 51, 62, 63, 64, 65
bias, 40, 43, 44, 48, 140, 183, 185, 282, 291, 314
binding, xi, 16, 39, 110, 111, 133, 135, 140, 141, 144, 194, 199, 209, 210, 214, 240
biochemistry, 42, 171
biodegradable, 295
biodegradation, 156
bioinformatics, 188
biological consequences, 164
biological macromolecules, 158
biological markers, xii, 27, 193
biological weapons, 267, 273
biomolecules, 152, 153, 156, 157, 303
biopolymers, 156, 166
biotechnology, 2, 221
biotin, 209, 210
birds, 267, 271
bison, 169
bleeding, 56, 118
blocks, 195, 223, 224
blood, viii, ix, x, 2, 3, 4, 5, 6, 7, 10, 11, 12, 13, 14, 15, 16, 17, 18, 20, 21, 22, 23, 26, 27, 28, 29, 30, 31, 32, 33, 34, 35, 36, 49, 56, 57, 73, 74, 75, 76, 79, 81, 85, 86, 87, 117, 119, 123, 138, 155, 180, 182, 197, 243, 246, 247, 279, 283, 304, 308
blood smear, 33
body fluid, 3, 4, 5, 7, 16, 27, 29, 31, 33, 118, 216

# Index

body temperature, 254
bonds, 111, 181, 204
bone marrow, 96, 283, 284
bootstrap, 260, 261
Bosnia, 113, 304
bosons, 310
bottleneck, 181
bottlenecks, 176
bounds, 110
bovine, 42, 95, 113
brain, 4, 7, 16, 18, 29, 169, 180, 248
Brazil, 262, 283
Brazilian, 282, 291
breakdown, 246
breathing, 251
breeding, 252, 264
British Columbia, 261
broad spectrum, 56
brothers, 87, 311
Buenos Aires, 291
buffer, 8, 81, 234, 286
Bulgaria, 53
burglary, vii, viii, 35, 36, 49, 53, 56
*Burkholderia*, 273
burn, xv, 293, 295
burning, 300, 302

## C

cadaver, 74, 78, 247
caffeine, 121
calcium, 4, 16, 33, 161, 234
Canada, 53, 54, 60, 62, 63, 196, 258, 260, 269
cancer, 32, 197, 198, 199
cancer treatment, 198
candidates, vii, 2, 17, 19, 29, 137, 145, 218, 221
capillary, viii, 2, 4, 5, 30, 35, 40, 42, 43, 48, 114, 136, 149, 203, 210, 214, 218, 222, 235, 267, 271, 273, 278, 287, 304
carbohydrate, 15
carbohydrate metabolism, 15
carbon dioxide, 264
carbonyl groups, 111
carboxylic, 111
carcinogen, 199
carcinogens, 199
cardiac muscle, 180
Caribbean, 277
carrier, 161, 165
case study, 149
categorization, xvi, 307, 308
category a, 68
cats, 268, 269

Caucasian, 213, 214, 218, 227, 228
cavities, 86, 119
cDNA, 9, 10, 11, 12, 13, 14, 15, 16, 17
cell, xi, 3, 16, 31, 32, 46, 74, 75, 77, 81, 83, 117, 118, 122, 123, 131, 134, 156, 180, 181, 196, 199, 204, 213, 256, 267, 270
cell lines, 196
cement, 300
cementum, 155, 300
Central America, 148
cereals, 246
certification, 89
cervix, 119, 126
channels, 205
charge coupled device, 208
chemical degradation, 156
chemicals, 4, 75, 76, 195
chemiluminescence, 75
children, 213, 242, 311
chimpanzee, 182
China, xvi, 53, 196, 247, 307, 308, 315
chloroform, xv, 7, 8, 21, 22, 23, 39, 81, 234, 258, 283, 286, 293, 296
chlorophyll, 272
chloroplast, xiv, 154, 265, 266, 270
chloroplasts, 269
chorionic villi, 241
chromatography, 156, 234
chromosomal abnormalities, 233
chromosome, xiii, xiv, xv, 84, 85, 86, 87, 123, 124, 126, 131, 143, 144, 146, 148, 194, 195, 197, 211, 212, 222, 224, 226, 227, 229, 232, 277, 278, 279, 280, 281, 282, 283, 291, 292, 304
chromosomes, 74, 85, 143, 144, 154, 158, 194, 219, 239
chronic disorders, 198
cigarettes, 199
circulation, 119, 125
CITES, 267
CJS, 55, 56, 58, 62, 63
classes, 227
classical, vii, ix, xiii, xiv, 1, 3, 27, 73, 80, 245, 254, 256, 265, 309
classification, 219
clay, 169
cleaning, 46, 76, 83
cleavage, x, 92, 94, 181, 201, 216
clinical diagnosis, 92
clone, 170
cloning, 169, 263
clusters, 64, 65, 92
coagulum, 16
codes, 123, 182, 194, 311

320 Index

coding, xii, 84, 85, 148, 174, 175, 176, 182, 186, 187, 189, 191, 194, 196, 213, 214, 227, 256, 257, 270, 314
codon, 194
codons, 310, 313, 314
coil, 115
coitus, 126
Coleoptera, 248, 249, 250, 251, 252, 254, 262
collaboration, viii, 2, 30, 142, 196
collagen, 155, 156, 157, 161, 169, 170
collateral, 163
Colombia, 283, 293, 303
colon, 7, 16, 18, 19, 26, 29, 198
colon cancer, 198
colonisation, 254
colonization, xv, 246, 254, 278
colonizers, 250
colors, 228, 248, 251, 295, 297, 310
commodities, 246
communication, 70
community, vii, ix, xiii, 1, 2, 3, 6, 28, 31, 44, 47, 51, 58, 69, 70, 123, 153, 154, 162, 196, 213, 216, 220, 221, 223, 231, 233, 237, 250, 261, 290
compatibility, 138, 141, 234, 235, 239
compilation, 263
complement, ix, 69, 73, 83, 139, 143, 144, 145, 182, 212, 213
complementarity, 311
complementary DNA, 200, 208, 209
complexity, xiii, 53, 69, 215, 231
components, 9, 16, 41, 43, 55, 92, 94, 122, 125, 155, 156, 157, 201, 207, 240
composition, 58, 113, 122, 176, 190, 266
compost, 94, 112, 113
compound eye, 248
compounds, 81, 92, 98, 110, 161, 251
computation, 242
concentrates, 39
concentration, 10, 39, 41, 44, 81, 94, 97, 98, 100, 101, 105, 106, 108, 109, 110, 111, 112, 121, 125, 146, 155, 204, 235, 286, 287
concordance, 87, 136, 137, 138, 139, 140, 141, 144, 145, 146
condensation, 159
condom, 76, 118, 126
confidence, 6, 206, 234, 297
configuration, 205
conflict, 57, 260
conjugation, 16
consensus, 38, 41, 44, 141, 142
consent, 119
conservation, 76, 152, 263
constraints, 68, 311

construction, 57, 278, 279, 290
consumption, 49
contaminant, 160
contamination, viii, ix, x, xii, 31, 36, 40, 41, 44, 45, 46, 50, 73, 74, 75, 76, 78, 88, 91, 92, 94, 123, 127, 140, 151, 153, 154, 158, 160, 161, 162, 165, 166, 168, 182, 189, 288, 304, 308
contracts, 249
control, ix, xii, xiv, xv, 5, 7, 10, 11. 16, 18, 19, 21, 23, 24, 26, 27, 29, 40, 45, 46, 54, 74, 88, 94, 114, 141, 173, 174, 176, 182, 183, 185, 187, 188, 189, 191, 209, 226, 227, 268, 269, 277, 278, 286, 288, 289, 291, 292, 293, 295, 296, 298
control group, xv, 293, 295, 296
Convention on International Trade in Endangered Species, 268
conversion, 15, 208
Copenhagen, 217
corona, 300
correlation, 153, 156, 157, 161, 185, 219, 247
correlation coefficient, 185
correlations, 195, 198
cost-effective, 205
costs, 61, 204, 222
cotton, 6, 10, 16, 17, 38, 76
Council of the European Union, 54
couples, 131
coupling, 7
courts, 36, 57, 256
covalent, 204
covalent bond, 204
covering, 54, 261
CPI, 242
CRC, 262, 274, 275
Crete, 165
crime, vii, viii, ix, x, xiv, 1, 2, 28, 31, 35, 36, 38, 39, 43, 44, 45, 46, 47, 50, 52, 53, 54, 55, 56, 58, 59, 60, 61, 62, 63, 64, 65, 66, 67, 68, 69, 71, 74, 75, 76, 77, 78, 83, 109, 117, 118, 119, 128, 138, 152, 181, 214, 219, 220, 221, 222, 223, 247, 266, 267, 268, 269, 271, 277, 290, 303, 311
crimes, vii, xi, 1, 27, 28, 52. 53, 54, 55, 56, 57, 58, 59, 61, 62, 63, 69, 70, 118, 121, 122, 124, 127, 308, 309
criminal activity, 67, 68
criminal justice, vii, 1, 6, 55
criminal justice system, 55
criminality, 65, 68, 70
criminals, 58, 65
criminology, 38, 246
Croatia, 53, 91, 96, 113, 114, 304
cross links, 159
cross-border, 54

cross-linking, 159, 181
crown, 295, 297, 299
crystallinity, 155, 157
crystals, 120
CTAB, 162, 258
Cuba, 282, 283, 291
culture, 266
cycles, 9, 41, 96, 97, 140, 161, 201, 235, 295, 296
cycling, 41, 96, 97
cysteine, 15
cytochrome, xiv, 171, 175, 246, 260, 263, 264, 267, 268
cytochrome oxidase, 260, 264
cytology, 121
cytometry, 225
cytoplasm, 213
cytosine, 158, 159, 167
cytoskeleton, 156
Czech Republic, 53

# D

data analysis, 154, 215
data generation, 185
data set, 260
database, viii, ix, xii, xiv, xv, 51, 52, 53, 54, 55, 56, 58, 59, 60, 61, 62, 63, 64, 65, 66, 69, 70, 71, 128, 129, 130, 141, 149, 173, 183, 185, 186, 187, 188, 189, 190, 196, 211, 217, 218, 229, 242, 259, 260, 261, 267, 272, 277, 278, 279, 280, 284, 286, 287, 290, 313
database management, ix, 51
dating, 154, 167, 174
death, xiii, 155, 245, 246, 247, 249, 251, 254, 255, 261, 262, 266, 268, 272, 273, 294
deaths, 266, 273
decay, 134, 155, 168, 190, 246, 251, 294
decision-making process, 66
decisions, 64, 66
decomposition, 134, 158, 165, 251, 254
decontamination, 46, 76
decontamination procedures, 46
defence, 56, 124
deficiency, 140, 144, 146, 149, 212, 232, 233, 237, 239, 240
definition, 152, 155, 156, 174, 232
degenerate, 141
degradation, x, 32, 81, 83, 91, 92, 94, 126, 134, 146, 152, 155, 156, 157, 158, 159, 160, 162, 165, 208, 256, 294
degradation process, x, 91, 134
dehydrogenase, xiv, 15, 246, 257, 268, 270
dehydrogenases, 175

denaturation, 8, 25, 43, 95, 98, 107, 108, 111, 161, 200, 235
Denmark, 53, 217
density, 123, 195, 196, 197, 225
dentin, 155
dentistry, 304
dentists, 283
deoxynucleotide, 208
deoxyribonucleic acid, 92, 113, 114, 168
deoxyribonucleotides, 202
Department of Energy, 195
Department of Energy (DOE), 195
Department of Justice, 31
deposition, 10, 28, 37, 155, 156
deposits, viii, 35, 37, 38
depression, 197, 252
derivatives, 159
desorption, 205, 206
destruction, xv, 76, 294, 299
detachment, 79
detection, viii, x, 3, 4, 6, 7, 10, 17, 18, 19, 20, 22, 23, 29, 30, 32, 33, 35, 38, 40, 41, 42, 43, 46, 90, 94, 95, 113, 114, 117, 118, 119, 120, 121, 127, 130, 134, 135, 140, 142, 157, 200, 201, 203, 204, 205, 206, 207, 209, 210, 211, 214, 216, 218, 222, 224, 225, 232, 267, 269, 272, 273
detection techniques, viii, 36
detention, 57
deterrence, 59
detoxifying, 199
developed countries, 53
diabetes, 197
diagenesis, xii, 151, 155, 156, 164, 165, 166, 167, 170
diagnostic markers, 195
diatoms, 272
diet, 152, 170
differentiation, xiii, 190, 213, 245, 256
diffusion, 7, 26, 42, 43
digestibility, 95
digestion, 98, 108, 109, 111, 122, 209, 286
dimerization, 22
dinucleotides, 181
direct measure, 155
disaster, xiv, xv, 92, 143, 150, 214, 218, 221, 277, 278, 284, 304
discipline, 62, 63, 64, 65, 66, 67, 68, 153, 247
discontinuity, 292
discrimination, 27, 134, 139, 141, 142, 144, 145, 148, 187, 190, 207, 209, 210, 213, 214, 216, 218, 221, 222, 225, 233, 268, 269, 271, 280, 283, 313
disease gene, 224
diseases, 197, 198

disequilibrium, 212, 224
displacement, 42, 48, 137
disseminate, 69
dissociation, 9
distilled water, 295
distribution, 66, 128, 148, 159, 191, 194, 212, 237, 238, 242, 253, 254, 282, 311
disulfide, 81
divergence, 258
diversification, xiv, 277
diversity, 148, 170, 174, 176, 183, 185, 191, 195, 224, 279, 290, 291
division, 60, 84
DNA damage, 158, 160, 168, 169, 221
DNA ligase, 170, 209
DNA microarray systems, 222
DNA polymerase, xv, 49, 94, 95, 112, 114, 115, 159, 161, 170, 181, 202, 204, 206, 207, 208, 235, 278, 287, 288
DNA sequencing, 209, 225
DNA testing, 124, 126, 146, 227, 232, 294, 304
DNase, x, 92, 95, 97, 98, 108, 109, 110, 111, 112
dogs, 268
domestication, 152
dominance, 149
donor, 2, 28, 37, 38, 45, 67, 68, 110, 123, 125, 126, 131, 215, 219, 220
donors, 21
doors, 112
draft, 26, 54
drainage, 126
dream, 152, 169
drinking, 36, 47, 56
dropouts, 40, 43, 138
*Drosophila*, 250, 256, 262
drowning, 266, 272
drug treatment, 198
drugs, 195, 197, 247
drying, 44, 76
duplication, 66, 68
dyes, 9, 95, 200, 201, 203, 205, 209, 236, 271

## E

ears, 37, 169
earth, xvi, 92, 155, 307, 309, 312, 313, 316
East Asia, 175, 282
ecological, 250
ecology, 247
Ecuador, 133, 147, 173, 283, 292, 303
egg, 15, 154, 171, 174, 249
ejaculation, 121
El Salvador, 148

elders, 310, 311
elective surgery, 121
electric field, 205, 226
electrochemical reaction, 205
electrodes, 204, 205
electrolyte, 204
electrophoresis, viii, 2, 3, 4, 5, 30, 35, 40, 42, 43, 48, 98, 108, 114, 136, 149, 203, 210. 214, 218, 222, 235, 267, 271, 273, 278, 287, 296, 304
elephant, 164
ELISA, 200, 225
elongation, 159
elytra, 249, 254
embryonic development, 211
emission, 94, 97, 207
enantiomers, 156
encoding, 154
endonuclease, 189
energy, 15, 200, 202, 206, 225
energy transfer, 200, 202
England, 96, 213
enthusiasm, 155
environment, 57, 64, 65, 111. 155, 156, 246, 248, 268, 286, 294
environmental conditions, 4, 28, 37, 134, 155, 156, 161, 181, 221, 249, 304
environmental factors, 155, 158, 159, 195, 197
environmental temperatures, 249
enzymatic, 27, 42, 127, 158, 169, 171, 199, 200, 209, 240
enzymes, 98, 110, 112, 121, 199, 207, 271
epididymis, 15
epithelial cell, viii, 15, 16, 28, 32, 35, 36, 37, 38, 44, 74, 75, 79, 90, 118, 122, 125, 130, 155
epithelial cells, viii, 15, 16, 28, 32, 35, 36, 37, 38, 44, 74, 75, 79, 90, 118, 122, 125, 130, 155
epithelium, ix, 73, 74, 80, 308
equality, 6
equilibrium, 140
*Escherichia coli*, 170
ESR, 41
estimating, 146, 246, 254, 255, 297
Estonia, 53
ethanol, 8, 38, 81, 295
ethical issues, 308
ethical standards, 314
ethnic groups, 147, 217
etiology, 266, 273
eugenics, 313
Eurasia, 175
Europe, 54, 56, 86, 141, 143, 147, 148, 247, 263
European Americans, 218
European Union, 54

# Index

Europeans, 219, 280, 281, 282, 283
evolution, 147, 153, 189, 191, 211, 212, 216, 262, 263, 270, 278, 291, 294
examinations, 46, 119, 234
exclusion, 46, 86, 87, 141, 233, 238, 241, 242, 243, 268
excretion, 198
exercise, 147, 149, 190, 228
exons, 21
exonuclease, 94, 95, 209
expert systems, 215
expertise, xiii, 87, 129, 223, 232, 254
exploitation, 69
exposure, 13, 15, 29, 159, 198
extinction, 309
extraction, viii, ix, x, xi, xv, 2, 4, 5, 7, 8, 12, 13, 15, 16, 17, 22, 23, 24, 25, 30, 31, 35, 38, 39, 43, 48, 49, 50, 73, 81, 88, 91, 92, 94, 95, 96, 98, 109, 113, 114, 118, 123, 126, 127, 130, 152, 157, 159, 161, 169, 170, 211, 234, 258, 266, 283, 286, 293, 294, 295, 303, 304
extraction process, xv, 5, 126, 159, 294, 303
eye, 47, 217, 219, 220, 223, 228, 248
eyes, 246, 248, 252

## F

fabric, 295, 297
failure, 58, 69, 129, 140
false positive, 75, 160
familial, 68
family, 86, 128, 154, 166, 167, 217, 218, 221, 222, 232, 236, 241, 248, 250, 251, 253, 304
family members, 218
fat, 78, 199
fatherhood, 233
fauna, 246, 247
FBI, 33, 53, 141, 183, 185, 188, 189, 243, 279
Federal Bureau of Investigation, 279
feedback, 64, 65, 67, 68
feeding, 60, 249, 250, 252
feelings, 57
feet, 79, 80
felony, 266
females, 83, 144, 212, 298, 310
femur, 86, 96
fertility, 190
fertilization, 15
fibrils, 169
fidelity, 164
film, 83
filters, 39, 200
filtration, 81, 234, 296

fingerprinting, 154, 294
fingerprints, 36, 47, 50, 67, 68, 168, 240
Finland, 53
fire, xi, xvi, 133, 136, 294, 307, 309, 310, 312, 313, 316
fixation, 81
flexibility, 155, 205
flight, 139, 146, 205, 206
flow, 67, 68, 204, 225, 282
fluctuations, 40
fluid, viii, 2, 3, 4, 5, 6, 7, 10, 11, 13, 15, 16, 19, 20, 26, 27, 28, 29, 31, 33, 118, 120, 121, 126, 216, 253
fluorescence, 4, 9, 83, 97, 114, 119, 200, 201, 202, 203, 204, 206, 207, 216, 225, 236, 271, 296
fluorescent light, 201
fluorogenic, 225
fluorophores, 9
foams, 81
follicle, 123
food, viii, 35, 56, 76, 246, 249, 266, 269
forceps, 76, 78, 79
formamide, 44
fossil, 153, 154, 155, 156, 157, 158, 163, 164, 165, 166, 167, 170, 171
founder effect, 176
fracture, 295, 300
fractures, 299
fragmentation, xi, 133, 134, 144, 158, 162, 181, 201
France, 33, 53, 54, 73, 86, 87, 89, 247, 315
fraud, 266, 269
free radical, 159
FTA, 26, 74, 77, 81, 86, 87, 283, 284
funding, 30, 53, 303
fungal, 160
fungi, x, xiv, 91, 246, 265, 272
fusion, 15

## G

gas chromatograph, 156
gel, 5, 7, 16, 43, 98, 108, 135, 234, 278, 296
gels, 2, 98, 225, 278, 296
GenBank, 9, 178, 181, 187, 259, 260, 267
gender, xv, 125, 144, 147, 294, 295, 300, 303
gene, xiv, 4, 5, 9, 10, 12, 13, 15, 20, 29, 30, 84, 113, 123, 144, 154, 165, 166, 169, 171, 194, 195, 197, 198, 203, 211, 220, 228, 229, 246, 257, 258, 260, 262, 263, 267, 270, 272, 280, 281, 304, 314
gene amplification, 12, 13, 29
gene expression, 4, 5, 9, 165
gene pool, 280, 281
gene transfer, 169

genealogy, xiv, 277
generation, 20, 30, 41, 50, 143, 152, 194, 204, 224, 270
genes, xii, xiv, 4, 10, 11, 15, 18, 26, 28, 29, 30, 85, 126, 145, 164, 174, 175, 182, 193, 194, 195, 196, 197, 198, 205, 219, 220, 224, 229, 246, 256, 257, 258, 261, 267, 268, 269, 270, 273
genetic code, 194, 262, 309, 310, 311
genetic diversity, 183, 185
genetic drift, 176, 212
genetic information, xi, 133, 134, 139, 156, 217
genetic marker, xiii, xiv, 141, 144, 218, 232, 265, 266, 267, 274, 291
genetic testing, 198, 269, 273
genetics, xi, xii, xiv, xv, 36, 39, 89, 92, 114, 133, 152, 154, 173, 174, 178, 181, 182, 188, 189, 191, 214, 218, 220, 221, 224, 228, 242, 262, 268, 271, 273, 274, 277, 278, 290, 291, 294
genome, viii, xii, xvi, 34, 35, 42, 48, 74, 84, 85, 148, 153, 154, 174, 176, 180, 181, 182, 187, 188, 189, 190, 191, 193, 194, 195, 196, 197, 201, 204, 212, 213, 216, 218, 219, 221, 223, 224, 225, 227, 228, 258, 270, 286, 287, 292, 308, 313, 316
genomes, 114, 182, 187, 188, 191, 200
genomic, xiv, 10, 20, 21, 30, 96, 97, 98, 109, 165, 170, 195, 209, 210, 216, 222, 246, 271, 313, 314
genomics, 146, 241
genotype, 122, 128, 141, 195, 196, 201, 228, 238, 239, 310
genotypes, 174, 197, 200, 204, 210, 228, 235, 236, 237, 238, 239
geochemistry, 155
germ cells, 125
Germany, 53, 54, 96, 97, 217, 295
gland, 7, 15, 20
glass, 37, 41, 75, 200, 201, 204, 216
gloves, 46, 49, 75, 79
glutamine, 111
glycol, 42
goals, 5, 119, 196
gold, 141, 313
gold standard, 141, 313
gonadotropin, 32
governance, 55, 58
government, 55, 273
gracilis, 149
grants, 31, 313
Greece, xvi, 165, 287, 307
Greenland, 292
groups, xiii, xv, 4, 28, 29, 81, 93, 98, 111, 136, 138, 147, 153, 159, 176, 195, 198, 215, 216, 217, 219, 236, 237, 240, 245, 248, 249, 250, 251, 255, 256, 267, 273, 293, 295, 296, 299, 308, 311

growth, xiv, 52, 53, 55, 58, 70, 240, 246, 254, 255, 256, 268, 277
growth rate, 254, 255, 256
guanine, 158
guidelines, 38, 44, 45, 124, 160, 162, 185, 233, 279, 287, 291
guilt, 47, 57
guilty, vii, 1, 247

# H

habitat, 246, 250, 268
hair cells, 286
hair follicle, 131
hallucinogenic mushrooms, 266
handling, 119, 159, 160, 161, 286, 302
hands, 30, 37, 46, 79, 80
handwriting, 46
haploid, 131, 134, 212, 256
haplotype, xii, 125, 128, 173, 178, 179, 183, 184, 185, 187, 188, 194, 195, 196, 211, 217, 223, 224, 228, 257, 260, 279, 287, 316
haplotypes, xii, xv, 125, 128, 134, 149, 173, 179, 183, 185, 186, 187, 190, 194, 197, 212, 213, 219, 260, 268, 269, 278, 279, 280, 281, 283, 290
HapMap, 196, 197, 210, 217, 224, 313, 316
hard tissues, 153
Hawaii, 262
health, 194, 196, 197, 266, 269, 310
heart, 4, 7, 16, 18, 29, 70, 197
heart disease, 197
heat, xv, 294, 297, 299, 302, 303
heavy metal, 81
height, 41, 42, 43, 44, 134, 220, 228
helix, 115
heme, 75, 113, 138
hemoglobin, 3, 16, 33
hepatitis, 4, 32
hepatitis C, 4
heterogeneity, xii, 92, 94, 158, 173, 176, 178, 181, 190
heterogeneous, 26, 92, 188
heterotrophic, 263
heterozygosity, 140, 218, 271
heterozygote, 140, 146, 149
heterozygotes, 224
high risk, xv, 278, 290, 313
high tech, 31
high temperature, 255
high-speed, 139
hip, 205
Hippocrates, 308, 309
Hispanic, 148, 213, 214

histochemical, 83, 156, 157, 166
histochemistry, 157
histological, 80, 130, 155, 157, 295
HIV, 4, 32
HIV-1, 32
HLA, 200, 232
holistic, 155
holistic approach, 155
Holland, 136, 148, 154, 168, 225, 290
Holocene, 170
homicide, 2, 27, 303
hominids, 286
homogeneity, 227
homology, 182, 267
homozygosity, 140, 240
homozygote, 44, 140
Honda, 147, 304
Hong Kong, 53
horse, 167, 269
host, 291
human behavior, 308, 314
human brain, 153, 166, 314
human chorionic gonadotropin, 32
human genome, xii, 74, 85, 114, 182, 188, 193, 194, 195, 196, 197, 212, 213, 219, 221, 223, 224, 225, 228, 313, 316
Human Genome Project, 195
human nature, 308
human resources, xiv, 277
humans, 152, 160, 162, 168, 174, 175, 189, 190, 197, 212, 228, 266, 308, 311, 314
humic acid, x, 91, 92, 93, 112, 113, 114, 115, 134, 138, 171
Humic acid, 92, 98, 108, 109, 110
humic substances, x, 91, 92, 94, 113
humidity, 79, 134, 221
Hungary, 53
hybrid, 199, 263
hybridization, 2, 114, 154, 157, 199, 200, 204, 205, 209, 210, 211
hybrids, 200, 226
hydrogen, 98, 110, 251
hydrology, 155
hydrolysis, 134, 158
hydrophobic, 81
hydroxyapatite, 155, 157
hygiene, 126
hypothesis, 112, 124, 175, 296

**I**

identity, 24, 25, 28, 92, 146, 202, 218, 221, 232, 240, 241, 283, 294, 303, 305

illumination, 98
imaging, 164
immigration, 168, 212, 232, 233
immunological, 266
implementation, viii, xiv, 51, 70, 136, 138, 139, 141, 226, 271, 272, 277, 278
impurities, 295
in situ, 139, 179, 213
in vitro, 96, 159, 169, 240
in vivo, 181
inbreeding, 218
incest, 139, 233
incineration, 294, 295, 298, 299
inclusion, xiii, 59, 60, 63, 64, 87, 88, 147, 161, 187, 231, 233, 241, 242
incubation, 25
independence, 204, 271, 272
independent variable, 296, 302
India, 54
Indian, 291
Indian Ocean, 291
indication, 36, 40, 125, 254, 255
indicators, 198, 254, 262
indirect measure, 219
individual character, xii, 173
individualization, 27, 28, 120, 217, 269, 271
Indonesia, 54
induction, 164
inert, 42, 49
infancy, 53
infections, 125
infectious, 266, 273
infectious disease, 273
inferences, 176
infrared, 83
infrastructure, 88
ingestion, 248
inheritance, 143, 212, 214, 219, 232, 314
inherited, 180, 213, 291
inhibition, x, 39, 42, 44, 91, 94, 95, 96, 98, 100, 101, 104, 105, 106, 107, 109, 110, 111, 112, 113, 115, 140, 153, 158, 162, 171, 174
inhibitor, 8, 11, 28, 95, 103, 109, 110, 111, 113, 170
inhibitors, xii, 10, 39, 40, 81, 92, 94, 95, 110, 111, 112, 113, 114, 134, 138, 140, 151, 161, 165, 221
inhibitory, 104, 108, 109, 110, 112, 115, 286, 288
injection, viii, 35, 43, 44
injections, 40
injuries, 56, 118
inorganic, 16, 95, 96, 98, 109, 155, 157
insects, xiii, xiv, 154, 164, 245, 246, 247, 248, 249, 250, 251, 252, 254, 255, 256, 257, 258, 259, 261, 266, 268, 271

insertion, 119, 178, 179, 182, 189, 194, 212, 280
instruments, 2, 4, 5, 119, 203
insults, vii, 1, 6, 12, 13, 29
integration, 62, 63, 67, 68, 190
integrity, 25, 49, 156, 215, 295, 297, 299
intelligence, x, xi, 53, 55, 56, 62, 63, 64, 65, 67, 68, 69, 117, 119, 133
intelligence gathering, 69
interaction, x, 5, 9, 20, 91, 95, 106, 107, 111, 112, 114, 215
interactions, 110, 215
intercalation, 95, 111, 112
interface, 205
International Trade, 267
interval, xiii, 125, 126, 127, 130, 131, 183, 245, 246, 247, 255, 263, 266, 295
intestine, 7, 16, 18, 19, 29
intrinsic, 159, 160, 200
intron, 20, 21
invasive, 216
inventiveness, 70
inversion, 313
investigative, 53, 56, 61, 62, 63, 64, 69, 217, 218, 219, 220, 241, 304
investment, 55, 59, 272
iodine, 7
ionic, 81, 199, 286, 288
ionization, 190, 205
ionizing radiation, 159
ions, 44, 81, 92, 94, 111, 161, 310
Ireland, 130
iris, 228
iron, 16, 75
isoenzymes, 120
isolation, viii, x, 2, 5, 24, 25, 30, 32, 81, 90, 91, 122, 131, 233, 273, 286, 298
Italian population, 146
Italy, 166, 193, 245, 262, 287

## J

Japan, 53, 145, 168, 196
Japanese, 127, 218
jobs, xv, 278, 290
joining, 181, 271
judge, 119
judges, 186
judiciary, 57
jumping, 159, 169
juries, 28
jurisdiction, 66
jurisdictions, 55, 58, 59, 62, 63, 65, 66, 69, 220, 221
jury, 28, 57

justice, vii, 1, 6, 65, 313
justification, 60
juveniles, 71

## K

Kenya, 189
keratin, 79, 123, 286
kidney, 7, 16, 18, 26, 29
killing, 247
kinetics, x, 91, 115, 165, 181
kinship analysis, 127, 129, 211, 212, 214
Korea, 54

## L

labor, 2, 3, 134
laboratory studies, 138
labor-intensive, 134
larva, 249, 251, 253, 255, 256
larvae, xiii, 245, 249, 251, 252, 253, 254, 255, 256, 268
larval, xiii, 245, 247, 252, 255, 256
laser, ix, xi, 4, 39, 73, 82, 83, 84, 90, 114, 118, 122, 130, 131, 203, 205, 206, 210, 241, 267, 271, 273
latex, 79
Latin America, xv, 268, 277, 278, 279, 280, 281, 282, 283
Latin American countries, xv, 278, 281, 282
law, 28, 53, 55, 58, 61, 62, 63, 66, 67, 68, 71, 129, 146, 179, 311, 313
law enforcement, 53, 55, 61, 63, 66, 67, 68, 71, 129, 146
laws, 54, 58, 272, 290, 310
lawyers, 186
legal issues, viii, 51, 58
legislation, xiv, 53, 54, 55, 58, 141, 277, 290
lenses, 83
LEO, 262
lesions, 158, 159, 160, 165, 166, 167
leucine, 258
Leukocyte, 232
leukocytes, 125
liberation, 7
liberty, 313, 314
life cycle, 249
life sciences, 207
lifecycle, xiii, 245
ligands, 95
likelihood, 44, 56, 63, 66, 134, 157, 170, 195, 197, 213, 219, 233, 268, 284, 313
limitation, xiv, 126, 134, 139, 181, 206, 265, 308

# Index

limitations, xi, 41, 47, 57, 63, 118, 122, 126, 205, 266, 273, 283
linkage, 154, 210, 212, 224, 229
links, 52, 53, 54, 55, 58, 60, 64, 65, 66, 67, 68, 69, 131, 159
liquefaction, 16
liquid nitrogen, xv, 283, 293, 295
Lithuania, 53
liver, 7, 16, 18, 29
loading, 60
location, 56, 57, 66, 120, 156, 157, 207, 247, 248
locomotion, 249
locus, vii, viii, xiv, 2, 35, 40, 84, 87, 98, 124, 134, 135, 139, 140, 141, 148, 149, 155, 194, 204, 210, 211, 213, 215, 236, 246, 258, 260, 261, 279, 290
London, 71, 165, 167, 170, 217, 262, 263, 315
long period, 286
losses, 39
low power, 134
low temperatures, 183, 249
luciferase, 208
luciferin, 208
luminescence, 216
lungs, 199
Luxembourg, 53, 54
lymphatic, 155
lysis, 25, 39, 50, 81, 122, 126, 127, 234, 286

## M

macromolecules, 92, 153, 158, 159
magistrates, 88
magnetic, 39, 81, 114
magnetic particles, 81
Maillard reaction, 159
maiming, 294
maintenance, 187
major histocompatibility complex, 15
malaria, 33
Malaysia, 54
males, xi, 21, 22, 118, 121, 124, 126, 132, 144, 211, 212, 279, 298, 310
mammal, 156
Mammalian, 9
mammals, 267
management, ix, 51, 53, 55, 59, 60, 64, 66, 67, 68, 70, 89, 196, 202, 291
manifold, 56
manipulation, 222, 286
mantle, 247
mapping, 66, 196, 206, 210, 224, 228
marijuana, 271
marketing, 271

marrow, 96, 283, 284
mask, 75, 164
mass spectrometry, 136, 146, 156, 187, 190, 205, 226
maternal, 74, 85, 86, 134, 174, 176, 198, 213, 241, 257, 281, 291
maternal inheritance, 257
matrix, 16, 38, 169, 204, 206, 295
Maya, 303
MDA, 42, 43
measles, 4, 33
measurement, 94, 216
measures, 162, 205, 207, 219, 274, 296
median, 185, 236, 237, 239
medical diagnostics, 195
Mediterranean, 170, 227, 287
meiosis, 123
melanin, 115
melt, 10, 20, 21, 22, 26, 27, 30
melting, x, 9, 26, 27, 92, 95, 107, 108, 111, 202
melting temperature, x, 9, 92, 111, 202
men, 32, 33, 125, 232, 242, 282, 296, 311
messenger RNA, 33
Mestizos, 147
metabolism, 15, 198, 314
metal ions, 92, 94
Metallothionein, 32
metals, 91
metamorphosis, 247
methanol, 118
metric, 61
Mexican, 291
Mexico, 283, 291
Mexico City, 283, 291
microarray, 204, 205, 213, 217, 222, 225, 226, 228
microarray technology, 203, 204, 226
microbes, 246
microbial, 16, 113, 114, 155, 156, 251
microfabrication, 204
microorganisms, xiv, 152, 265, 266, 267, 273
microsatellites, 84, 147
microscope, 80, 83, 90, 92, 122, 131, 248
microscopy, x, 27, 117, 121
Middle East, 219
migration, 2, 175, 211, 212, 225, 280
mimicking, 182
mineralized, 156, 164
minerals, 169, 310
miniaturization, 274
minisatellites, 84, 154
Miocene, 166, 169
misidentification, xiii, 245, 254
misleading, 144, 182, 313

Missouri, 262
mitochondria, 74, 81, 174, 180, 181, 292
mitochondrial, xii, xiv, xv, 43, 74, 78, 89, 90, 114, 134, 135, 148, 152, 153, 154, 166, 167, 169, 173, 174, 182, 188, 189, 190, 191, 194, 214, 222, 227, 240, 256, 260, 262, 263, 264, 265, 266, 267, 268, 269, 277, 278, 279, 280, 281, 286, 287, 288, 290, 291, 292, 303
mitochondrial DNA, xii, xiv, xv, 74, 78, 114, 134, 148, 152, 153, 154, 166, 169, 173, 174, 182, 188, 189, 190, 191, 194, 214, 240, 260, 262, 263, 264, 265, 266, 267, 268, 269, 277, 278, 279, 286, 288, 290, 291, 292, 303
mixing, 8, 125
mixture analysis, 144
MMP, 5
mobility, 65, 66, 69, 203, 209, 210
model system, 95
models, xv, 55, 57, 58, 59, 60, 62, 63, 67, 68, 69, 70, 111, 255, 294, 296
modus operandi, 66, 68
moisture, 251
molecular biology, 36, 46, 71, 88, 92, 114, 154, 204, 256, 303, 309, 313
molecular markers, xiv, 277
molecular mass, 206
molecular mechanisms, 168
molecular weight, 127, 143, 203, 205, 206, 207
molecules, xii, 6, 39, 81, 110, 111, 112, 134, 151, 153, 156, 157, 158, 162, 164, 166, 180, 202, 204, 205, 206, 207, 213, 256
Møller, 292
monocytes, 32
morphological, xiii, xiv, xv, 83, 245, 256, 261, 265, 266, 268, 294, 302
morphology, 249
Moscow, 243
mosquitoes, 33
mothers, 174
mouth, 76, 249
movement, 60, 161, 247
mRNA, vii, 1, 3, 4, 5, 6, 10, 16, 18, 19, 20, 28, 29, 30, 31, 32, 33, 308, 314
mtDNA, xii, xiii, xiv, xv, 134, 139, 144, 145, 148, 152, 153, 154, 157, 158, 165, 173, 174, 175, 176, 177, 178, 180, 181, 182, 183, 185, 186, 187, 188, 189, 190, 191, 193, 212, 213, 214, 218, 227, 228, 232, 246, 256, 257, 258, 260, 277, 278, 279, 280, 281, 282, 283, 285, 286, 287, 288, 289, 291, 292
MUC4, 30
mucin, 30
mucous membrane, 80
multidisciplinary, 308

multiples, 308
multiplexing, vii, 2, 5, 6, 19, 29, 136, 203, 206, 215, 221, 222
mumps, 33
murder, 71, 74, 79, 89, 154, 167, 246, 269, 271
muscle, 153, 180
muscles, 74, 79, 86
mushrooms, 266, 272
mutant, 200, 202
mutation, xii, 85, 86, 140, 148, 173, 174, 176, 178, 180, 181, 186, 188, 189, 190, 191, 193, 194, 195, 202, 203, 211, 212, 213, 214, 216, 218, 221, 223, 224, 225, 229, 233, 240, 256, 280, 304
mutation rate, xii, 173, 174, 176, 178, 180, 181, 186, 188, 189, 190, 191, 193, 195, 212, 213, 214, 216, 218, 221, 256
mutations, xiii, 86, 126, 139, 140, 144, 158, 176, 180, 181, 182, 183, 184, 185, 195, 202, 203, 204, 215, 225, 226, 231, 233, 240, 280, 287
Mycobacterium, 273
myopic, 69

# N

NADH, xiv, 175, 246, 257, 268, 270
National Academy of Sciences, 165, 169, 170, 171
National Institutes of Health, 195
Native American, 189, 191, 280, 281, 282
Native Americans, 281, 282
natural, xii, 155, 181, 193, 253, 286, 309, 311
natural environment, 286
Netherlands, 35, 41, 47, 53, 54, 228
network, 155, 185
networking, 66, 68
New York, 31, 41, 136, 138, 146, 167, 225, 243
New Zealand, 41, 51, 54
next generation, 84, 85, 159, 174
nicotinamide, 16
Nielsen, 147, 157, 165, 166, 169, 170, 228
Nigeria, 196
NIH, 195, 196
NIST, 142, 146, 213
nitrogen, xv, 93, 110, 283, 293, 295
noise, 188, 204
non-human, xiv, 144, 265, 266, 267, 272, 274
non-immunological, 16
non-random, 212
normal, xvi, 101, 104, 120, 125, 187, 228, 250, 251, 308, 314
normal curve, 101, 104
North America, 258
Northern Ireland, 44, 46, 71
Norway, 53

nose, 246
nuclear, xi, xiv, 4, 32, 74, 78, 97, 113, 114, 133, 138, 149, 154, 158, 164, 166, 171, 176, 181, 182, 183, 185, 189, 194, 213, 240, 257, 260, 263, 265, 266, 268, 269, 270, 273, 302, 310
nuclear genome, 154, 176, 181, 182, 189
nuclease, 8, 9, 200, 225
nuclei, 80, 118
nucleic acid, viii, 2, 25, 26, 30, 81, 155, 159, 165, 171, 225, 226
nucleotide sequence, 185, 191, 199, 208, 262, 311
nucleotides, 5, 9, 20, 139, 140, 181, 184, 185, 202, 206, 208, 214, 270, 310, 313, 314
nucleus, 16, 74, 81, 182, 190, 213
null hypothesis, 296
nylon, 38, 200

# O

obligation, 89
observations, 60, 92, 181, 261
offenders, 52, 56, 59, 60, 62, 63, 65, 66, 68, 71
Office of Justice Programs, 31
oils, 37
oligonucleotide arrays, 225
oligonucleotides, 201, 204, 209, 210
omission, 59
online, xii, 131, 174, 185, 187, 201, 217, 227
on-line, 6
operating system, 96
operator, 286
opposition, 75, 183, 185, 310, 311
optical, 95, 205
optimization, 30, 170, 286
oral, 16, 33, 122
oral cavity, 16
organic, xv, 7, 25, 81, 92, 94, 95, 98, 127, 155, 156, 165, 181, 293, 296
organic compounds, 92, 94
organic matter, 165
organic solvent, 7
organism, 89, 123, 248, 257, 258, 260
orientation, 194
osteoblasts, 155
osteocalcin, 155, 157, 165, 169
osteocyte, 164
osteocytes, 155, 156
osteonectin, 155
outsourcing, 57
oversight, ix, 51, 64, 66
ownership, 54
oxidation, 134, 158, 162
oxidative, 15, 159, 174, 182, 267

oxidative damage, 159
oxygen, 16, 93

# P

packaging, 119, 157
packets, 64
pairing, 260
paleontology, 168
pandemic, 273
paradoxical, 310
paraffin-embedded, 214, 241
paramagnetic, 210
parasite, 33
parasites, 250
parentage, xiii, 141, 147, 214, 231, 232, 234, 241, 242, 243
parents, 232, 240, 311
Paris, 89, 90, 167, 315
particles, 81, 210
partnership, 20
passive, 205
paternal, 143, 198, 211, 212, 235, 236, 282, 291
paternity, xiii, 74, 87, 139, 144, 147, 148, 211, 212, 214, 221, 222, 226, 227, 231, 232, 233, 234, 236, 237, 238, 239, 241, 242, 266, 268, 269
pathways, 152, 156, 158, 159
patients, xv, 198, 293, 295
pedagogical, 314
pedigree, 269
penis, 77, 119
Pennsylvania, 219
peptide, 16, 81
peptides, 93, 111
perception, 127, 248, 290
perceptions, 310
periodontal, xv, 293, 295
periodontal disease, xv, 293, 295
peripheral blood, 32, 283
permafrost, 152, 155, 159, 171
permeation, 205
permit, ix, 27, 31, 74, 122, 123, 139, 199, 204, 210, 212, 213, 218, 222
pH, 8, 81, 92, 134, 155, 156, 158, 181, 235
pharmaceutical, 195, 196
pharmaceutical companies, 196
pharmaceuticals, 195, 197
phenol, xv, 8, 21, 22, 23, 24, 25, 26, 30, 39, 234, 258, 283, 286, 293, 296
phenolic, 93, 98, 111
phenotype, 85, 176, 195, 219, 220, 228, 310
phenotypes, 219, 310, 311

phenotypic, xii, 193, 195, 216, 219, 220, 223, 310, 313, 314
philanthropy, 196
philosophical, ix, xv, 52, 307, 308, 309
phosphatases, 119, 120
phosphate, 7, 15, 16, 181, 270
phosphodiesterase, 33
phosphorylation, 15, 174, 267
photons, 310
phylogenetic, xii, xv, 152, 161, 166, 174, 176, 177, 178, 179, 184, 185, 189, 258, 259, 260, 263, 278, 286
phylogenetic tree, 174, 177, 260
phylogeny, 174, 176, 179, 181, 182, 264
physical abuse, 246
physiological, 158, 181, 309, 310, 314
physiology, 85, 195, 308
phytoplankton, 272
plague, 273
plankton, 266, 272
plants, xiv, 152, 265, 266, 269, 270, 271, 272
plasma, 16, 32, 33
plasma proteins, 33
plastic, 37, 39
platforms, xiii, 10, 193, 216, 217, 223, 274
platinum, 204
Plato, 308, 309, 315
play, x, 28, 37, 117, 118, 145, 157, 199, 217, 223
PLC, 196
Pleistocene, 169
point mutation, 139, 140, 148, 225
poisoning, 272
poisonous, 266
poisonous plants, 266
Poland, 53, 241
polarity, 111
polarization, 207, 226
polarized light, 207
police, 46, 48, 51, 53, 54, 55, 58, 61, 62, 63, 64, 65, 66, 68, 70, 127
policy makers, 61
pollen, 270
polyacrylamide, 2, 278, 296
polyethylene, 42
polygenic, 198
polymer, 42
polymerase, x, 2, 32, 33, 41, 42, 43, 91, 92, 94, 96, 97, 101, 102, 103, 104, 105, 106, 107, 109, 110, 111, 112, 113, 114, 115, 127, 140, 153, 159, 162, 169, 170, 171, 200, 202, 203, 234, 236, 240, 263, 287
polymerase chain reaction, 2, 32, 33, 92, 113, 114, 127, 153, 169, 170, 171, 235, 240, 263

polymers, 92
polymorphism, 2, 84, 85, 124, 148, 186, 194, 216, 220, 225, 226, 228, 234, 236, 258, 267, 269, 270, 291
polymorphisms, xii, 33, 92, 143, 154, 174, 181, 193, 194, 195, 196, 209, 212, 213, 214, 215, 219, 221, 224, 225, 227, 228, 268, 270, 314
polypeptide, 15, 194
polypeptides, 311
polypropylene, 96
polysaccharides, 111
polyvinylpyrrolidone, 162
pools, 226
poor, 45, 58, 81, 137, 188, 200, 218
population, xiv, xv, 2, 37, 54, 58, 59, 61, 87, 92, 140, 143, 144, 145, 146, 147, 148, 174, 176, 180, 181, 183, 185, 186, 187, 188, 189, 190, 191, 194, 198, 210, 211, 212, 214, 215, 216, 217, 218, 219, 221, 223, 227, 228, 233, 235, 240, 242, 243, 261, 262, 272, 277, 278, 279, 280, 281, 286, 287, 290, 291, 292, 311, 312, 313
population group, 176, 215
population size, 194, 212
porosity, 155, 160
porous, 37
Portugal, xi, 53, 118, 127, 129, 148, 173, 268
postmortem, 95, 113, 166, 181, 182, 188, 247, 262, 263, 266, 294
powder, 38, 295
power, 6, 120, 134, 139, 141, 142, 143, 144, 145, 160, 186, 187, 213, 215, 216, 218, 221, 222, 227, 228, 232, 233, 243, 268, 269, 270, 271, 280, 283
precipitation, 16
predators, 254
prediction, xii, 193, 216, 219, 220
preference, 158, 278
pressure, 57, 58, 90, 131
prevention, 46, 161, 191
primacy, 311
primates, 169
prior knowledge, 270, 272
PRISM, 94, 95, 97
probability, xiii, 42, 66, 87, 88, 126, 131, 139, 217, 231, 232, 235, 236, 237, 238, 239, 242, 256, 271, 279, 280
probe, 2, 9, 10, 27, 29, 94, 97, 100, 101, 103, 104, 123, 199, 200, 201, 209, 210
production, ix, 36, 41, 52, 85, 86, 159
professional development, 57
professionalism, 63
progenitors, 233
program, 9, 53, 263, 270, 273, 287
property crimes, 60

prosecutor, 28
prosperity, 311
prostate, x, 4, 15, 16, 32, 117, 120, 125
prostate cancer, 32
prostate gland, 16
prostate specific antigen, x, 117, 120
prostrate, 15
protection, 79, 153, 169
protective clothing, 50
protein, 3, 15, 16, 85, 86, 113, 155, 157, 159, 164, 165, 167, 169, 175, 194, 198, 199, 220, 232, 256, 266, 272, 295, 310
protein sequence, 169
proteinase, 8, 25, 39, 81, 234
proteins, 16, 31, 32, 33, 81, 123, 155, 156, 159, 171, 174, 182, 194, 198, 199
proteomics, 31
protocol, xv, 8, 9, 25, 26, 30, 41, 75, 94, 97, 152, 187, 203, 286, 287, 293, 295
protocols, xiv, xv, 43, 88, 89, 96, 97, 114, 119, 123, 152, 187, 243, 265, 266, 278, 287
protons, 310
prototype, 26, 27, 33
proxy, 156
PSA, 10, 11, 16, 17, 18, 21, 29, 121
pseudo, 240
public, 46, 58, 195, 196, 197, 217, 267, 290
pulp, 303, 304
pulse, 206
pupal, 255
purification, viii, 35, 43, 44, 48, 50, 83, 94, 113, 159, 162, 202, 216, 234, 283, 287
PVP, 162
pyrolysis, 156
pyrophosphate, 208, 225

## Q

quality assurance, ix, 74, 263
quality control, 183, 184, 185, 186, 187, 188, 190
quartz, 96
query, 54, 227, 259
quinone, 50, 93

## R

race, 36, 87, 132, 310, 314
racemization, 156, 164, 165, 169, 303
racism, 314
radiation, 134, 159, 181, 191
radical mechanism, 159
radius, 65

random, xiii, 8, 40, 42, 126, 159, 198, 214, 231, 235, 236, 237, 238, 239, 270
randomly amplified polymorphic DNA, xiv, 246
range, viii, xii, xiv, 4, 16, 17, 26, 27, 28, 35, 40, 56, 59, 60, 64, 65, 66, 92, 110, 111, 139, 147, 152, 182, 193, 210, 214, 236, 237, 238, 255, 261, 268, 271, 277, 295, 297, 299, 310
RAPD, 270
rape, 119, 120, 121, 125, 126, 132, 246
reactants, 42
reactivity, 3, 20, 21, 26, 29, 30
reagent, 11, 12, 14, 15, 32, 160, 161
reagents, 39, 92, 124, 161, 202
real time, 32, 113, 154, 171
reasoning, 314
reception, 119
receptors, 248
recidivism, 70
recognition, 69, 205, 266, 270, 304
recombinant DNA, 113
recombination, xi, xii, 118, 126, 143, 159, 173, 174, 184, 185, 211, 212, 218, 223, 257
reconstruction, x, 117, 118, 174, 176, 211, 217, 219, 220, 221, 280, 295
recovery, 37, 39, 47, 49, 90, 113, 127, 131, 138, 143, 152, 153, 154, 156, 157, 214, 263, 294
recurrence, 186
red blood cell, 16, 75
red blood cells, 16, 75
reducing sugars, 165
redundancy, 5
regression, xv, 97, 185, 294, 296, 302
regression line, 97
regular, 159
regulation, 158, 209
regulations, 268
relationship, 6, 85, 124, 234, 240, 258, 260, 262, 280, 309, 310, 311
relationships, 66, 156, 157, 242, 263, 314
relatives, 134, 233, 242, 243, 246, 260, 261, 283, 285
relevance, 59, 64, 65, 156, 160, 168
reliability, viii, 36, 83, 211, 216, 234, 236, 237, 238, 239, 240
religions, 310
repair, 158, 159, 164, 166, 168
reparation, 84
repetitions, 137, 271
replacement rate, 180
replication, 154, 163, 174, 175
reptiles, 267
research and development, 223
reservoir, 154
residential, 49

residues, 295
resin, 81, 94, 95, 96, 99, 304
resolution, ix, xiv, 52, 54, 59, 152, 165, 187, 206, 213, 223, 224, 232, 266, 277
resources, xiv, 10, 28, 31, 56, 63, 66, 196, 277
respiratory, 249
restorations, 294
restriction enzyme, 98, 112, 271
restriction fragment length polymorphis, 2
retention, 57
retirement, 142
returns, 75, 260
reverse transcriptase, 8, 32
RFLP, 2, 174, 177, 199, 205, 232, 258, 259, 263
Rhodophyta, 149
ribonucleic acid, 256
ribosomal, xiv, 246, 257, 260, 268, 269, 270, 272, 273
ribosomal RNA, xiv, 246, 257, 260, 268, 269, 270, 272, 273
rings, 92, 111
risk, xv, 44, 48, 59, 85, 88, 139, 160, 183, 197, 198, 233, 278, 290, 304, 313
risk factors, 198
risks, 46, 241, 242
RNA, vii, 1, 3, 4, 5, 7, 8, 9, 10, 11, 12, 13, 14, 15, 18, 20, 21, 22, 23, 24, 25, 26, 28, 29, 30, 31, 32, 33, 34, 39, 194, 256, 257, 270, 273
robbery, 74
robotics, 2
robustness, 16, 136, 138, 139, 142, 176, 204, 278
Roman Empire, 152
Romania, 53
room temperature, 4, 6, 8, 10, 11, 12, 13, 14, 15, 16, 17, 21, 22, 23, 28, 29, 76, 77, 119, 249
root hair, 78
rubella, 33
Russia, 235, 243, 303
Russian, 303

## S

salaries, 57
saliva, viii, x, 2, 3, 4, 6, 7, 16, 17, 18, 19, 20, 21, 22, 23, 24, 25, 26, 27, 28, 29, 30, 31, 32, 33, 34, 35, 44, 49, 50, 95, 117, 119, 123, 138, 268
salmon, 39
salt, 81, 98, 181, 205, 248, 272
salts, 43, 44, 81, 97, 111, 206
sampling, 31, 40, 58, 60, 75, 76, 120, 190, 260
San Salvador, 148
sanctions, 55, 58
SAP, 206

satellite, 170, 304
saturation, 183, 190
scientific community, 153, 154, 162, 261
SDS, 39, 97, 234, 286
search, 31, 54, 59, 121, 164, 259, 260
searches, 19, 52, 140, 141
searching, 54, 55, 68, 196, 217
seasonality, 262
Seattle, 137, 242
second generation, 224, 316
secretion, 5, 22, 23
sediments, 112, 113, 152, 167
seeds, 152, 271
selecting, 70, 200
SEM, 164
semen, x, 4, 7, 12, 15, 16, 17, 18, 19, 20, 21, 22, 23, 24, 25, 26, 27, 28, 29, 30, 31, 32, 33, 36, 44, 56, 57, 74, 75, 81, 117, 118, 119, 120, 121, 123, 125, 127, 130, 131, 132, 182
semiconductor, 204
semiconductors, 225
seminal vesicle, 125
sensitivity, vii, 2, 16, 17, 28, 29, 31, 40, 41, 46, 49, 88, 136, 138, 139, 140, 142, 202, 222, 272, 273
separation, 67, 68, 81, 113, 122, 123, 139, 159, 161, 162, 203, 216, 225
sequencing, xii, 81, 86, 140, 154, 159, 165, 166, 169, 171, 173, 174, 182, 185, 186, 187, 189, 191, 202, 207, 222, 224, 260, 263, 266, 267, 270, 272, 273, 287, 288, 292, 314
series, 43, 56, 61, 63, 64, 65, 66, 109, 200, 204, 249, 263, 290
serum, 15, 42, 95, 113, 115, 232
serum albumin, 42, 95, 113, 115
sex, xv, 114, 123, 128, 144, 236, 268, 294, 296, 304
sex chromosome, 304
sex ratio, 128
sexual assault, xi, 2, 27, 28, 31, 74, 77, 81, 118, 119, 120, 121, 122, 123, 124, 125, 127, 129, 130, 211
sexual assaults, xi, 118, 119, 127, 130
sexual contact, xi, 117, 118, 121
sexual intercourse, 118, 125, 126
sexual offences, x, 56, 117, 128
sexual violence, 127
shape, 95, 101, 104, 248, 249, 253, 254, 287, 300
sharing, 54, 174, 218, 233, 235, 238, 239, 242
sheep, 262, 264, 269
short period, xii, 52, 174, 278
short tandem repeats, 2, 92, 131, 144, 146, 154, 214, 304
short tandem repeats (STRs), 2, 214
sibling, 233, 241, 242
sickle cell anemia, 170

silica, 39, 81
silver, 2, 149
similarity, 130, 236, 260, 267
simulation, 40, 233
Singapore, 53
single nucleotide polymorphism, 85, 154, 174, 196, 209, 212, 214, 221, 224, 225
single test, 4
single-nucleotide polymorphism, 194, 195, 225, 314
singular, 65, 68, 143
sites, xi, 26, 92, 111, 133, 135, 140, 158, 165, 191, 203, 204, 205, 210, 240, 247, 253, 259, 271
skeleton, 304, 305
skin, 7, 16, 18, 21, 23, 26, 29, 36, 37, 50, 79, 80, 118, 132, 217, 219, 220, 223, 228, 249, 267, 310
slave trade, 280
Slovakia, 53
smoking, 121
social roles, 311
sociological, 309
sociologists, 309
Socrates, 308
sodium, 7, 8
software, 9, 20, 21, 22, 23, 26, 27, 97, 185, 190, 204, 206, 235, 259
soil, 39, 92, 94, 98, 113, 114, 134, 155, 273
soils, 92, 112, 113
solvent, 207
solvents, 38
somatic cell, 123
South Asia, 219
South Carolina, 262
Southeast Asia, 175, 292
SPA, 224
space-time, 310
Spain, 53, 54, 133, 151, 173, 193, 217, 265, 268, 287
Spaniards, 280
spatial, 81, 92, 203, 310
species, xiii, xiv, 3, 4, 160, 166, 178, 194, 245, 246, 249, 250, 251, 252, 253, 254, 255, 256, 258, 259, 260, 261, 262, 263, 264, 265, 266, 267, 268, 269, 270, 271, 272, 273, 274
specificity, vii, 2, 5, 10, 16, 18, 19, 22, 23, 29, 31, 42, 49, 125, 199, 200, 210, 272, 273
specter, 314
spectrophotometer, 98
spectrum, xi, 3, 56, 151, 152
speculation, 44
speed, 8, 45, 106, 107, 139, 207
sperm, ix, xi, 4, 15, 16, 17, 18, 19, 20, 21, 30, 31, 39, 47, 73, 74, 76, 86, 90, 117, 121, 122, 125, 126, 127, 130, 131, 174, 183, 308

spermatozoa, x, 4, 16, 33, 77, 83, 90, 117, 121, 122, 123, 127
spheres, 59
spin, 8, 94
St. Louis, 196
stability, vii, 1, 4, 28, 33, 95, 111, 164, 199, 294
stages, xiii, xiv, 44, 61, 64, 65, 160, 245, 246, 249, 251, 252, 254, 255, 256, 299
standard error, 185
standardization, 178, 268, 269, 274
standards, 54, 96, 138, 185, 188, 269, 274, 313, 314
statistical analysis, ix, xiv, 64, 73, 87, 122, 140, 277
sterile, 8, 16, 38, 96, 160, 161, 286
stochastic, 40, 44, 48
storage, 4, 11, 12, 13, 14, 15, 21, 22, 23, 46, 119, 157, 160, 247
strategies, 37, 41, 60, 64, 65, 69, 131, 143, 152, 158, 160, 161, 168, 170, 221
stratification, 210, 228
strawberries, 271
strength, 57, 81, 155, 199, 205
streptavidin, 200, 209, 210
stress, xv, 307
STRs, xi, xiii, 41, 43, 48, 84, 85, 118, 123, 124, 125, 128, 131, 132, 133, 134, 136, 138, 139, 142, 143, 144, 145, 146, 147, 148, 149, 158, 193, 203, 212, 214, 215, 223, 227, 229, 232, 233, 241, 269, 270, 271, 272, 279, 283, 290, 291, 292, 308
structural changes, 164
structural gene, 225
sub-cellular, 122
substances, 92, 94, 120, 161, 266, 269, 272
substitution, 176, 178, 190
substrates, 36, 37, 207, 208, 210
success rate, viii, 35, 36, 38, 39, 47, 138, 141, 144, 150, 202
sugars, 7, 93, 159, 165, 181, 310
suicide, 246
summer, 263, 310
sunlight, 221
supernatant, 8
suppression, 200
surprise, 256
surveillance, 33, 57
survival, 156, 157, 158, 165
survivors, 283
suspects, xv, 47, 52, 58, 60, 66, 74, 76, 79, 218, 247, 266, 269, 294, 302, 308
sweat, 37
Sweden, 53
Switzerland, 41, 51, 53
synthesis, 159, 166, 169, 207, 243, 304
systematics, xiv, 246, 262, 263, 264

## T

Taiwan, 54
tandem repeats, 2, 92, 131, 144, 146, 154, 214, 304
targets, xiv, 5, 20, 30, 95, 199, 210, 246, 269
taxonomic, xiii, 92, 245, 248, 256, 258, 260, 270, 286
taxonomy, 260, 312
T-cell receptor, 15
teaching, 39
technical change, 3
technician, 75
technological progress, 221
teeth, xii, xv, 78, 79, 86, 92, 113, 149, 151, 152, 153, 155, 156, 160, 161, 166, 168, 171, 240, 293, 294, 295, 296, 297, 299, 302, 303, 304
temperature, xiii, xv, 4, 6, 8, 9, 10, 11, 12, 13, 14, 15, 16, 17, 21, 22, 23, 28, 29, 76, 77, 79, 81, 98, 107, 108, 111, 119, 134, 155, 157, 158, 181, 182, 199, 207, 245, 249, 254, 255, 294, 295, 296, 297, 299, 300, 302, 304
temporal, 152, 155, 310
terrorism, 54, 273
terrorist, 212, 273
terrorist attack, 212, 273
terrorist groups, 273
testimony, 28, 57
Texas, 136
Thai, 243
Thailand, 54, 189
thalassemia, 33
theft, vii, viii, 35, 36, 53, 89
thermal denaturation, 95
thermal stability, 199
thermoplastic, 83
thinking, 60, 61, 310
Thomson, 48, 233, 242
thoracic, 249
thorax, 248, 249
threat, 54, 314
threshold, 22, 23, 30, 36, 44, 48, 94, 97, 134, 135
thresholds, 41, 64
thymine, 256
time periods, 45
tissue, vii, ix, xi, 1, 3, 4, 6, 16, 18, 20, 23, 24, 26, 27, 28, 29, 30, 31, 32, 44, 73, 96, 118, 122, 152, 166, 168, 170, 186, 251, 284, 295, 304
titration, 30
TMRCA, 176
tobacco, 199
Tokyo, 49, 243, 290, 303
tolerance, 85
toxic, 266
toxicology, xiv, 265, 266
toxins, 195
trade, 266, 268, 280
training, xiv, 31, 45, 57, 60, 63, 124, 139, 277
traits, xii, 193, 219, 220, 221, 313
transactions, 165, 167, 170
transcriptase, 8, 32
transcription, 4, 5, 8, 9, 185, 194
transcription factor, 194
transcripts, vii, 1, 5, 6, 9, 20, 21, 30, 33
transfer, 37, 45, 46, 49, 50, 75, 79, 83, 119, 124, 132, 169, 185, 200, 202
transformation, 113, 156
transglutaminase, 16
transition, 3, 31, 107, 108, 155, 178, 179, 280
transitions, 159, 178, 179, 182, 186
translation, 174
transmission, xii, 134, 173
transport, 16, 46, 86, 119, 160
transportation, 83, 119, 198
trauma, 118, 247, 295
travel, 65
trees, 85, 191
trial, 44, 61, 62, 63, 234
triggers, 211
troubleshooting, 10
TSC, 196
tsunami, 180, 189
tuberculosis, 273
turnover, 180
two-dimensional, 204
typology, xv, xvi, 307, 308, 314

## U

UAE, 173
Ukraine, 53
uncertainty, 45, 176, 178
uniform, 66
unions, 282
United Arab Emirates, 188
United Kingdom, 45, 46, 196
United States, 31, 165, 169, 170, 171, 196, 273, 279
universe, 310, 311
updating, xii, 174
urban population, 240
urinary, 86
urine, 3, 6, 26, 199
UV, 83, 95, 98, 111, 134

## V

vagina, 119, 120
vaginal cells, 118, 122
validation, 5, 45, 123, 132, 149, 160, 204, 206, 212, 215, 222, 226, 261, 267, 269, 272, 274
values, 92, 98, 100, 101, 105, 106, 107, 109, 139, 155, 178, 207, 235, 236, 237, 238, 239, 296
variability, xii, 193, 196, 212, 267, 271
variable factor, 314
variables, xv, 47, 294, 296, 299, 301
variance, 176
variation, xii, 5, 37, 38, 40, 45, 56, 58, 85, 121, 125, 126, 139, 140, 141, 147, 178, 179, 182, 188, 189, 190, 193, 194, 196, 197, 204, 214, 219, 220, 224, 228, 257, 259, 290, 291, 295, 313
vasectomy, 16, 121
vein, 297
Venezuela, xiv, 277, 278, 279, 280, 290
Vermont, 1, 7
vertebrates, 267
*Vibrio cholerae*, 114
victim profiles, 130
victims, xi, xv, 74, 76, 77, 79, 92, 113, 118, 125, 127, 128, 129, 136, 148, 189, 214, 241, 242, 266, 269, 273, 278, 283, 285, 304, 308
Victoria, 54
violent, x, 56, 117, 119
violent crime, x, 56, 117, 119
violent crimes, 56
virus, 32, 76
viruses, 4, 195
viscosity, 207
visible, 7, 44, 66, 68, 75, 85, 208
visualization, 49, 202
vulva, 119

## W

war, 92, 113, 241, 242, 311
water, xvi, 8, 9, 38, 39, 81, 92, 94, 199, 248, 272, 286, 295, 307, 309, 310, 312, 313, 316
water-soluble, 199
wavelengths, 31, 95
weakness, 186
Weinberg, 140
wells, 7, 209
wet-dry, 38
whites, 310, 311
wild type, 202, 205
wild-type allele, 200
Wisconsin, 49, 146
wisdom, 314
witnesses, x, 58, 117, 118
women, 213, 282, 296, 311
wood, xvi, 37, 307, 309, 312, 313, 316
workload, viii, 35, 55
workstation, 48
World Health Organization, 33, 125
worms, 246
writing, 47, 70, 89, 112, 130, 145, 164, 188, 223, 240, 261, 274, 290, 315

## X

X chromosome, 85, 143, 144, 148, 194, 211, 212
X-linked, 149

## Y

Y chromosome, xi, 85, 86, 118, 124, 126, 128, 136, 143, 144, 148, 149, 194, 211, 212, 218, 281, 291
yang, xvi, 307, 310, 311, 313, 314, 316
Y-chromosomal, 125, 144, 149, 304
yeast, 113
yield, vii, 1, 2, 3, 24, 25, 39, 49, 126, 156, 213, 222
yin, xvi, 307, 310, 311, 313, 314, 316
young men, 311
young women, 311

## Z

zinc, 32